# OPTIC NERVE IN GLAUCOMA

# OPTIC NERVE IN GLAUCOMA

edited by

Stephen M. Drance
and
Douglas R. Anderson

Kugler Publications bv/Amsterdam / New York

**Library of Congress Cataloging-in-Publication Data**

Optic nerve in glaucoma / edited by S.M. Drance.
p. cm.
Includes bibliographical references.
ISBN 9062991238
1. Optic nerve--Diseases. 2. Glaucoma--Complications. 3. Optic Disk--pathology. I. Drance, Stephen M.
[DNLM: 1. Glaucoma--etiology. WW 280 061 1995]
RE727.O66 1995
617.7' 41--dc20
DNLM/DLC
for Library of Congress 95-8861
CIP

ISBN 90-6299-123-8

The publication of this title has been made possible by Alcon.

Distributors:
For the U.S.A. and Canada:
Kugler Publications
c/o Demos Vermande, Order Department
386 Park Avenue South, Suite 201
New York, NY 10016, USA
Telefax (+212) 683 0118

For all other countries:
Kugler Publications bv
P.O. Box 11188
1001 GD Amsterdam, The Netherlands
Telefax (+31.20) 638 0524

DR. FREDRICK FELDMAN

89 Ames Circle · Don Mills, Ontario ·
445-6076

# Table of Contents

# PREFACE

STEPHEN DRANCE

Welcome to Venice. The concept of this meeting is to resurrect the Josiah Macy Foundation glaucoma meetings. We wanted the setting to be like those meetings in the sixties where people assembled who had things to say to each other in groups small enough that speakers not only *can* be interrupted but *should* be interrupted with comments and questions.

Our first meeting, held in Bermuda, was precisely that. The format has some drawbacks, one of which is that to permit editing and publication of the discussion, you have to identify yourself on the microphone. Therefore, while we hope the discussion can be very informal, if you can remember to tell us your name, we would appreciate it. The whole meeting will be transcribed, and you will, of course, have an opportunity of adding or editing your section, and also the discussion that pertains to your particular subject and presentation.

For this meeting, Dr. Anderson and I asked Drs. Quigley, Caprioli, and Flammer to organize the three topics that we want to discuss. We are delighted to see so many of our colleagues from other fields have accepted the invitation to be here. To orient our non-glaucomatologist colleagues and set the stage for the meeting, Dr. Anderson circulated in advance an introduction to what glaucoma is all about. It will appear as the first chapter in the published transcription. We would love our colleagues to challenge some of the concepts that we hold as dogma in glaucoma, so that we can learn from the tremendous expertise that you have as to what we should be thinking of and how we should be going about solving our problems.

I want to thank Drs. Przydryga and Mr. Crewe of Alcon for the excellence of the arrangements and for bringing us together.

## LIST OF CONTRIBUTORS

Anderson, D.R. - Bascom Palmer Eye Institute, 900 N.W. 17th Street, Miami, FL 33136, USA

Baumbach, G.L. - Department of Internal Medicine, E 317-B, University of Iowa, College of Medicine, Iowa City, IA, USA

Bray, G.M. - Center for Research in Neurosciences, McGill University, 7855-1650 Cedar Avenue, Montreal, Quebec H3G 1A4, Canada

Browder, S. - Alcon Laboratories, Glaucoma Research, 6201 South Freeway, R2-41, Fort Worth, TX 76134-2099, USA

Cantu-Crouch, D. - Alcon Laboratories, Glaucoma Research, 6201 South Freeway, R2-41, Fort Worth, TX 76134-2099, USA

Caprioli, J. - Yale University Eye Center, 330 Cedar Street, New Haven, CT 06510-8061, USA

Choi, D.W. - Washington University, School of Medicine, Box 8111, 600 South Euclid Avenue, St. Louis, MO 63110, USA

Clark, A.F. - Alcon Laboratories, Glaucoma Research, 6201 South Freeway, R2-41, Fort Worth, TX 76134-2099, USA

Costa, E. - Fidia Georgetown Institute for the Neurosciences, 3900 Resevoir Road S.E., Washington, D.C. 20007, USA

Drance, S.M. - Department of Ophthalmology, University of British Columbia Hospital, 2211 Westbrook Mall, Rm F-197, Vancouver, B.C. V6T 2B5, Canada

Flammer, J. - University Eye Clinic Basel, Mittlere Strasse 91, CH-4056 Basel, Switzerland

Haefliger, I.O. - Department of Ophthalmology, University Hospital, Kantonsspital Basel, Petersgraben 4, CH-4031 Basel, Switzerland

Hoffman, P.N. - Wilmer Ophthalmological Institute, The John's Hopkins University School of Medicine, 601 North Broadway, Maumanee Bldg., Baltimore, MD 21205, USA

Kapin, M.A. - Alcon Laboratories, Glaucoma Research, 6201 South Freeway, Fort Worth, TX 76134-2099, USA

Langer, S.Z. - Synthelabo Recherche (L.E.R.S.), B.P. 110, 31 Avenue Paul Vaillant-Couturier, F-92225 Bagneux Cedex, France

Lüscher, T.F. - Kardiologische Abteilung, Medizinische Universitätsklinik, Inselspital, CH-3010 Bern, Switzerland

McCartney, M.D. - Alcon Laboratories, Glaucoma Research, 6201 South Freeway, R2-41, Fort Worth, TX 76134-2099, USA

Meyer, P. - Department of Ophthalmology, University Hospital, Kantonsspital Basel, Petersgraben 4, CH-4031 Basel, Switzerland

Morrison, J.C. - Oregon Health Sciences University, Casey Eye Center, 3375 S.W. Terwilliger Blvd., Portland, OR 97201-4197, USA

Pyeritz, R.E. - Department of Human Genetics, Allegheny Singer Research Center, 320 East North Avenue, Pittsburgh, PA 15212-4772, USA

Quigley, H.A. - Dana Center for Preventative Ophthalmology, Wilmer Eye Institute, 120-600 North Wolfe Street, Baltimore, MD 21205, USA

Ransom, B.R. - Yale University, Department of Neurology, School of Medicine, 333 Cedar Street, 702 LC1, New Haven, CT 06510, USA

Siesjö, B.K. - Laboratory for Experimental Brain Research, Department of Neurology, Experimental Research Center, University Hospital, S-221, 85 Lund, Sweden

Steely, H.T. - Alcon Laboratories, Glaucoma Research, 6201 South Freeway, R2-41, Fort Worth, TX 76134-2099, USA

Wilson, K. - Alcon Laboratories, Glaucoma Research, 6201 South Freeway, R2-41, Fort Worth, TX 76134-2099, USA

Zeiher, A. - Department of Cardiology, Medizinische Universitätsklinik, Hugstetter Strasse XX 55, D-7800, Freiburg, Germany

Zeimer, R. - Wilmer Ophthalmolological Institute, John's Hopkins Medical Institute, Woods Research Bldg., Rm 355, Baltimore, MD 21205, USA

# 1. GLAUCOMA, ITS TERMINOLOGY AND FUNDAMENTAL NATURE

DOUGLAS R. ANDERSON, M.D.

## Introduction

The participants in this symposium, and readers of its proceedings, are not equally familiar with the clinical and pathophysiologic features of glaucoma. The purpose of this introduction is to orient scientists from other disciplines with the disease under discussion and with some of the terminology they may expect to encounter while discussing glaucoma with those whose clinical and scientific efforts have centered on this condition. The description represents my summary perspective of the disease, but others participating may debate some details or the emphasis placed on certain highlighted aspects.

## Anatomy of the eye

The wall of the eye has three layers. The outer layer consists of the clear cornea anteriorly, through which light is admitted, and the white sclera, which completes the structural wall of the eye. The iris, ciliary body, and choroid form a continuous second layer, together called the uveal tract. An opening in the iris, the pupil, transmits light to the lens and the cavity posteriorly, which is filled with vitreous humor. The root of the iris inserts into the ciliary body. The ciliary body lies within the anteriormost part of the sclera and contains the ciliary muscle, which is responsible for changing the shape of the lens. This allows the eye to focus on objects at varying distances, or to accommodate. The inner epithelial lining of the ciliary body produces aqueous humor by a combination of ultrafiltration and active transport. The aqueous humor bathes the lens, passes through the pupil, and exits mostly through the trabecular meshwork located in the peripheral cornea just anterior to the iris insertion into the ciliary body. The third part of the uveal tract is the choroid, a pigmented highly vascular tissue that lies under the retina and provides nutrition to the outer retina.

The retina is the innermost layer of the ocular wall. The retina receives and detects the light that has been focused into an image by the optics of the cornea and lens. Light is detected by photoreceptors, which are in the outer retina, separated from the choroid only by the retinal pigment epithelium. Visual information is processed through neural interconnections in the retina. The innermost retinal neurons, the ganglion cells, transmit the partially processed visual information via axons that traverse the inner retina toward the optic nerve head, where the axons form the optic nerve, which conducts the impulses from the retina to the brain.

Within the eye, the lens lies directly behind the pupil. It is suspended from the ciliary body by zonular fibers, and as already noted, change in the lens shape (accommodation) is controlled by muscles in the ciliary body. In front of the iris and lens is the anterior chamber filled with aqueous humor. Behind the lens is the vitreous cavity. The space in front of the vitreous, but behind the pupil and iris, is the posterior chamber; it contains the lens and the aqueous humor that surrounds it.

*Optic Nerve in Glaucoma, pp. 1–14*
*edited by S.M. Drance*

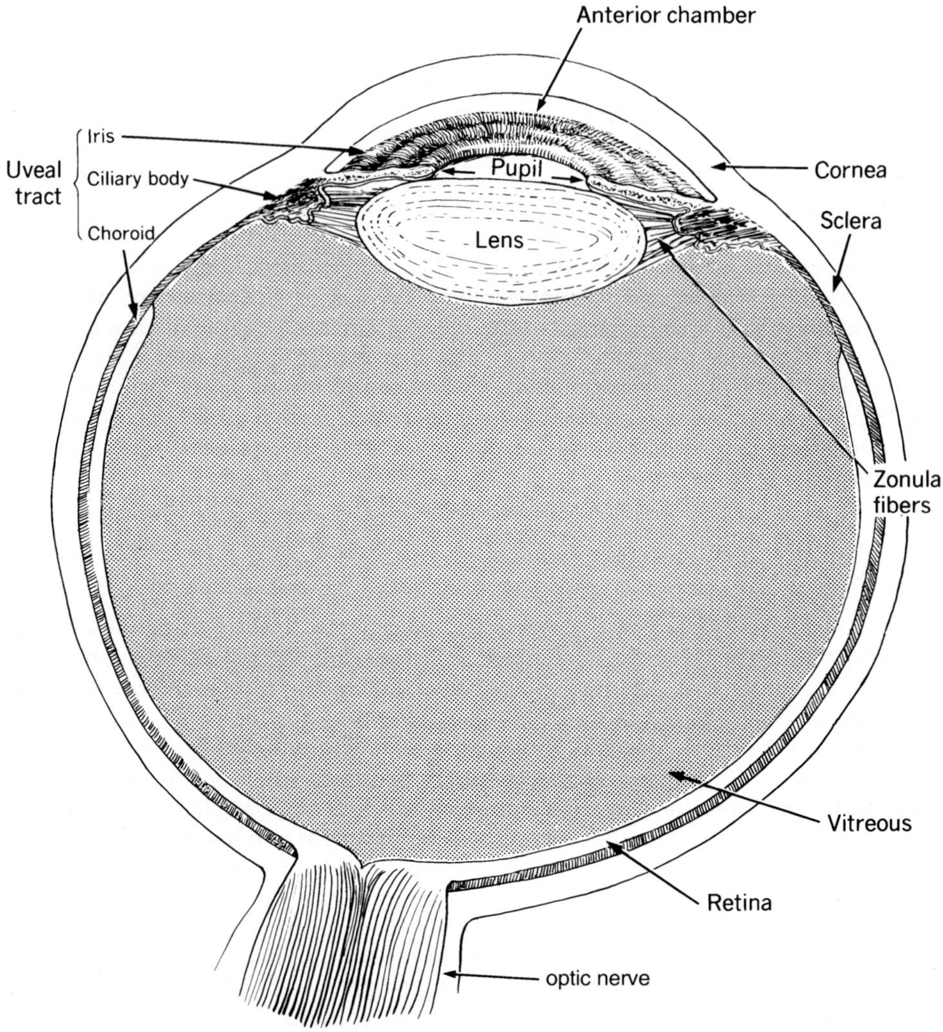


*Fig. 1.* Cross section of the eye. (Reproduced with permission from: Anderson, DR: *Testing the Field of Vision.* St. Louis: The C. V. Mosby Co, 1982, pp 18-19.)

## Definition of glaucoma

In a broad sense, glaucoma is a condition of the eye in which intraocular pressure (IOP) damages the eye and its function in some manner, or threatens to do so. Usually the IOP is high, *i.e.*, outside the statistical range of usual "normal" pressure (higher than 21 mm Hg, because 95% of individuals have IOP that is lower).

However, included in the definition of glaucoma are cases of "normal-tension glaucoma" (sometimes called "low-tension glaucoma"), in which the IOP is not elevated outside the normal range, but the normal IOP is high enough to produce damage to an eye particularly sensitive to the harmful effects of pressure. It is to be presumed that glaucoma-like damage to the optic nerve in the presence of normal IOP (normal-tension glaucoma) is nonetheless a pressure-induced glaucomatous phenomenon in which the "normal" level of intraocular pressure is, being higher than atmospheric pressure, one of the participating pathogenic factors. Evidence on this point is that (1) when intraocular pressure is different in the two eyes (though in the normal range in both), damage is greater in the eye with the higher pressure (although there may also be other asymmetric factors to produce asymmetric degrees of damage), and (2) therapeutic lowering of intraocular pressure to a subnormal range seems to reduce the rate of damage to the optic nerve.

In the context of clinical diagnosis, patients with "ocular hypertension" are often kept separate from the definition of glaucoma. These are individuals who, without apparent cause, have an abnormally high IOP. The IOP is high enough to produce symptoms or to be damaging to some eyes, but has not done so, at least to this point in time, in this person. There is an inconsistency in everyday usage of the diagnostic term "glaucoma" in that if the cause of IOP elevation is known (that is, it is not idiopathic), the patient is said to have glaucoma even if the elevated IOP has not produced harm. In the limited context of ocular hypertension (asymptomatic idiopathic elevation of intraocular pressure without pressure-induced damage), the presence of abnormally high IOP is considered a risk factor for the future development of glaucoma, which is diagnosed only if there later develops pressure-induced damage. Individuals with ocular hypertension, as well as those who have some other risk factor for future development of glaucoma (for example, a family history of glaucoma), are sometimes called "glaucoma suspects".

In the present scientific context, in which we are attempting to understand the role of IOP and of other factors in the production of optic nerve damage (and resultant visual loss), we must consider all these groups, no matter what we call them. In assessing the role of elevated IOP, we must study those who have damage without elevated IOP ("normal-tension glaucoma") and the inverse situation of high IOP without damage ("ocular hypertension"). Similarly, in understanding other factors that contribute to glaucomatous optic nerve damage, we must consider those with and without migraine, with and without family history, etc., etc., with and without optic nerve damage.

## Intraocular pressure

The eye, enclosed by the cornea-sclera ocular coat, is a closed cavity with a certain hydrostatic pressure within it, which keeps the eye inflated. There are only slight differences between certain tissue compartments (examples: the pressure in the suprachoroidal space is not quite the same as in the vitreous cavity, and under circumstances of relative pupillary block there may be some difference in pressure on the two sides of the iris leaf). These small pressure differences may be important to certain aspects of intraocular physiology, but these pressure differences within intraocular compartments are small compared to biologic variation in the intraocular pressure as a whole. The optic nerve is exposed to the pressure in the vitreous cavity, and this is not meaningfully different from the intraocular pressure in the anterior chamber, which is measured clinically.

Ignoring for the present purposes the slight differences in pressure between various compartments, the intraocular pressure is determined as an equilibrium balance between the rate of aqueous humor secretion and the resistance to its outflow from the eye. Aqueous humor is formed by the double epithelial layer of the ciliary body by active transport of a number of solutes with net water entry determined by osmotic forces. The rate of active secretion is lower during sleep, perhaps related to a lower general sympathetic tone (beta-adrenergic blockers lower the daytime IOP by reducing aqueous humor secretion rate, but then do not lower the aqueous humor secretion or IOP during sleep). The rate of this active secretion is not much influenced by the level of intraocular pressure and 2 μl per minute is a convenient round number estimate of human daytime aqueous humor inflow ($F_i$). The slight reduction of aqueous humor inflow as intraocular pressure is elevated and is, for historical reasons, called "pseudo-facility". The details of this physiology are not important in the present discussion.

In contrast to the active, relatively pressure-independent formation of aqueous humor, the exit of aqueous humor through the trabecular meshwork, Schlemm's canal, and collection channels into episcleral veins is a passive process dependent on the pressure difference between the intraocular pressure ($P_o$), the pressure in the episcleral veins ($P_e$) into which the aqueous humor drains, and on the resistance to flow between these two pressure compartments. The outflow ($F_o$) equals the outflow pressure ($P_o - P_e$) divided by the resistance (R). Under circumstances of equilibrium the outflow must equal the inflow, and aqueous humor dynamics are standardly described by the Goldmann equation: $F_i = F_o = (P_o - P_e) / R$ [Sometimes the equation is expressed in terms of facility of outflow (C) where facility is the reciprocal of resistance ($C = 1/R$). Then $F_o = C (P_o - P_e)$.]

A reasonable round number for normal outflow facility is 0.2 μl/min/mm Hg, and for episcleral venous pressure is 8 mm Hg. At equilibrium $F_i = F_o$, and if $F_i$ is 2 μl/min $P_o$ will equilibrate to 18 mm Hg.

## Uveoscleral outflow

An alternate channel of aqueous humor outflow is via uveoscleral outflow. Approximately 90% of the aqueous humor exits the eye through the "conventional" outflow channels by the physiology described in the preceding section, that is, through the trabecular meshwork, Schlemm's canal, and collector channels, into the episcleral veins. In humans, under physiologic circumstances, the remaining 10% exits through the interstitial spaces of the uveal tract, passing through the ciliary body into the choroid toward the optic nerve. Along the entire pathway posteriorly through the uveal tract, this fluid exits across the scleral wall into the orbital tissue, driven by the intraocular pressure.

Material contained within the aqueous humor is drawn with the bulk flow into the uveal tract. It is exchanged with the bloodstream in accordance with the relative concentration between the aqueous humor and blood, and other factors that affect exchange of materials between the interstitial fluid of the uveal tract and the blood (for example molecular size and permeability of the blood–tissue barrier to the substance in question). Thus, fluorescein in the aqueous humor flows into the ciliary body but is equilibrated with the bloodstream rapidly, so not much is carried very far posteriorly. Large molecules are carried further into the choroid (in decreasing concentration because of exit across the sclera along the way), and microspheres are carried as far back as the optic nerve.

This uveo-scleral pathway, not often highlighted in discussions of glaucoma, is mentioned here as it may come up in the discussion at this symposium and should be among the background information provided to participants. This pathway is relevant to glaucoma in at least three ways. First is the production of uveal edema. The bulk flow of fluid across the sclera is pressure-dependent, and the volume that must be transported across the sclera is dependent on the amount of non-absorbable solute (for example protein that crosses the choroidal capillaries into the interstitial space), which can not be absorbed back into the bloodstream, and is not carried away by lymphatics, which are absent within the eye. Under conditions of very low pressure (so transscleral exit is reduced), inflammation (with increased exudation of interstitial protein), or increased transscleral resistance, excessive fluid may collect in the choroid to produce clinical conditions of uveal effusion and choroidal detachment. This may occur spontaneously and produce angle closure glaucoma, or may occur as the result of hypotony and inflammation after glaucoma surgery. Secondly, drugs that are administered topically to the eye and enter the aqueous humor will be carried into the uveal tissue. Depending on the concentration that is carried posteriorly, there are potential pharmacologic effects in the posterior choroid and even in optic nerve. Thirdly, enhancement of uveal scleral outflow is of potential therapeutic benefit in lowering the intraocular pressure; it is the apparent mechanism of pressure lowering by prostaglandins, presently under development for this purpose.

## What causes high IOP? How are the glaucomas classified?

An elevation of intraocular pressure is caused by impairment of aqueous humor outflow through the channels that drain the anterior chamber angle. Clinicians classify the glaucoma into diagnostic types according to the mechanism that obstructs the aqueous humor outflow and produces an abnormally high intraocular pressure. "Angle closure glaucoma", for example, refers to the type in which the peripheral iris obstructs aqueous humor outflow by closing the anterior chamber angle. Glaucoma may occur secondary to inflammation, in which inflammatory products and debris or tissue swelling obstructs aqueous humor outflow. Each type may additionally be labeled acute, subacute (intermittent), or chronic, depending on the suddenness of onset of the pressure elevation or of the symptoms. The glaucoma is called a "secondary" glaucoma if some other ocular disease (vascular obstruction, inflammation, tumor) has produced the obstruction of aqueous humor outflow. In the absence of such specific causes, the glaucoma is called a primary glaucoma, either of the angle closure or open angle type (and there is a primary infantile glaucoma as well). Primary open angle glaucoma is "idiopathic" (mechanism of IOP elevation unknown). It is due to as yet undefined biochemical or structural changes at the submicroscopic level that increase the resistance to outflow through the trabecular meshwork and Schlemm's canal. The idiopathic abnormality, whatever it is, has a familial tendency and increases with age.

The broad definition of glaucoma does not specify the nature of the pressure-induced symptoms or harm. When the intraocular pressure is very high, the anterior segment, including the iris and ciliary body, becomes ischemic, producing pain, corneal edema, impairment of iris and ciliary body function, conjunctival hyperemia and edema, and permanent damage to the ciliary body, iris, and lens (cataract). The eye may become red and painful, and the vision affected by corneal edema and cataract formation. However, most cases of glaucoma do not have such a high pressure that this type of damage and pain occur. Excluding "ocular hypertension", the most frequent clinical manifestation of glaucoma is a mild or moderate idiopathic pressure elevation that over time produces painless damage to the optic nerve with progressively increasing visual loss, and ultimately perhaps total blindness. The vast majority of cases of glaucoma are of this chronic slowly progressive type. In everyday usage in clinical circles, if the term "glaucoma" is used without specifying a type, this common type is meant; more explicitly, it is called chronic open angle glaucoma or primary open angle glaucoma (POAG), in former times called chronic simple glaucoma or glaucoma simplex.

## Clinical features of glaucoma

Before primary chronic open angle glaucoma ensues, the intraocular pressure is "normal", varying from hour to hour according to physiologic circumstances. A typical daytime mean IOP is 17-18 mm Hg, with 95% of eyes with a pressure under 21-22 mm Hg. With age an increasing number of individuals develop gradual (over months or years) rise in the fluctuating intraocular pressure, with very few developing an intraocular pressure greater than 30 mm Hg and even fewer greater than 40 mm Hg. Many with elevated IOP remain as "ocular hypertensives" without pressure-induced damage, but a minority of individuals with pressures above 22 mm Hg develop damage to the optic nerve axons, recognized by a visible loss of reflection in the retinal nerve fiber layer, by a visible alteration in the optic nerve head configuration, or by a change in some component of visual function (in clinical practice, determined by testing "differential light sensitivity" in representative locations within the field of vision, called "perimetry", or "visual field test").

A feature of note is variability in the degree of harm to the optic nerve for any given pressure level. In some people the pressure may become quite high (even 40 or 50 mm Hg) without producing damage, at least on the short term. An intraocular pressure of 35 mm Hg has usually produced harm in about half of the individuals when their elevated IOP is discovered. Intraocular pressure in the 20's will harm some eyes, and of particular note is that an IOP in the normal range (under 21-22 mm Hg) may produce harm in a few eyes. Eyes with ocular hypertension (no damage despite distinctly elevated IOP) and those with normal-tension glaucoma are at opposite ends of the spectrum with regard to the optic nerve's susceptibility to harm. Because eyes with normal intraocular pressure so greatly outnumber those with abnormally high pressure, somewhere between 10% and 35% of individuals with glaucomatous optic nerve damage have a pressure in the normal range ( 21 mm Hg), at least on a single random reading. The average intraocular pressure of all individuals who have glaucomatous optic nerve damage is about 23-24 mm Hg (see Fig. 2).

This is not to say that IOP is unrelated to disc damage. Intraocular pressure is a causative factor (evidence: producing elevation of pressure experimentally or by elevation of IOP naturally by secondary mechanisms produces optic nerve damage, and lowering of IOP therapeutically will halt optic nerve damage). However, the wide variation in susceptibility to damage from IOP signifies the equal importance of "susceptibility factors" of epidemiologic importance that make the optic nerve vulnerable to pressures that are only slightly elevated or even normal. Susceptibility to harm from pressure increases with age, with genetic make up (race and family history are risk factors), and with certain diseases (for example, a relationship to migraine and other vasospastic conditions has been noted).

The fact that an individual has not yet suffered harm ("ocular hypertension") is to some degree a clinical sign that the susceptibility factors are not predominant, and such individuals tend to do reasonably well (1% per year, or 10% in a decade, develop evidence of nerve damage and field loss). However, such individuals are naturally at higher risk than those who do not have elevated intraocular pressure (whose risk is less than 1% per year). Thus, those with "ocular hypertension" are "glaucoma suspects",

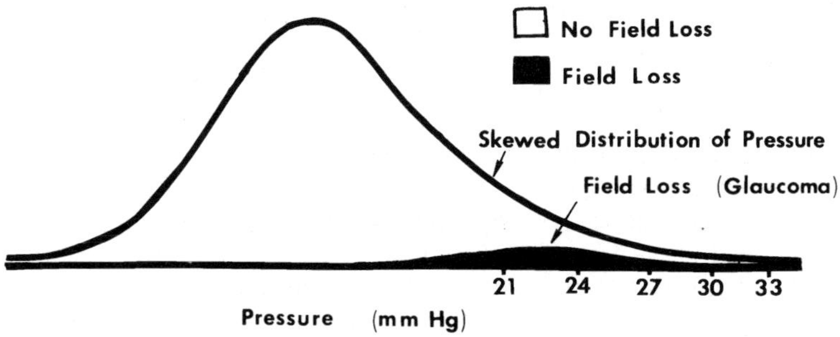


*Fig. 2.* Frequency curve of IOP with superimposed frequency curve of IOP-induced field loss. Note increasing proportion with field loss with higher IOP, but peak IOP with field loss is 23-24 mm Hg. (Reproduced with permission from: Anderson DR: The management of elevated intraocular pressure with normal optic disks and visual fields. I. The disk-field status as a risk predictor. *Surv Ophthalmol* 21:479-489, May-June, 1977.)

the broad term to indicate people whose risk of developing fully manifest glaucoma with glaucomatous optic nerve damage and visual field loss is higher than those without risk factors. The broad category of glaucoma suspects should also include others who are at risk, for example those who have a strong family history of glaucoma-caused blindness, those who have an anatomically narrow anterior chamber angle that is at risk of closing, and those with pseudo-exfoliation of the lens capsule, dispersion of iris pigment, or other states that might one day lead to elevation of intraocular pressure and resultant optic nerve damage. When we understand the mechanism of optic nerve damage, those with the degree of increased risk for each factor may become known, but at present the epidemiologic data are insufficient to do so.

## Types of optic nerve cupping

With the above background and the general nature of glaucoma in mind, it is the intent of this symposium to focus on pressure-induced damage to the optic nerve and its axons.

When the eye of a patient with glaucoma is examined, attention is drawn to the location where the optic nerve is formed by retinal nerve fiber layers converging to the site of exit from the eye toward the rest of the brain. This visible portion of the optic nerve is anatomically called the optic nerve head. By virtue of its ophthalmoscopic appearance during clinical examination it is often called the optic papilla, or the optic disc, the latter being the most commonly used term at present in the United States. The prominent feature by ophthalmoscopy is an excavation of the optic nerve head, usually called "cupping", due to a loss of axons passing through the region, as well as collapse and outward bowing of the lamina cribrosa, the perforated support structure through which the optic nerve fibers exit from the eye. Other visible features of the disease process include small splinter-shaped hemorrhages that occur from time to time within the disc or crossing the margin of the disc into the adjacent retina. Of uncertain relevance to the process is that the retinal pigment epithelium and choroid near the optic disc is attenuated or depigmented as a mild congenital abnormality or acquired atrophy. Peripapillary depigmentation occurs more frequently in patients with glaucoma than in others, and by virtue of its ophthalmoscopic appearance may be called a peripapillary crescent or halo.

Although it does not seem possible to classify glaucomatous cupping into distinct types, there is a spectrum of anatomic configuration of the glaucomatous excavation. Greater prominence of one feature in some cases and some other feature in others has suggested that separate pathogenic factors dominate in different cases, or at least some factors may be of more consequence in certain patients than in others. It is the details of these factors and interactions that we intend to discuss at this symposium.

Clinically, individuals in the early decades of life, often have a secondary type of glaucoma with strikingly elevated intraocular pressure. Perhaps because of the higher intraocular pressure in these secondary glaucomas or greater elasticity of the tissue in youth, or both, there is often a very deep, concentrically enlarged, excavation at the center of the disc. If the intraocular pressure is lowered in such cases, the disc may "fill in" with disappearance of the central excavation ("reversibility of cupping"). It is as if the elevated intraocular pressure bowed the elastic lamina cribrosa backward and perhaps stretched the scleral canal sideward with the neuroretinal tissue squeezed against the sides of the volumetrically enlarged walls that confine the optic nerve head. This created the concentrically enlarged cup. Permanent damage to the axons may be minimal, manifest by normal or nearly normal visual function when the intraocular pressure is successfully relieved, and the elastic stretching of connective tissue is relieved.

In the more common glaucoma of older patients with mildly elevated intraocular pressure, the excavation is not so deep and has a greater tendency to be localized (with the excavation extending often toward the lower temporal border of the disc and to a lesser extent to the upper temporal border of the disc in preference to other locations). Some cases are characterized by a crescent or halo of absent or depigmented retinal pigment epithelium surrounding the disc. Sometimes the localized character of the excavation is so marked that there appears to be a notch or a pit at the margin of the disc where the excavation is deepest. Small hemorrhages may occur within the disc tissue or across the disc margin, forming a splinter shape as it extends among the axons of the nerve fiber layer.

The exact anatomy of the glaucomatous excavation must also depend on the normal anatomic configuration that preexisted the development of glaucoma, which is variable. "Physiologic cupping" is highly variable, dependent in part on genetic factors, some of which relate to refractive error, but most often is quite similar in the two eyes. The size and shape of the normal excavation in the center of the optic disc ("physiologic cupping") depends in part on the size of the scleral opening for exit of the optic nerve axons and the obliquity of the canal for exit through the sclera of the lamina cribrosa. Except infrequently in cases of unilateral glaucoma (in which it can be assumed that the optic nerve configuration of the two eyes was the same) or in cases in which a photographic image of the optic nerve happened to be available before the onset of glaucoma, there is not much opportunity to be certain of the nature of the anatomic configuration before it was altered by glaucoma.

## Visual loss in glaucoma

As the axons of the optic nerve are compromised they may be present but poorly functioning for awhile, but ultimately they disappear and do not regenerate. The visual consequence is a change in many aspects of visual function. In the usual slow chronic case of insidious onset, there is a patchy dimming of visual sensation, perhaps with loss of contrast and loss of color intensity. This visual loss is typically not noticed by the afflicted individual (or else is considered by him to be the natural consequence of aging) until a major portion of the optic nerve fibers have been lost. A number of aspects of visual function have been tested in scientific studies, for the most part in an effort to determine what visual test might reveal the damage at its earliest stages in clinical testing, but in part also to understand the nature of the quietly progressive damage. In the clinical setting, the visual function that is standardly tested to recognize the presence of damage, and to quantify it so that it can later be determined if it is worsening, is "differential light sensitivity". The test determines how different in intensity a spot of light must be from its background to be perceived at various locations within the visual field. This clinical examination is called "perimetry", or a "visual field test". A Goldmann perimeter was used to conduct the test manually for many years, replacing the earlier tangent screen method. In the recent decade automated perimetry has taken over, with the Humphrey and Octopus instruments being the ones used most frequently. Although perimetry tests the ability to perceive minimal contrast at various portions in the visual field, it is not to be confused with a different test called "contrast sensitivity testing", a test of global contrast sensitivity, which also becomes abnormal in glaucoma, along with virtually any other test of visual function.

## Microscopic anatomy of the optic nerve head

To discuss at a basic level the pathophysiologic events, the anatomy of the optic nerve head and its blood supply must be reviewed. The optic nerve head (optic papilla, optic disc) is the location where retinal nerve fibers converge and make a turn before exiting the eye through a perforated lamina cribrosa at the level of the scleral coat. Numerous astroglia provide support for the axons of the optic nerve head as they turn posteriorly to form the optic nerve. After turning, as they pass posteriorly, the axons traverse the lamina cribrosa. Although the lamina cribrosa at first glance seems to be simply a perforated region of the sclera, it is in fact a more complex specialized tissue that spans the scleral opening through which the nerve fibers pass. As will be described in this symposium, the connective tissue of the lamina cribrosa is of somewhat different composition from the connective tissue of the sclera, with which it is continuous, containing abundant elastin, among other things.

The optic nerve head thus consists of unmyelinated nerve fibers, a glial support structure that interfaces with the collagenous lamina cribrosa, and blood vessels that form a network within the glial and collagenous connective tissue. In Figure 3, the relationship of the connective tissue elements and the glia is shown. In the next section, the blood vessel anatomy is described.

## The blood vessels

The central retinal artery enters the optic nerve and courses anteriorly at the core of the nerve (Fig. 4). Although it provides some branches to the intraorbital portion of the nerve (but note, not the optic nerve *head*), its main destination is the inner retina.

Most of the blood supply to the optic nerve in its orbital course is from various orbital branches that penetrate the dura mater, spread over the pia mater, and send branches into the septa of the optic nerve. The posterior ciliary arteries penetrate the

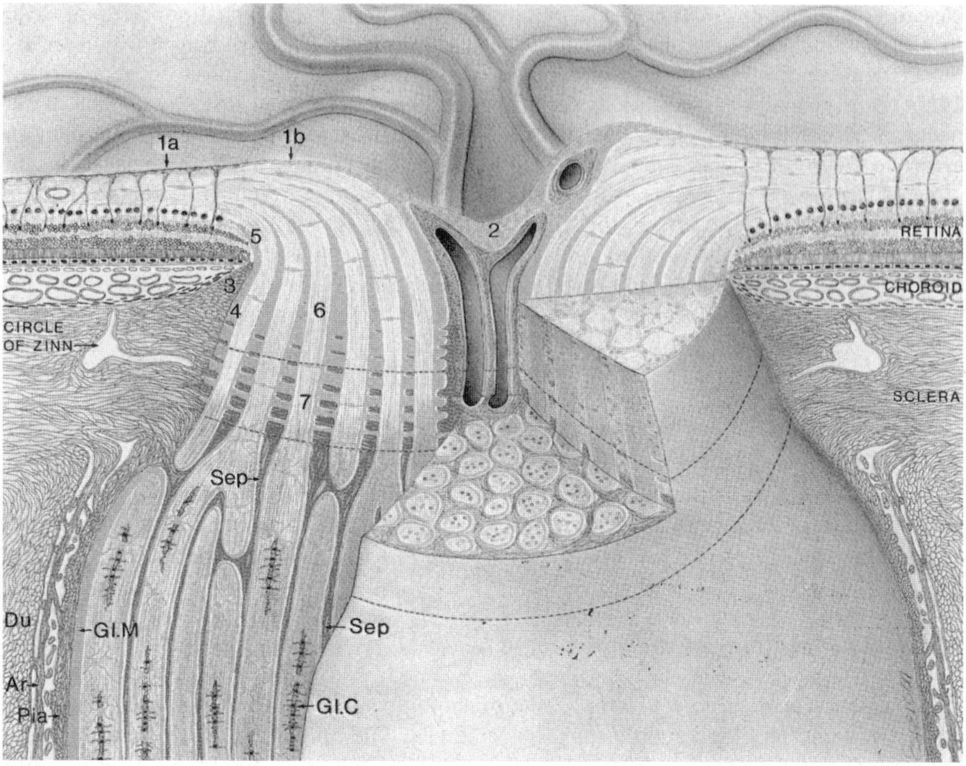


*Fig. 3.* Microscopic anatomy of the optic nerve head. (Black and white reproduction of color figure. Reproduced with permission from: Anderson DR and Hoyt WF: Ultrastructure of intraorbital portion of human and monkey optic nerve. *Arch Ophthalmol* 82:506-530, October, 1969.)

sclera, sending branches both to the choroid and to the optic nerve. The branches to the optic nerve spread to the optic nerve head anteriorly, to the lamina cribrosa, and via retrograde divisions to the pia mater and the optic nerve immediately behind the globe. The arterial supply has been studied in considerable detail because of the presumed relevance to the pathophysiology of glaucomatous optic neuropathy. There has been debate about some of the anatomic details, in part because of apparent individual variations in anatomy, as well as differing interpretations of the physiologic implications of the anatomic features.

Venous drainage is into the nearby central retinal vein. Some have observed minor tributaries into the adjacent choroid, or anastomoses with choroidal veins, some of which seem to form shunt vessels after occlusion of the central retinal vein, but others have denied the importance of tributaries toward the choroid, or even their existence. Details of the venous drainage have not been considered relevant to the process of glaucomatous optic nerve damage.

Branches of the posterior ciliary artery that enter the choroid break up into the capillary network of the choriocapillaris, with its fenestrated endothelium. This capillary layer lines the outer retina, separated from the photoreceptors by a connective tissue layer (Bruch's membrane) and the retinal pigment epithelium.

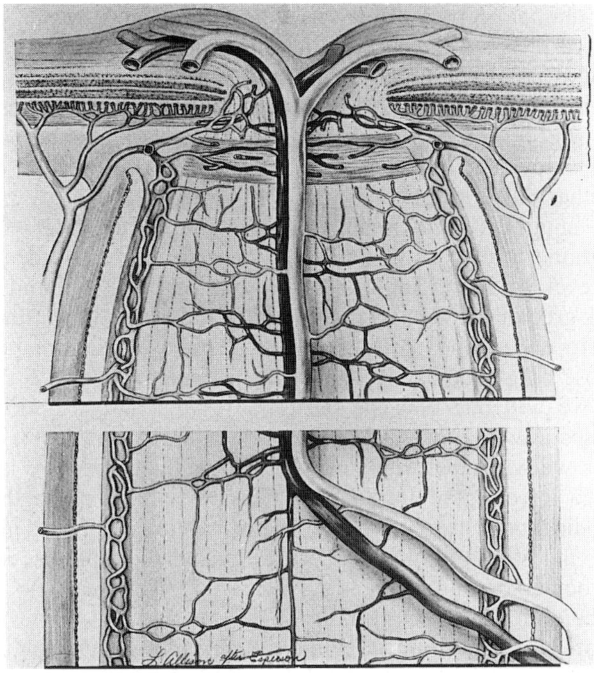

*Fig. 4.* Vascular supply and drainage of the optic nerve. (Reproduced with permission from: Anderson DR and Quigley HA: The Optic Nerve. In Hart WM Jr. (ed), *Adler's Physiology of the Eye.* St Louis: Mosby Year Book, 1992, 9th edition, pp 616-640.)

However, the branches of the posterior ciliary arteries that enter the optic nerve form a capillary bed that has the morphology of central nervous system (CNS) vasculature. Pericytes (mural cells) engulf the capillaries, and the non-fenestrated endothelium has tight junctions. Because of these fundamental anatomic differences, the physiology of the microvasculature in the optic nerve head may differ from that of the choroidal vessels, even though they share an arterial source. Specifically, the optic nerve vessels share with those of the retina (and of the CNS in general) the physiologic properties of autoregulation and the presence of the blood–tissue barrier.

## Pathogenic mechanisms of optic nervc damage

None of us doubt that intraocular pressure is a pathogenic factor in glaucomatous optic nerve damage. However, the apparent variation and susceptibility to intraocular pressure noted epidemiologically, as well as the differing manifestation of the optic nerve excavation, related at least in part on the level of intraocular pressure, emphasizes that other pathogenic factors are involved. As mentioned above, these factors in one sense determine the susceptibility of the optic nerve to intraocular pressure. However it would be just as accurate to say that the level of intraocular pressure determines the susceptibility to these other factors, and thus the other factors must be considered of equal importance. Part of our discussion may center around whether or not there are cases in which intraocular pressure by itself may produce damage, and if so by what mechanism. Conversely, are other cases in which the damage occurs determined by the other, non-pressure factors? Studies of normal tension glaucoma suggest that even in these cases the intraocular pressure is involved; if an intraocular pressure of 24 mm Hg can be harmful, why not 18 or 19 mm Hg, which is also higher than atmospheric pressure (0 mm Hg). However, it would only be fair to state that the question has been raised as to whether or not pressure is involved in all cases that we presently call glaucoma. There is suggestive statistical evidence that in patients with some form of vasospasm (migraine headaches, Raynaud's phenomenon, etc.), the degree of damage relates to the level of intraocular pressure, but in those without any evidence of vasospasm the degree of damage seems unrelated to the level of intraocular pressure.

While trying to understand the mechanism of optic nerve damage in cases that we presently diagnose as glaucoma, we must not get sidetracked into the argument as to whether or not we will one day use the term "glaucomatous optic atrophy" to refer only to those cases in which intraocular pressure interacts with other factors to produce damage. Perhaps we will label those in which intraocular pressure is not a pathogenic factor (and hence lowering of intraocular pressure will be of no therapeutic benefit) into a different diagnostic category, one of the several other non-glaucomatous optic atrophies. But in the present day we call cases glaucoma if the disc has the appearance of glaucoma, whether or not there is elevated IOP, if there is no evidence of some other cause of the optic nerve abnormality.

The subject of the symposium is to understand how glaucomatous damage occurs. The theme will certainly be to understand how intraocular pressure damages the axons, or at least interferes with their function, ultimately killing them. The intended search will be for factors that interact with the intraocular pressure or add to its effect in producing harm through changes in the collagenous structures or alteration of blood flow. We may challenge the basic tenet that pressure is the sine qua non for the definition of glaucoma by considering damage from pressure-independent factors, exploring the relationship to the types of optic nerve damage that we do not identify as glaucoma, such as pits or dehiscences of the optic nerve and anterior ischemic optic neuropathy (AION). There are, incidentally, two types of AION, one related to giant cell arteritis affecting the posterior ciliary arteries (called arteritic AION), and another (called non-arteritic AION) of some other undefined cause. You may hear these terms used in the course of the discussions at this meeting.

Broadly, the current main concepts of what happens with elevated IOP and glaucomatous damage is as follows. The connective tissue along with astroglia form a structural support at the point of exit of axons from the inner coat of the eye, and it is logically a vulnerable point at which there is a hydrostatic pressure gradient of the intracellular substance as the axon passes from within the eye (where the tissue pressure is the intraocular pressure) to the orbital portion of the optic nerve (enclosed within the meninges, and hence with the tissue pressure equal to intracranial pressure). With elevation of intraocular pressure there is a stretching of the sclera and an elastic outpouching of the lamina cribrosa, as well as an increased pressure gradient along the axon. The degree to which the openings of the several sheets of lamina cribrosa become misaligned, kinking and distorting the axons, is uncertain. The distortion may compress blood vessels in the region. Differences in the rigidity or compliance of the connective tissue may account in part for individual differences in susceptibility to IOP-induced damage.

At the same time, the intraocular pressure compresses the veins at their most downstream intraocular location (or at least the veins are collapsed just outside the eye by a

Bernoulli effect) so that the venous pressure is necessarily somewhat higher than the intraocular pressure within the boundaries of the globe. The rise in venous pressure is a challenge to blood flow, reducing the difference of pressure between arteries and veins. Under physiologic circumstances there is obviously a compensatory change in the resistance of the arteriovenous pathway, because the blood flow in the retina and optic disc are minimally affected as the intraocular pressure becomes elevated. The process of adjustment is known as autoregulation, the general term for local control of blood flow (as opposed to remote control through hormones or autonomic nerves). One hypothesis about glaucoma is that an inadequacy of the autoregulatory mechanism in the optic nerve of some individuals is a susceptibility factor that accounts for individual differences in the damage from a given level of IOP.

In the context of this symposium we must remind ourselves that there are already several known varieties of optic atrophies (conditions in which optic nerve axons are destroyed with consequential visual loss) that are not glaucomatous. In particular we have already noted that there are two identified varieties of anterior ischemic optic neuropathy (AION): one related to giant cell arteritis involving the posterior ciliary arteries, and another related to acute ischemia of the optic nerve head due to a different, but unidentified mechanism. As we discuss whether or not IOP-induced ischemia is part of the process of glaucomatous optic nerve damage, among the questions to be considered is what in the mechanism of producing ischemia accounts for the different clinical presentation of AION and glaucoma and the different appearance of the optic nerve after AION has occurred and glaucoma.

Axons challenged by mechanical forces and ischemia may have imperfect function for awhile, so that when intraocular pressure is successfully lowered, occasionally some portion of visual function improves, but ultimately the axons (and their retinal cell ganglion bodies) drop out to leave a permanent loss of the visual function they served. Along with the neuron loss the retinal nerve fiber thins, the optic nerve head develops a cavity (cup, or excavation), the sheets of lamina cribrosa become thin and stretched outward, and paths of capillaries are absent by fluorescein angiography in the regions where there is no longer any glial tissue to serve. The jury is hung with regard to whether the connective tissue damage, the microvascular damage, or both, when observed at this late stage, represent primary pressure-induced effects (with axon damage and loss of axons as consequence), represent pressure-induced damage that accompanies (but is independent of) pressure-induced axon damage, or represent atrophic change that follows as a consequence of the loss of axons in the region.

## Implications of understanding pathogenesis

Thus, in trying to understand the mechanism of damage of the optic nerve, the subject of this symposium, intraocular pressure is a contributing factor, and is the one that has been most clearly demonstrated to be so. We have clues about the other contributions, but the relationships have not been so clearly defined. Apart from scientific curiosity, there are some practical reasons for making an effort to understand the mechanism of optic nerve damage in glaucoma. One is the potential assessment of future risk of an individual. We can quantify the intraocular pressure in an individual and project that the higher the pressure the greater the risk he has of developing visual loss over the next period of time. If we could similarly quantify other factors involved, we could more accurately quantify the risk, and this better diagnostic ability would lead to better decisions concerning who needs treatment or who needs more aggressive treatment than they are presently receiving. A second practical result of understanding the mechanism would be the potential to treat to correct the other abnormal factors besides the intraocular pressure.

## Structure of the symposium

As we consider the mechanisms of optic nerve damage, the symposium is divided into three sessions. In one session the mechanical aspects of the connective tissue in the region of the optic nerve are considered. It is to be recognized that the connective tissue of the lamina cribrosa is not simply a portion of the sclera perforated by the passage of bundles of nerve fibers, but is a connective tissue of different composition from the sclera. An elevated intraocular pressure stretches the sclera, but also (and seemingly to a greater degree) stretches the lamina cribrosa outward. Histologically as glaucomatous cupping proceeds, there is collapse and disruption of the connective tissue that makes up the lamina cribrosa. The degree to which these phenomena of stretching and collapse are responsible for harming the axon (as opposed to being coincidental manifestations of elevated intraocular pressure) is unsettled. Perhaps the collapse contributes to but is not the exclusive cause of axon damage. The stretching and collapse of the lamina cribrosa may pinch axons, or pinch the vascular tree, challenging the circulation, compounding the challenge of IOP-induced elevation of venous pressure.

Another session of the symposium will concentrate on the potential contribution of ischemia to the local tissue damage, and in particular on the interaction of intraocular pressure with other physiologic or pathologic contributions to local ischemia. The ultimate result may simply be a compounding of the challenges produced by vasospasm and intraocular pressure, for example, but the question of why the clinical manifestation of low-tension glaucoma differs from that of acute ischemic optic neuropathy must be addressed.

Another session has to do with agonal changes in axons, how irreversible injury occurs and what might be done to minimize it. In the end, it is the axon that suffers, and its suffering is responsible for the visual loss we hope to prevent.

# 2. OVERVIEW AND INTRODUCTION TO SESSION ON CONNECTIVE TISSUE OF THE OPTIC NERVE IN GLAUCOMA

HARRY A. QUIGLEY, M.D.

We have decided to shuffle the order this morning a little bit. As I understand it, we are going to have three sessions, one of which deals with connective tissues, one with ganglion cells, and the third is circulation. I do not know that you can actually keep the subjects separate. Glaucoma is a subject matter where we are going to slop back and forth and hopefully be talking about all three of those things at the same time, and I am going to give an introductory talk to show you why I do not really think you can separate the topics with total independence, even though we will be breaking things up into pieces and asking each of the experts to talk about the thing about which they know most.

Typically, someone stands up at the start of a conference on glaucoma and says: "Well, you know, glaucoma is this terrible disease that we just can not even come to a definition of, do not even know what it is." I get really tired of hearing that, because it is wrong. I think those of us in this room who take care of glaucoma have a pretty good idea of what this disease is, so I am going to define it for us. We could spend the rest of the morning arguing about that definition if you wanted to, but I doubt that that is a useful exercise.

Glaucoma is a disease in which there is the loss of visual field, typically in the midperipheral visual field in preference to the center or the far periphery, and in which there is a characteristic appearance of the optic nerve head, an appearance I am going to call excavation (Figs. 1, 2). It is a particular way in which the substance of the optic nerve loses its tissue, leading to the rim of the optic disc having the appearance that you could stick your finger in under the edge of it as in this patient over here, in under there. Now that is distinct from other diseases of the optic nerve or of the retina in which you lose nerve fibers, but this thing called excavation does not happen.

So what actually we are going to talk about this morning in this connective tissue session actually is this phenomenon of excavation, why it happens in glaucoma, what it is due to, and if that is the particular defining feature of the disease as I am going to propose it to you, then how does it happen in glaucoma and what specifically does its occurrence lead us to in terms of understanding the varying susceptibility of patients to being injured by the disease.

Let us look at the contrast of glaucoma with a different disease. These are some pictures Doug Anderson should remember because they were from his patient (Fig. 3). This is ischemic optic neuropathy, and it happens to be a person who had a photograph of the optic nerve on the left taken before the person had the disease and the picture on the right taken after the person had the disease. Were you to see the loss of side vision in this patient it would qualify for what I just said about glaucomas: the loss of side vision, as in glaucoma, was in the midperipheral field. The center of vision in this person happened to have been preserved, and the periphery of the vision was also preserved, so if I showed the results of the field test to you on a chart, you would say, "Well, that looks like a glaucomatous field defect." But I think you can see this affected optic disc is pale, and this companion unaffected optic disc is not pale. There is a lot of nerve fiber loss in the right-hand picture. What is not present is excavation: it does not

*Optic Nerve in Glaucoma, pp. 15–36*
*edited by S.M. Drance*

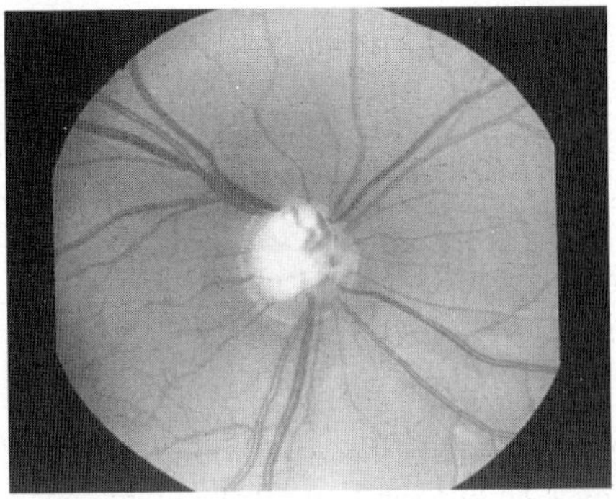

*Fig. 1.*

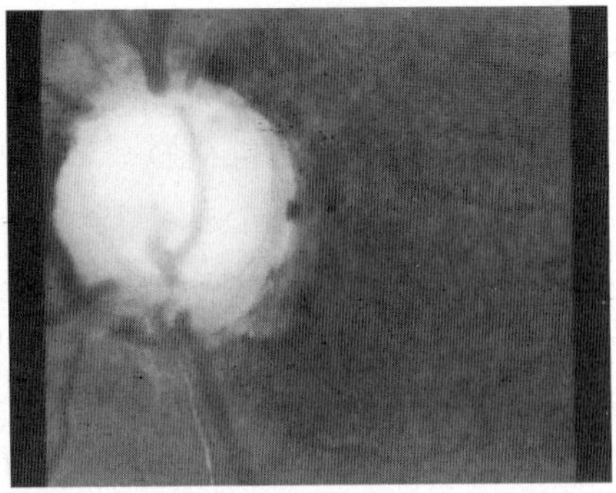

*Fig. 2.*

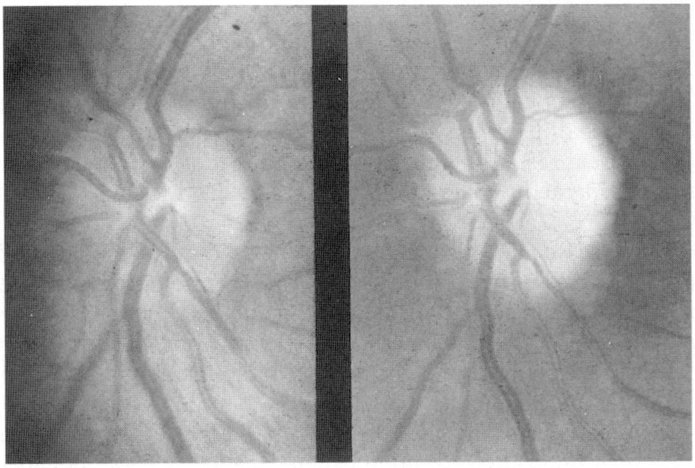

*Fig. 3.*

appear that I could get my finger in here anywhere. That is, the surface of the optic disc has subsided, but there is not a physical deepening and an undermining of the rim. So, what I propose is that the big difference between what disease this person had (ischemic optic neuropathy) and the disease the two people in the preceding pictures had (glaucoma) is this physical appearance of the optic nerve head.

So let us spend a moment looking at the general histology in glaucoma. John Morrison a little bit later in this session is going to talk more about the ultrastructure and the detailed structure of changes that occur in the optic nerve head. But let me first show you grossly where that appearance comes from. These are two histological pictures of monkey optic nerve head (Figs. 4, 5). In this picture, we have a normal monkey optic nerve head with the surface of the optic disc, the central retinal artery and vein, the neural tissue before and after it is myelinated as it leaves the back of the eye in the normal monkey. That is the vitreous cavity, and of course, this is retrobulbar optic nerve. In this picture over here we have caused the eye pressure to be elevated in this monkey's eye by lasering the trabecular meshwork to elevate the eye pressure, and the pressure had been up in this animal for, say, a year or so in the range that is typical

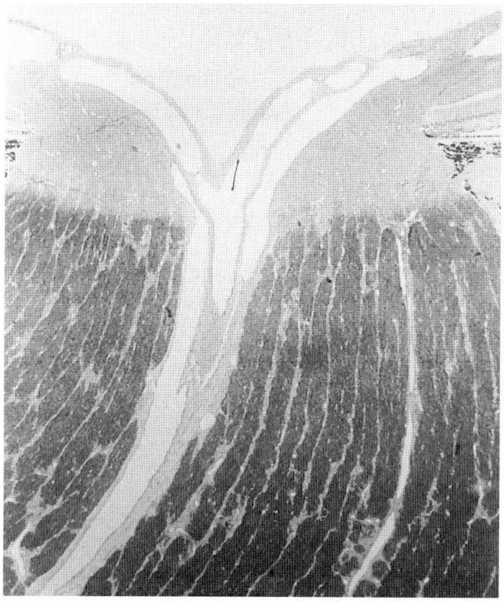

Fig. 4.

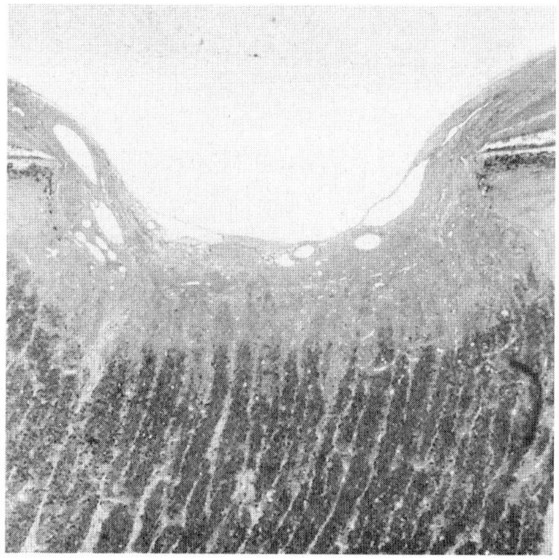

Fig. 5.

for exfoliation glaucoma, 35 mm Hg. You can see two or three things that are different between the normal and here. First, the neural rim of tissue is narrower. The nerves as they went into the optic nerve head are fewer. They used to be over here and now they have receded to that point. You can also see that what you would call the floor of the optic nerve head, which formerly sat up here, and this picture, of course, filled by the vessels, has also subsided downward, so the thing looks deeper.

Now, if we look at another picture, a much further along stage of glaucoma, these now happen to be human optic nerve heads, the one on the left is a beautiful normal, lots of neural tissue going over the rim (Fig. 6). There is the edge of the retina, the end of Bruch's membrane, myelinated nerve would be right back down here somewhere, and here you see excavation. This is the end of the pigment epithelium right at the optic disc, so this is the entry zone inlet to the optic disc. That is the last remaining blood vessel hanging on the rim. There is not a nerve fiber going over the edge of here, and look how you could put your finger in underneath here, into what essentially looks like an undermined, a dug-out area behind the disc. In other words, light coming this way would strike here, actually the light could hit an empty space if it could get by the pigment epithelium and Bruch's membrane. To see these a little better, some years ago we began doing a digestion preparation where we essentially erased the nerve tissue and the glial tissue with a detergent and then did scanning electron microscopy of the optic nerve head.

The left side is a normal adult human optic nerve head prepared in this particular way (Fig. 7a,b). The vitreous cavity would be up there, this is the myelinated optic nerve back here, and this, the lamina cribrosa, the area where the nerve bundles dive through 300 to 500 holes, which leave through the eye wall. And here is the engineering problem, an engineering problem: How do you get a million axons out of a pressurized cavity without a significant enough leak that the eye can not keep itself inflated? And, with those nerve fibers not being hurt or destroyed or kinked in some way, such that through 75 years or so of life they do not drop dead? This disorder probably is a

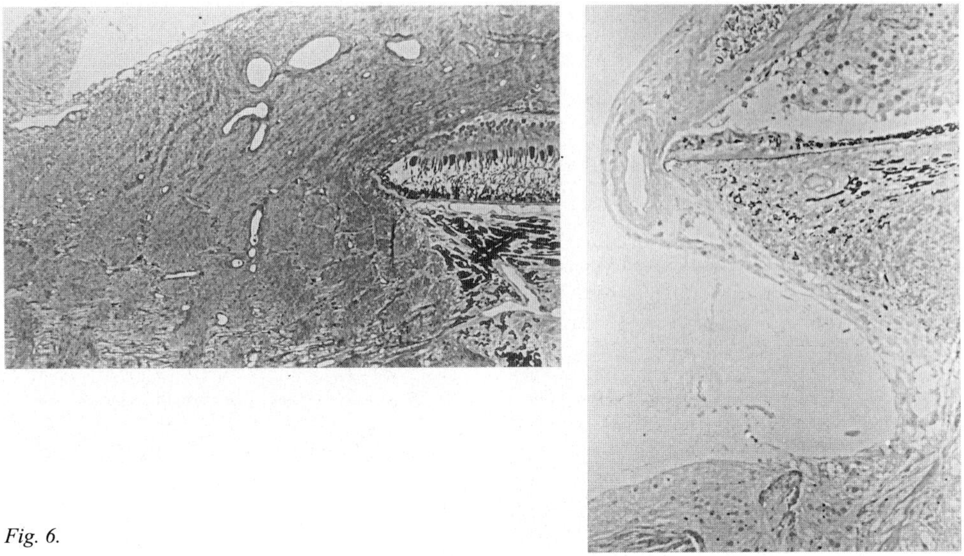

*Fig. 6.*

failure of that particular engineering solution, and that is why the axons die in one way or another.

Figure 7c shows a person who had glaucoma during this person's life. We have this person's name and history, we know what the visual field finding was, but I show you the picture only to show you the change that occurs grossly in the optic nerve head. You can see that it looks as if the lamina cribrosa has been sagged backward. We like to joke that it looks as if someone sat on it. And this is the lower and the upper pole of this optic disc, the nasotemporal axis was through here. Once again, the vitreous cavity is up there and the optic nerve head has been sectioned across straight through.

If we were to look in detail at how this structure, the lamina cribrosa (it is an apt analogy in Italy) is a colander, the thing in which you drain spaghetti. The lamina cribrosa is like a series of 8 or 10 colanders stacked on top of each other, with the holes not exactly in register and in fact, with not exactly the same number of holes going through at any one level. They branch, they get actually a little wider as you go upward or narrower as you go downward, downward meaning toward the retrolaminar optic nerve. I am showing you this picture to show you the insertion zone of the lamina cribrosa here into the sclera, that is what it hangs on to at the edge. To put it another way, vector forces in the eye wall that would be generated by the eye pressure changing or by the eye pressure under normal circumstances would be pulling on this thing, there would be circumferential tension in the eye wall. In addition, if the eye pressure were actually high enough that it could displace the lamina cribrosa, it would displace it in a vector in this direction (anteroposteriorly). So we could think that there might be two forces acting on this structure which itself of course is not as strong as the overall sclera. The sclera is a millimeter and a half thick; this lamina cribrosa is about 300 or 400 microns thick, and is full of holes. Of course, the holes are full of nerve fibers.

You can see the insertion of the lamina in this zone, in the glaucoma eye now, has done two things. First, it actually looks like it is going backward this way instead of being more orthogonal. See how the sclera here has a little notch in it, but it basically looks like it is sort of a straight up and down thing. It has moved outward, and the

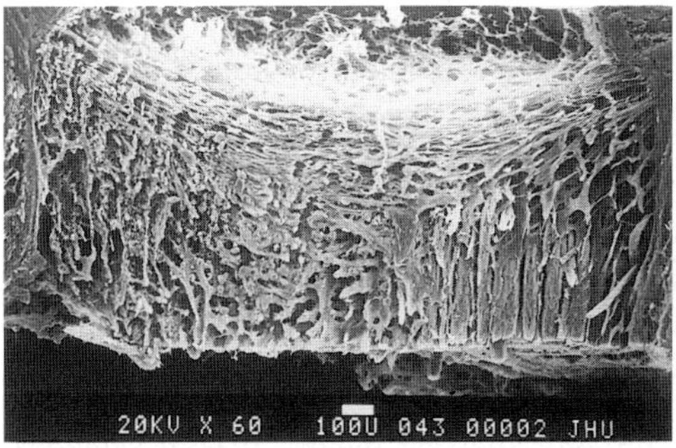


a.

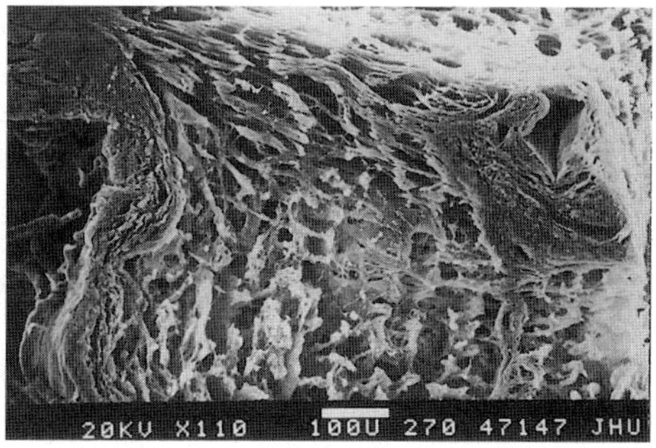


b.

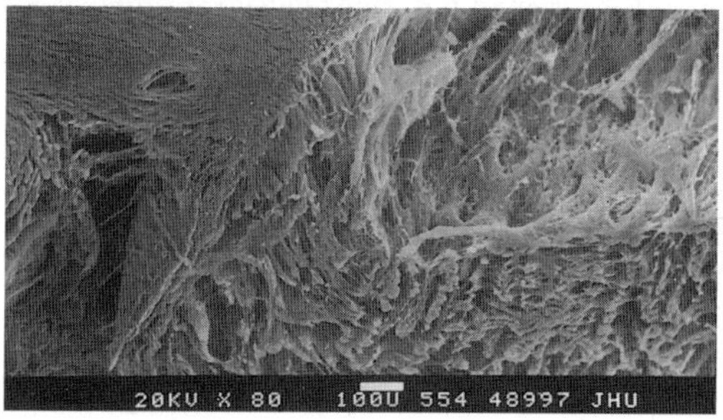


c.

*Fig. 7.*

lamina heads south before it comes across the optic nerve head inlet. And this, in fact, is where you put your finger in under, this is excavation.

**Dr. Anderson**: I will start the process of interruption and questioning. You said earlier the lamina cribrosa was like a series of colanders with the holes not perfectly aligned. My recollection from the old anatomy books, and I wonder if you had new information since the old anatomy books, was that the lamina cribrosa was, in fact, completely and nicely aligned at this place where there is a pressure gradient it has to go through. I thought that the misalignment did not occur until you got outside of the eye into the retrolaminar part of the optic nerve. I wonder if in the normal circumstances the holes are completely aligned, and it is only in the abnormal circumstance where the pressure becomes elevated and each of these layers are put on stretch that they become misaligned.

**Dr. Quigley**: Well, it is an excellent question, and the reason I can give you some kind of an answer, Doug, is that over the last 10 years on three different occasions we have tried to do histomorphology of the pores as they go through. Comparing people in different racial groups was one thing that we did in an attempt to look at it. We set someone busy doing serial sections in this plane, so we were cutting through essentially in the plane of the scleral wall, trying down through the lamina cribosa. Now, if all the pores were aligned and if in fact our plane of sectioning was following the perpendicular to that alignment, we would be able to take one pore and just follow it right on through the lamina. The first reason I can tell you that it is not aligned is that the structure has a natural backward curve to it. In other words, it is like a hammock going across a hole. And that also makes a bunch of good physical sense, because if you try to stretch a string across an opening, or hold a string like this, you have to put tremendous force on it to have it be straight, it wants to curl downward a little bit. In the string case, of course, it is gravity that is making it go down. In the case of this eye wall thing, you have got a spherical structure, so that to have something be actually straight across there would be rather ridiculous, and it would not be the way the tissues would naturally hang due to the forces that are on them. The eye wall tension is trying to pull it straight; the inside out pressure, whatever vector that provides, the eye pressure being in the range of 15 and the pressure outside being somewhere between 0 and 8, depending on what you read. There is a difference inside and out, so the thing is curved. And that means, if you wanted to say, are the pores all aligned, you would have to cut it perpendicular to the eye wall, and when you do that, and we have done that on either side to some degree, you still find that these pores branch and coalesce and go somewhat diagonally through.

Now to answer your question another way, Doug, I am not sure what is true in the real life eye. I am only sure what I can see histologically. If some of our friends who are now doing laser tomography of the disc can get pores in their sights, maybe they can find out in live eyes what it is like. But I think you can see here (Fig. 8a), here is one that looks kind of orthogonally arranged and then it sort of takes a turn to this side, see that? This is actually one of the pores going through. We were completely frustrated in attempting to say, for example, let us follow one pore right on through the lamina, because of that particular business, they dive off obliquely and they branch. So no, I do not think anybody who wrote a textbook that says they are all straight and they are all aligned normally was right.

**Dr. Anderson**: I guess that when we tried to look at that sort of thing we found that we could follow individual channels. It may, as you say, take a diagonal course rather than being perfectly straight, but at least it did not branch, and so that there was no exchange of nerve fibers from one bundle to another, until it was beyond the lamina cribosa. And in these kind of preparations, of course, the eye was fixed at a time when there was not the pressure gradient that is normally present. So, if you fix the eye with a pressure of 15 in the eye and then made sure that later on there was no elasticity or change, this picture, for instance, represents the eye with zero pressure within it, as opposed to one that has the physiologic pressure within it.

**Dr. Quigley**: You are probably aware that we have done some recent stuff looking at elastin. If John Morrison does not cover it, I will, I have got the extra slides here. What we found out or what we learned, at least from the general literature, was that elastin is a neat molecule in that you can fix it with aldehydes and it still has some spring to it. So we pressurized eyes to pressures between 15 and 75, then fixed them with aldehyde fixative running into the vitreous at that pressure, then froze the eye, so that even if the elastin wanted to change shape after all that, after that fixation, it would be frozen in position, then we cut frozen sections and used the fuchsin stain, a thing called Luna stain, which is like the Verhoeff-van Gieson's, for those who like histopathology. It still looks like this.

**Dr. Anderson**: Where we separate on the point, really, is only this: that if we are going to talk about the mechanical effects of the pressure and what it does to these holes, and therefore the support for the axons, it is important to know in detail what is happening here. It certainly is different at the level of the lamina cribosa from the

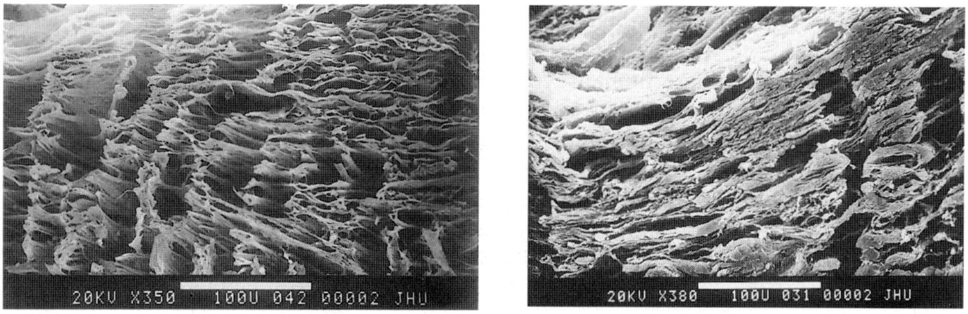


*a.* *b.*

*Fig. 8.*

situation further back, where the support structure is very different. It is a different support structure in this particular place where there is a pressure gradient, and we should make sure that we understand exactly what the anatomy is.

**Dr. Quigley**: Point well taken.

**Dr. Zeimer**: Could you elaborate more on what you mentioned about fixation at high pressure. I know that you did the microhistology; did you also do gross anatomy so the same structure of the lamina cribrosa, the curvature, the hammock, ....

**Dr. Quigley**: If one looks at eyes fixed at different pressures there are no differences in the pore sizes with the present limitations of measuring.

**Dr. Zeimer**: Not the pore, but did you see that hammock?

**Dr. Quigley**: Yes, it does not change much, not in the limits that you can see histologically.

Let me move on because we do not want to get hung up on my presentation because we have a lot more things that we want to do. This eye was fixed at atmospheric pressure (Fig. 8a). Here are pores coming through, there is one coming through, and in the plane in which this was cut, you can see that pore dived off that way, because here you can see it disappear. Here is the near side wall as that pore went thataway. Here is a pore and again, you see this one coming down and then it dives off that way, this one more or less stayed in alignment, then it went off diagonally in this direction coming through. That is the normal.

This is glaucoma (Fig. 8b). And you can see what has happened here is, it looks like somebody took an accordion and closed it. And in fact, we can do measurements for the glaucoma versus the normals fixed at the same pressure, and in this case atmospheric pressure, of the relative height of this portion from myelinated optic nerve to the upper portion that contains connective tissue. Further up anterior in the optic nerve head there is no collagenous connective tissue, no elastin, there is only collagen type IV around capillaries up here. But this structure here is half the height of the normal laminar position, taking account again, these are dead eyes fixed at atmospheric pressure. So the whole structure is undergoing three things. This is the schematic of it.

**Dr. Van Buskirk**: Was that in the monkey model?

**Dr. Quigley**: No those are human eyes. The glaucoma one I pointed to on the right was one of a series of about 15 with known glaucoma histories that we did. The monkey looks generally the same. In terms of Koch's postulates, you can generate the appearance that I have talked about as characteristic of glaucoma in a normal non-human primate eye, simply by raising the eye pressure. We will hopefully not get hung up on unitary theories of disease. We hope that anyone who still thinks that glaucoma comes from one cause will be corrected. Glaucoma comes from many causes. One of them certainly has to do with the eye pressure. Later in the meeting others will deal with other aspects than the ones we will talk about here.

**Dr. Kaufman**: Are we going to have a discussion at some point as to why it seems to happen so much faster in the monkey, at least that is my impression, than it does in the human, even at comparable elevated pressures?

**Dr. Quigley**: Well, Paul, now, having had about 100 monkeys devote themselves to this model in our lab, we have now seen animals who my lab people call supermonkeys, who will demonstrate to us that a pressure of 35 to 40 can happen to some of these monkeys for 18 months while they eat our chow, and no damage happens. So there is a variety of damage possible, even in the monkey, and I wish I could study animals in such detail that I could find out why supermonkey is different. We have a couple of them that we are trying to look at carefully. I do not know that we know whether monkeys and humans are different or the same.

**Dr. Hoffman**: Harry, what happens when you reverse the gradients, for instance, with raised intracranial pressure. Do you have any idea whether or not things bow forward instead of being pushed back?

**Dr. Quigley**: There is some evidence. I think Mike Yablonski attempted to study this in cats. What he did was essentially he cannulated the front of the eye and changed the intracranial pressure. It was an interesting experiment and produced some evidence that it appears to move in the other direction.

The things I am showing you here, though, Paul, are things that are physically fixed by the time you are looking at them. That is, I am not talking about watching it move actually in the material I just showed you. Certainly there is actually viscoelastic movement of the nerve head. We will talk about it after Ran's talk a little bit, because we are now measuring it in vivo in animals, as he has measured it both in vivo and in dead eyes. But most of the change we are talking about at this moment is something that took a long time to happen, and John will show you some of what it is that is actually going on. The laminar beams are actually breaking and rehealing, and they are, by and large, fixed in position. The structure gets very stiff or gets stiffer.

So excavation (Fig. 9a,b) from a biological, from a histological standpoint, consists of compressing together of these laminar plates, rotation of the insertion of the lamina at its edge in the sclera, and probably a widening of the whole optic nerve head behind Bruch's membrane, but not a widening of the optic disc as we view it clinically, because the part we view clinically is actually the terminal edge of Bruch's membrane as a limiting factor to the opening. And Bruch's membrane is a very rigid structure. It will crack and break as we see in pseudoxanthoma elasticum

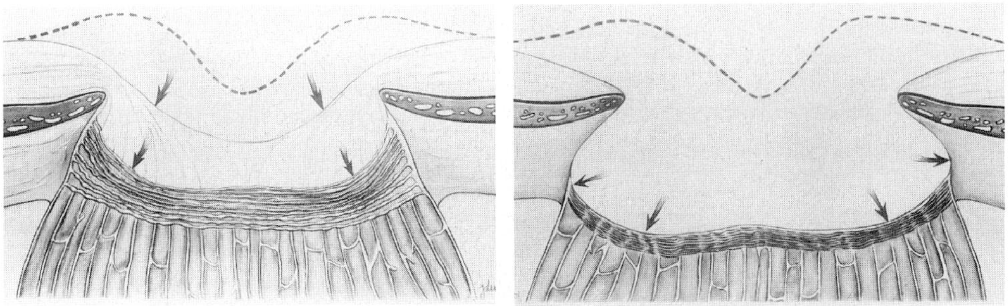

*Fig. 9.*

with angioid streaks or in lacquer cracks in high myopia. But Bruch's membrane, once formed in the adult, does not change much. So it is, in fact, the knife edge against which everything else might physically wind up, I have no idea whether it actually compresses axons or not. But from a clinical standpoint, the disc rarely gets bigger than this point I am pointing at right here, which is actually the edge of Bruch's membrane.

And finally, of course, there is loss of nerve tissue. But that is not what is unique to glaucoma, since any optic neuropathy loses nerve tissue. As one of my favorite examples that shows physical events going on within the optic nerve head, this is the optic disc of the same person about 12 years apart (Fig. 10). He is a man who by this point had developed an eye pressure in the 35 to 40 range. His momma had glaucoma, he had developed his first field defect at the time of this particular picture. He happened to have been in the collaborative glaucoma study, and he had some old records. He dug up his old optic nerve pictures, and it almost does not look like the same optic nerve head. You can see what has happened is not only cup enlargement and deepening, but the disc is actually physically rotated that way. You would say, well, that is a typical tilted myopic optic disc, the clinicians here would recognize that. The problem is, he did not use to have it, and this was when he was an adult, he was 30 years old here and about 43, 44 there.

So physical changes are going on at the back of the eye. Joe Caprioli was one of the people who first pointed out that the way to determine the remaining nerve fibers might be to measure the neural rim, Stephen had published measurement of the neural rim, and one of the things that they both detected was that we do not all have the same number of nerve fibers. Different optic discs appear to have different amounts of nerve rim area, if you measure this area, which is presumably the neural tissue leaving the eye. If you could summarize that area in actual square millimeters, you would have essentially an objective measurement of how many nerve fibers there are. And what we want to know in glaucoma is, if we are losing nerve fibers, how many do we lose? And the problem is illustrated by the two discs that I have on these two pictures (Fig. 11a,b). What Joe detected, and also Britton, working with Stephen, was that discs are bigger and smaller, and the bigger the disc is, the more nerve fibers you seem to have. That is, the bigger the neural rim area. And one of the big variables we have to deal with in glaucoma is disc size.

On the left and on the right is a 95% confidence interval for normal disc size in humans. It is a histological study that we did in which we got a bunch of normal eye bank eyes and measured their size. We did a number of other things with them, but this is how big or how small the 95th percentile and the 5th percentile are for size.

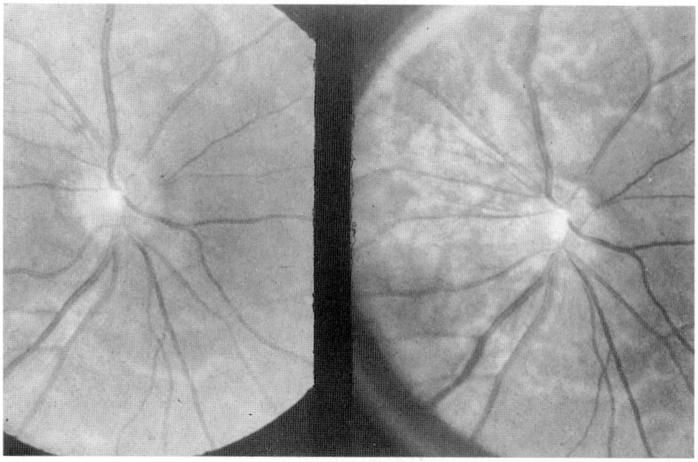

*Fig. 10.*

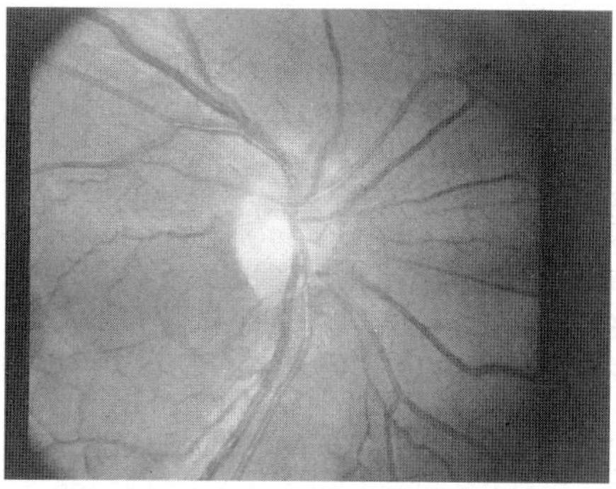

*a.*

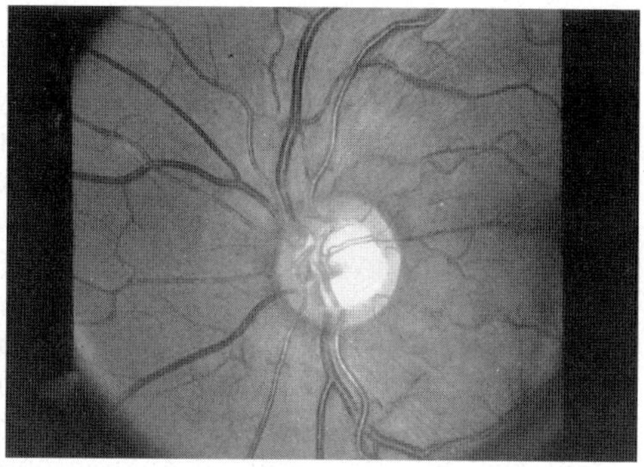

*b.*

*Fig. 11.*

There is quite a variation. And I used to give a lecture on this subject and I would say, now, different discs are different sizes but we all have about a million axons. We do not. People with this size disc have closer to 500,000 or 600,000 axons, and people with that size have about 1.4 million or 1.5 million. There is a tremendous variation in the number, and in fact, the number of fibers is directly related to the area of the optic disc.

This (Fig. 12) is a histological study in monkeys, this is about the same slope of increasing number of nerve fibers per disc size that Joe and the Drance group found when they used image analysis to measure nerve rim area from clinical photographs of the optic disc.

Now, if you were a physicist or an engineer, you might say, well, if I have a big hole in the back of the eye and you are talking about some kind of a biomechanical problem, the bigger the hole, the worse off the person would be. Because it is even a bigger problem to fix a flat tire when you have a bigger hole in it than when you have a pinpoint hole. From the physics stance, that makes sense, but when you study glaucoma eyes, you find that whether you study them by image analysis or you look at them histologically, larger optic disc size is not a risk factor for glaucoma visual

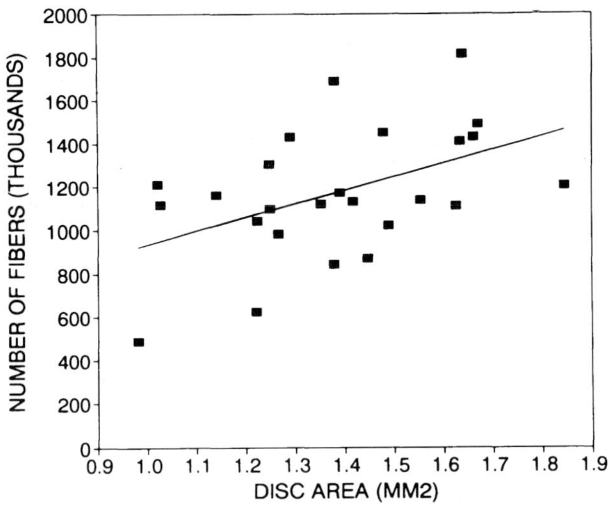


*Fig. 12.*

field loss. I do not know why that is. We might, in fact, kick that around a little bit later on or now, why that is, but I will just throw that fact into the pot.

I want to give you two more pieces of information, and then I will open it up for further discussion. Sure, Doug?

**Dr. Anderson**: I was going to ask you what your evidence was for that last statement that larger disc size was not a risk factor.

**Dr. Quigley**: Well, I believe that Joe, I know that Jonas, and probably Drance's group, probably have, using various forms of photography, taken pictures of the optic disc on cross-sectional, clinic based samples of patients and compared them to a normal age-matched group. You find that the mean and the distribution of the size of the optic disc in adult human eyes with glaucoma is identical to the control group. Now, that does not necessarily mean there are not some extreme large discs which got that way, and got glaucoma, because they were larger, but what it means in terms of biostatistics is that having a larger disc is not a risk factor for glaucoma field loss. The histology I pointed to is we have measured the size of the disc in a series of human eyes, histological fixed tissue at atmospheric pressure, compared to age-matched control eye bank normal eyes, and the distribution of size is the same. Now, what that leads you to is two conclusions. First, if the glaucoma disc was more likely to become a glaucoma disc because it was bigger, it would still be bigger in the histological fixed tissue, and is not. And second, if glaucoma caused the whole disc to get bigger, measured at the inlet of Bruch's membrane, then it would be bigger after field loss has happened. So two things are true: larger discs are not at greater risk for glaucoma, and glaucoma does not cause the disc, as we measure it, to get larger. Now, it does get larger behind Bruch's membrane, where I have been pointing to this excavation.

**Dr. Zeimer**: My question to you is, clinically you talk about the size of the disc according to the size of Bruch's membrane; however, if you want to look at forces, you have to look at the size of the sclera and canal. I have two questions, one is...

**Dr. Quigley**: Back there it is wider, right there it is not.

**Dr. Zeimer**: Right, so then when you do histology do you find a correlation, some kind of a risk factor of the size of the scleral canal, is the size of the scleral canal larger in glaucoma eyes than in normals?

**Dr. Quigley**: Yes, because the sclera and lamina cribrosa are stretchable.

**Dr. Zeimer**: And my other question is, when does Bruch's membrane, at what stage of development, become mature compared to the maturation of the optic nerve?

**Dr. Quigley**: That is an excellent question, and I do not have the answer to it. I know in adults it is a rather thick structure, but I do not know whether it is continuously still being added to with time after, say, teenage. I know the overall optic disc, including Bruch's membrane, gets wider in infants in the first year of life. Both the phenomenon of reversible cup change and of expansion of the optic disc and the whole eyeball in children suggest that they have not laid down all their collagen yet and the collagen is not cross-linked, and so the whole structure creeps against the increased force of eye pressure.

**Dr. Zeimer**: Could it be that Bruch's membrane matures first, before the lamina cribrosa matures?

**Dr. Quigley**: A worthwhile study to do. Have not done it. You want to do it?

**Dr. Zeimer**: Could you relate it to my previous question regarding the size of the scleral canal in glaucoma?

**Dr. Quigley**: The scleral canal posterior to Bruch's membrane here is excavated and wider in eyes that were known to have field loss during the person's life. I have no way of knowing whether that was wider prior to the damage, because we have a one point in time view of the histology.

**Dr. Drance:** It cannot be seen, of course, by any methods we currently use clinically.

**Dr. Quigley**: No, but I would love to know with the people who have such a thing as the Heidelberg instrument or other instruments, can they measure the width of the scleral canal through Bruch's membrane, as opposed to the inlet at Bruch's membrane.

**Dr. Zeimer**: Is it true that you can not see it clinically? I mean, would not you assume that if you have a Bruch's membrane that is fixed, and the scleral canal is large, you would see some kind of excavation or backward or peripheral direction of the blood vessels even before the damage.

**Dr. Quigley**: You might assume that, but I would have to prove it by some kind of a correlative study.

**Dr. Zeimer**: But what is your impression clinically? I mean, are there discs that you see the nerve fiber.

**Dr. Quigley**: My impression clinically is worthless, and I have no data.

**Dr. Kaufman**: My understanding, at least in the monkey and I think, in the human, is that with age there is a loss of elastic tissue, at least in the anterior portion of the elastic lamina, of what is called the elastic lamina of Bruch's membrane. I have an interest in this not so much from the standpoint of glaucoma but from the standpoint of presbyopia and the ciliary muscle, but there is pretty good histologic evidence that there is almost a collagenalization, for want of a better term, of the elastic lamina of Bruch's membrane, at least anteriorly, and I wonder whether if you lost some degree of play in the system posteriorly as well, whether this might enter into some of the changes that we are going to talk about later.

**Dr. Quigley**: John Morrison, you want to comment on elastin and the lamina cribrosa with age?

**Dr. Morrison:** Harry, I think you have been working on that more than I have, as far as...

**Dr. Quigley**: John did a lovely study as a fellow in the lab, showing us that as elastin develops in other tissues, it first lays down a fibrillar matrix. Reed is going to talk about this. The major alpha elastin, the "springy stuff itself", actually just keeps getting fatter looking with age, and then starts sort of looking kind of moth-eaten. Adult humans do not look like their elastin is falling apart in the lamina, I do not know about Bruch's membrane.

**Dr. Caprioli:** Harry, you have shown nicely the compression of the laminar plates and distortion of the pores and so forth, and backward bowing. What is the evidence that these are primary changes rather than secondary changes simply because the axons have dropped out and now the laminar plates have collapsed?

**Dr. Quigley**: Yes, it is a key thing. How do we know that this is not simply something that happened after the axon was dead? In the first thing that we reported, where we took human eyes that we knew had a history of glaucoma, we looked at the degree of optic nerve damage that they had, categorizing them into 25% loss of the optic nerve, 50%, 75%, and the whole thing, and then looked at the changes in the lamina quantitatively, to see, were the changes in the lamina lagging behind the optic nerve damage, were they seemingly running parallel to it, or, if we got lucky, did it actually seem to be happening before the nerve damage. Now, you can imagine that because of variability, with 20 eyes, you could not really read it very finely. There is compression of the lamina and rotation on its insertion at the stage where the optic nerve has lost about 25% of its fibers, which would be considered clinically a relatively early stage of the disease. But I can not deny that if you said, "But that is just because 25% of the nerve disappeared and now you have measured 25% compression which happened after the nerve fibers were lost", absolutely true, I can not tell.

**Dr. Anderson**: How about in optic atrophy which is non-glaucomatous? Could you learn anything by looking at the lamina in those cases where you have lost the axons and therefore determine whether or not the lamina cribrosa secondarily has changes just from loss of axons?

**Dr. Quigley**: Well, I learned as a fellow in the laboratory of Doug Anderson how to transect the optic nerve from Barry Davis, whose picture is sitting right here. We have used such a model, and John Morrison has studied the details of collagen 1, 3, 4, and some other things. Comparing the experimental elevated eye pressure in monkey model to the optic nerve transection model and looking at the lamina cribrosa. Doug, it is very different. John is going to show you what it looks like. It leads you to the conclusion that raising the eye pressure does something different than just killing off nerve fibers.

**Dr. Caprioli**: But also, there are cases of non-glaucomatous cupping. They are relatively unusual, but even compressive injuries to the optic nerve may produce cupping. I think you have pointed out that the arteritic variety of ischemic optic neuropathy can also cause excavation. So, excavation is not purely glaucomatous.

**Dr. Quigley**: I never saw a disorder that was absolutely completely different from everything else. So, there are clearly going to be examples of other diseases that look like the disc is excavated, and those of us who clinically look at optic discs know that you can get fooled. If you look at a population of people, you do not get fooled distinguishing glaucoma from normal except in about 5% of the examples. We are in the midst right now of looking at the Baltimore Eye Survey population – based sample of optic disc photography, which is simultaneous stereo. The normal data are being reported in a paper this year and the glaucoma data are going to be presented at ARVO. Some other previous work, in fact, John Trobe got together a group of optic disc pictures that Joel Glaser and Doug and others had collected, and showed them to a bunch of glaucoma experts, and sort of made monkeys out of them, and I would have been just as bad a monkey, because they were discs that looked like glaucoma. Doug, you remember examples we saw of cupping in cases that were pituitary adenomas and meningiomas. Joe, you are absolutely right, but it is unfair, I think, to take a crowd of highly selected photographs and show them to someone and say, now, see there, you can not tell glaucoma from something else. Because what they did was to pick, in a sample from the population, the 1% presenting into a tertiary center that someone thought looked just like glaucoma, took a picture of it and keep it in a file, you know. I mean, how many pictures did they take of all the pituitary adenomas that just had plain pale discs?

The arteritic study is an interesting one, because we looked at non-arteritic ischemic neuropathy, and it is really uncommon for those to simulate glaucoma, though the occasional one does.

**Dr. Anderson:** It is occurring to me that we may not be able to put everything in one basket. That is to say, there may be both pressure-induced changes and changes secondary to axon loss. Obviously, when the pressure is elevated this elastic tissue stretches. Obviously also when axons are lost, in the lamina cribrosa, even if not stretched, there is going to be some rearrangement of the tissue because there is not a cavity that develops. The support tissue collapses into the space where the axons are gone. There may be a reaction in the type of connective tissue material which is manufactured during any healing stages following either loss of axons or prolonged stretch with rearrangement. Therefore we may have to consider what features of glaucomatous cupping are found when you have simple optic atrophy, that is, loss of axons due to some other condition other than pressure-induced loss, optic atrophy from pituitary tumors and other things like that. In contrast, what happens in the optic disc of an ocular hypertensive patient who is subjected to high pressure and has chronic stretch of the lamina cribrosa but no axon loss as a result, and how do those two conditions differ. We may have to not look at connective tissue damage as one package, but look at the individual elements of that package and which ones correlate with what by looking at these other conditions as controls.

**Dr. Quigley**: I think what you have said is very wise, I would only add one thing to it, and I think we should stress, especially for those who are not as familiar with glaucoma as a clinical entity. You said, under the influence of elevated eye pressure. I absolutely detest the word elevated eye pressure. It has led to very poor identification of this disease in the population, because as most of us know, 20 to 25% of people with glaucoma have never in their lives had an elevated pressure. Stephen tried to point this out to all of us for years. I used to think he was absolutely wrong, that we just had not caught these people having an elevated pressure. It is quite clear, however, that people who have an eye pressure of 15 have quite a number of vector forces acting on this optic nerve head. It is not true that at normal pressure that there is no force on the nerve head. So those who develop this disease at a pressure of 15, or 12, may in fact simply have (as one hypothesis) connective tissue that stretches under those forces that are present in the normal eye, whereas for the rest of us it does not. I am essentially extending your point, Doug, by saying yes, there may be a variety of responses; some of them are connective tissue responses, some are vascular responses, others are nerve responses. And I actually want to make one more 5-minute point, and then we will move on to Reed's talk, continuing the discussion, I do not want to shut down the discussion but I do want to actually keep each one of us to about a 45-minute slot. Does anybody want, any quick comment before I give you my last point, which is which nerve fibers die? Reed.

**Dr. Pyeritz**: I am just a simple country geneticist, Harry, and I tend to look at life in terms of pedigree, so something you said intrigued me, and that is the size of the opening in Bruch's membrane. If there is that much variability, does it run in families?

**Dr. Quigley**: Does anybody have evidence on it?

**Dr. Drance**: The answer is yes, it does. There is evidence; all you need to do is to go to an Inuit settlement and look at their normal discs. You can almost tell who the parents are of a particular individual who has, for instance, a huge normal cavern in a normal disc. But I do not think it has actually been done in a way that would satisfy you genetically, as a simple country geneticist.

**Dr. Quigley**: I was going to hold back, but yes, simple country population study in Baltimore shows, as Joe and others have demonstrated, Black Americans have substantially larger discs, on average, than do White Americans. They do not, however, have more or fewer optic nerve fibers, judged by the rim area in their optic disc on a population basis.

**Dr. Drance**: Harry, one very quick question, if I may. The question of the size of the optic nerve always bothers me. What does the individual's optic nerve look like in cross-section who has a huge disc and an 0.9 cup with a normal neuroretinal rim and is a healthy individual? What does that lamina look like? To be specific, could we make it somebody with a huge nerve, one of about 2%, maybe 1% of the population, who have large nerves, absolutely normal, an 0.9 cup. What would that lamina look like if that individual developed very early glaucoma? He would start off by having a cavern. If you would be able to watch the thickness of that lamina, would it go backwards?

**Dr. Quigley**: I would love to have that histology. We are actually trying right now to get our hands on nothing more complicated than myope nerve heads, people who were more than -4 during their lives...It is extraordinarily difficult to get that into your hands. Paul Kaufman?

**Dr. Kaufman**: Harry, just to finish the sentence, which you did not finish, about your simple country study in Baltimore. The black people with the large disc do not have more or fewer nerve fibers, but they sure do have more glaucoma.

**Dr. Quigley**: You got it. They have bigger discs and they have got more glaucoma, and one might suspect it is because they have got bigger discs, but in fact, when you look at the black persons who have glaucomatous field loss, they do not have any bigger discs than the white persons who have glaucomatous field loss.

Now for my final point. There is a certain zone of the field that is damaged first, and the axons that go from that visual field area down to the optic disc live in a particular place in the optic disc. In a patient from Bascom Palmer that was the first of the human examples I studied the cross-section of the optic nerve behind the eye (Fig. 13) which shows preserved fibers here and here in a bow-tie configuration, and a loss selectively of fibers shaped like an hourglass, the upper and the lower pole of the optic nerve head. And the reason I am bold enough to suggest to you that the connective tissue change in glaucoma has something to do with glaucoma is that the normal pattern of the lamina cribrosa looked at from the front (Fig. 14) looks just like that pattern over there. In this micrograph the holes that go through, which Doug and I were talking about before, are seen from the front. If what you do is you put it in a histological measuring device and you measure the open space at any single level going down, there is more open space in the upper and lower quadrants than there is in the nasal and temporal quadrant, as you can see qualitatively by looking at this picture.

This is the normal pattern of the lamina cribrosa in the normal human eye, and to my knowledge is the only regional anatomical or physiological feature of the optic nerve head that fits with that pattern of neural loss in glaucoma. So one of the features of the eye's normal anatomy leads you to an intuitively obvious statement that the weaker place in the optic nerve head gives first, for whatever reason, because of lousy connective tissue or because of the influence of the forces generated by eye

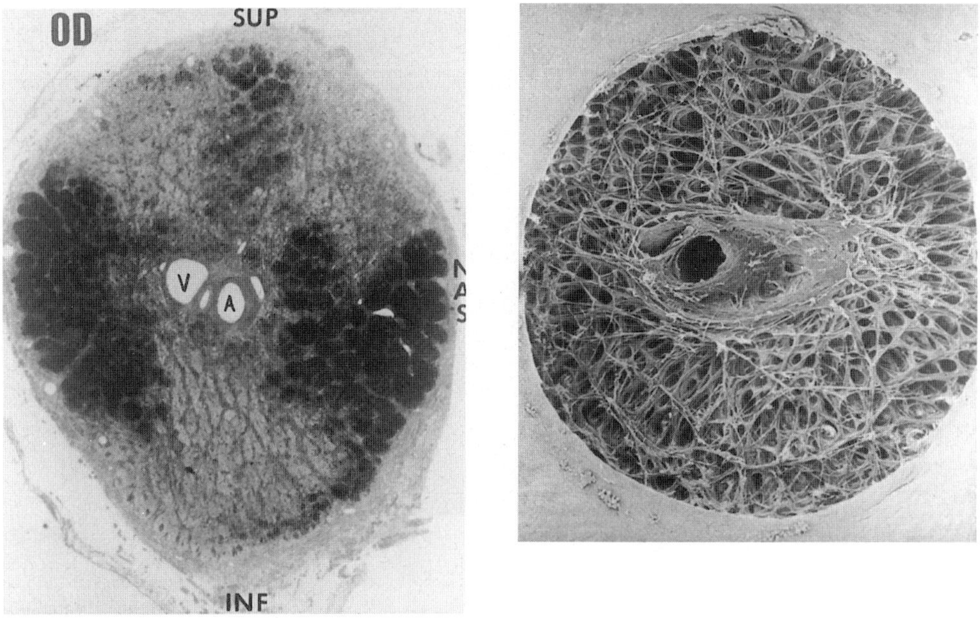


*Fig. 13.*

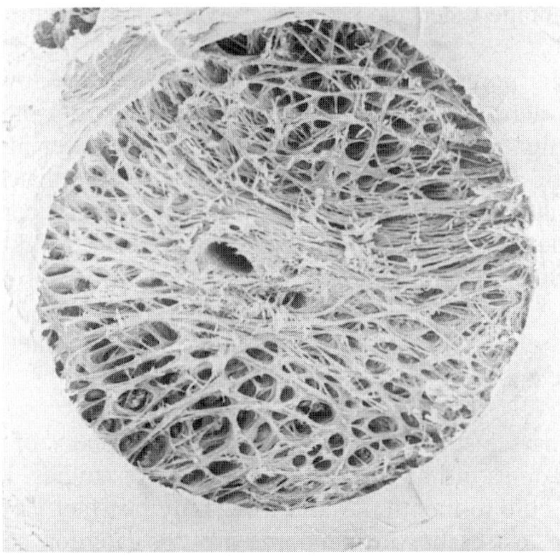

*Fig. 14.*

pressure – not *elevated* eye pressure, just eye pressure. This is a quantitative study, which happened to have been in monkeys, showing you that the most damaged areas quantitatively in the optic nerve actually were in this hourglass shape (Fig. 15).

Now, so that by the time we get to blood flow on our third session somebody would not say, you cut out all the blood flow, here is where the capillaries live within the connective tissue beams of the lamina cribrosa. They live actually within the beams (Fig. 16). There are no capillaries in the nerve bundles themselves. So if

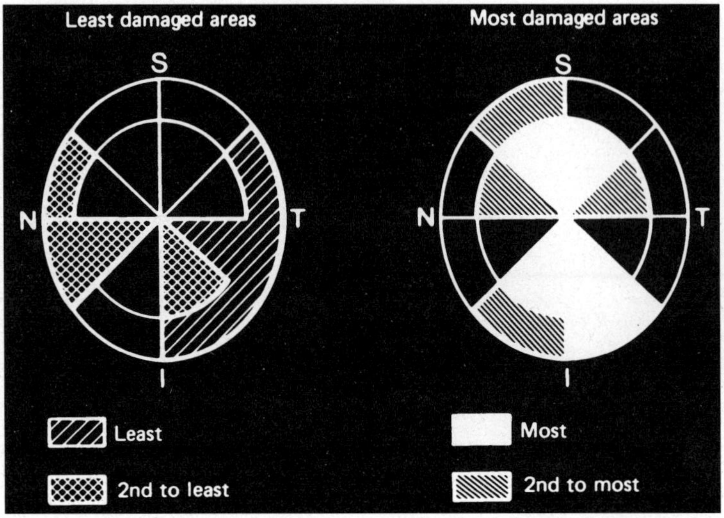


*Fig. 15.*

the connective tissue is undergoing some sort of change or stretch or movement, the poor capillary sitting in the middle of this connective tissue beam is at some very substantial disadvantage when the beam is moving and stretching and even breaking, as we will see.

In addition, if the pores are bigger at the upper and the lower part of the nerve head, the distance across the nerve bundle is much greater at the upper and lower part, so that you might say the density of capillaries is lower in the more susceptible portions of the optic nerve. Now, whether that is a feature that is important, whether there is a diffusional constant that is suddenly exceeded at a certain pore size, so the center of the bundle should really be starving for oxygen, we do not know. But those are features of regional anatomy.

**Dr. Zeimer**: Would you talk about the relation between the first fibers lost and Bruch's membrane and periphery of the lamina cribrosa?

**Dr. Quigley**: The fibers lost are not in the furthest periphery of the optic nerve. It is not a feature that comes out of any of our quantitative studies. However, there is one more regional attribute to mention – and this is my last fact. My last fact is that ganglion cells that are lost earlier in glaucoma are the ganglion cells that are larger diameter ganglion cells. The first work in that regard came from our looking at the cross-sectional diameters of axons (Fig. 17), there is about 1.2 million axons in the human; we did a Gallup poll sampling method with histomorphometry to look at them. You can see the sort of variety of sizes of axons here, and if you happen to design the system well enough you can read that in a quantitative fashion.

You also can look at the ganglion cell bodies themselves. These are whole mounts of the retina of a human glaucoma patient whose history we knew. The patient had more field loss corresponding to this retinal area (Fig. 18b) with fewer ganglion cell bodies than to that retinal area in which you can see more ganglion cells (Fig. 18a). We did a quantitative study of the number of cells remaining, and their sizes (Fig.

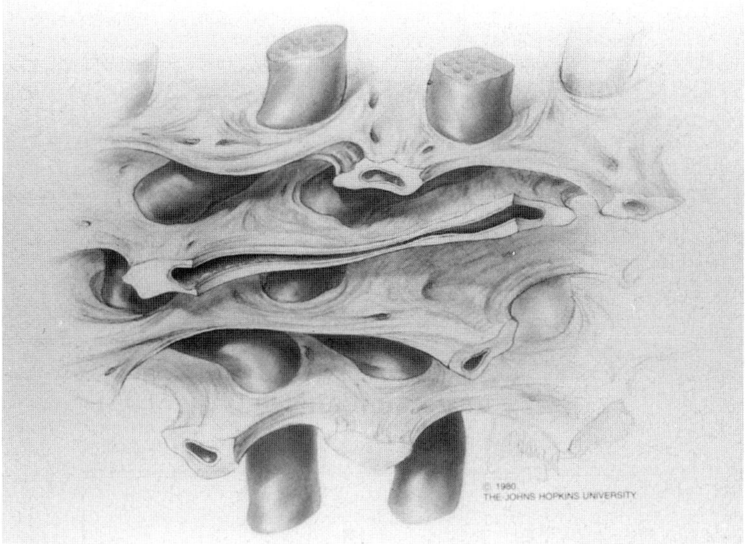


*Fig. 16.*

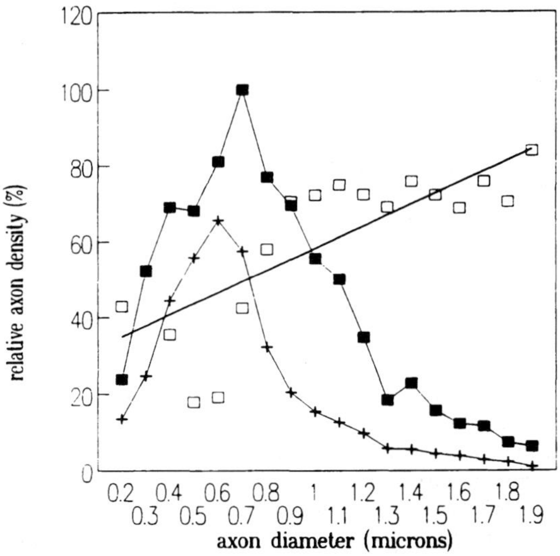


*Fig. 17.*

19). This was in the glaucomatous damaged area; this happens now to be in an elevated pressure monkey, this particular slide. And this is the normal distribution of cell size, showing the relative proportion of cells of the various sizes, small to large. And you can see that in the glaucoma case, you have proportionately lost more in these bundles down here, and greater loss of larger cells compared to the smaller cells. Likewise in the cross-section of the optic nerve, it is the larger diameter axons that disappear first. In the system of our vision, we have essentially two large divisions in the ganglion cells of the retina, the M system and the P system. M cells are

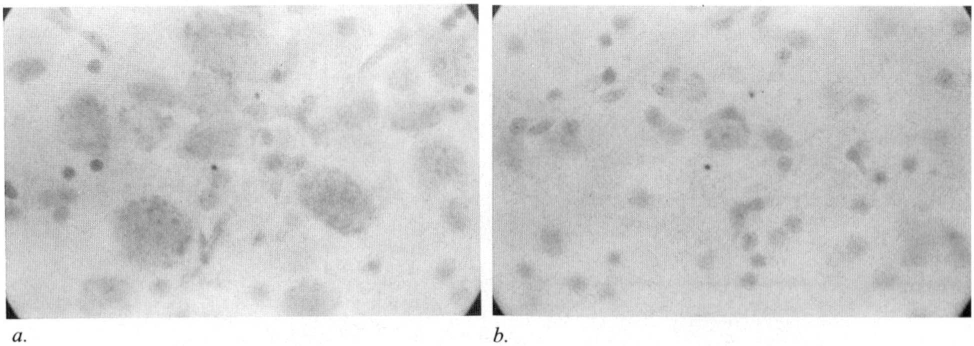


*Fig. 18.*

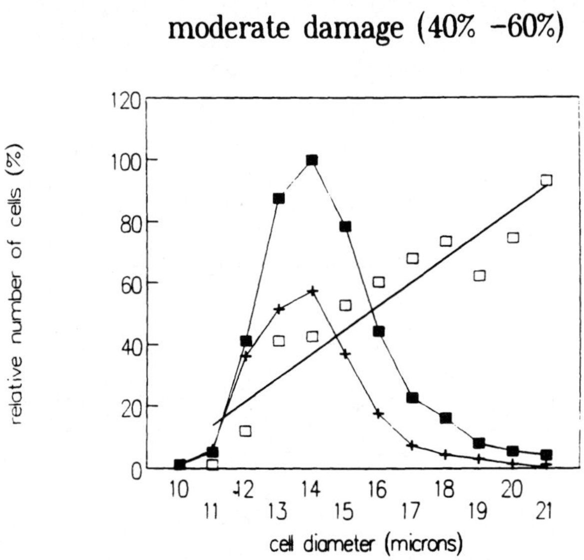


*Fig. 19.*

the bigger, fatter ones. P cells are the smaller ones. The M cells are the minority in the optic nerve, and they are axons who do luminance and motion detection and they tell you whether the room lights are dim in here or not. The smaller ones, who are the majority, do a lot of things, but they do among other things, your color vision and your acuity. As we looked at cross-sections of optic nerves you can also see the selectively greater loss of axons in the larger bins compared to the smaller bins. In terms of mean axon diameter, the mean axon diameter in glaucoma eyes, whether it is human or monkey, is smaller than in non-glaucomatous eyes.

One of the things we worried about was, what if while they are dying they are getting smaller? It would look as if all the big ones disappeared simply because as they start to get sick they shrink. In fact, Paul Hoffman was one of the first to challenge us to prove that was not true in our data. If it were true we might, for example, see the glaucoma distribution all shift this way, and it does not. One of the nicest pieces of additional information was suggested by Anita Hendrickson, and that was to look at the lateral geniculate body. In the lateral geniculate body you have the first way station for axonal synapse going up to other brain centers that are higher. These P

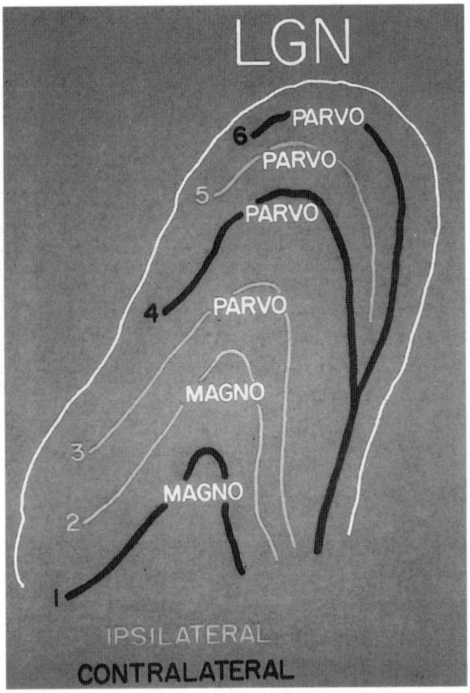


*Fig. 20.*

cell and M cell groups are divided into layers at the lateral geniculate body, so there are two large cell layers, M cells or magnocellular layers, one for each eye on each side of the brain, and four parvo or smaller cellular layers, two from each side (Fig. 20). And as we looked quantitatively at what happens – in monkeys, this is now only possible to be done in our hands in experimental monkey eyes – if you feed radioactivity to the ganglion cells in the eye and then you do an autoradiogram some time later, you find the magnocellular and the two parvocellular layers from that injected eye are lit up by axonally transported material, which has gone up to the lateral geniculate body (Fig. 21a). If at some point in the process of experimental elevated eye pressure in the monkey you do the same thing to a glaucomatous eye, you see radioactivity arriving at two parvocellular layers but not at the magnocellular layer corresponding to the glaucomatous eye (Fig. 21b). And actually, there is a recent study now from a group at Harvard who looked at autopsies of human eyes from persons who had glaucoma and suggest that the lateral geniculate cells in the magnocellular layers – these are not the ganglion cells, these are cells on which the ganglion cells would have synapsed – seemed to be fewer in the magnocellular layers, as if there was some transsynaptic degeneration going on. I was delighted to see it, it is the first corroboration of all this stuff that we have done for a long time about the large cells going first. There are some functional, some testing consequences of this. If you want to design a test for glaucoma you might want to design it, if you were looking for early glaucoma, to target the functions of these larger cells, and several of us are trying to do that.

Those are the features I wanted to talk about, I wanted to get actually to more connective tissue things.

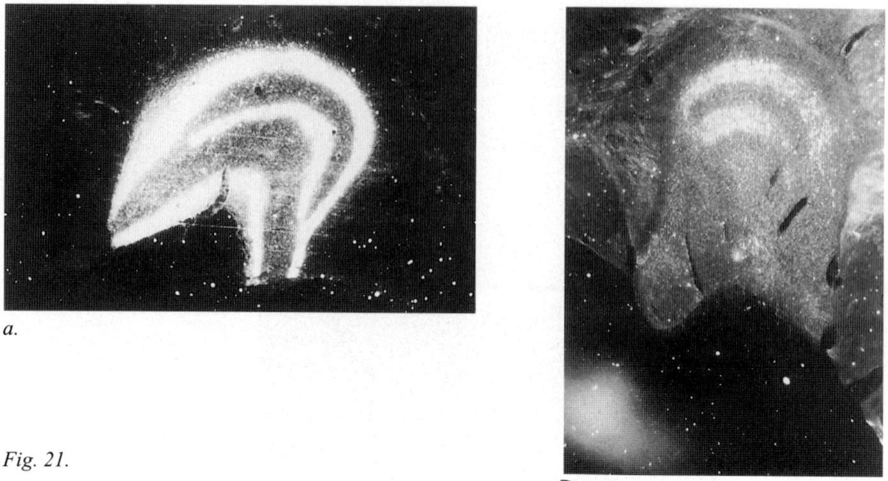

a.

Fig. 21.

b.

**Dr. Anderson**: I wanted to just point out that what you have done very nicely is to pose several questions that are up for discussion in the next few hours here. And I just want to remind our resident biostructural engineer who is going to speak a little later that he must address the question that you posed, or the situation where you pointed out the correlation between the size of the holes occurring at the vertical poles of the disc being much larger than those that are in the bow-tied center. While that correlation is very suggestive that there may be a cause and effect relationship, it would be nice to know what is the nature of that cause and effect. Is it really true, having looked at some Gothic architecture in the last few weeks, that smaller or bigger holes are weaker or stronger to lateral forces, circumferential forces around the globe, and just exactly what is the nature of the stress there. We are talking about forces which tend to stretch the circular hole and tend to push things out. Is it really true that they are weaker and what kind of distortion happens from such a weakness?

For the neurobiologists who come later, they might answer the question of what kind of challenge, what kind of physiologic challenge is likely to be more injurious to the larger ganglion cell than to a smaller cell. Are they an innately weaker kind of cells, or are they subject to certain specific challenges physiologically, such as ischemia, or kinking, or whatever else we might thing of. Why should a larger cell be the first one to go. You have presented the fact, now we need an explanation for that from some of the people who are here as our guests. I just want to make sure that the people who are coming later are reminded that they need to answer those questions for us.

# 3. BIOLOGY AND PATHOBIOLOGY OF THE EXTRACELLULAR MATRIX

REED E. PYERITZ, M.D., Ph.D.

This presentation addresses three topics. The first is the underlying biochemistry and molecular biology of the extracellular matrix (ECM). The second is the biophysical properties of connective tissue. The third is some of the human disorders associated with known variation in components of the extracellular matrix.

In a standard histologic section of virtually any organ, the extracellular matrix occupies the space between the structures that we recognize, epithelium, blood vessels, parenchymal cells, and so forth. Extracellular matrix is produced by cells that are derived from mesenchyme, be it from mesoderm or neural crest. Mesenchyme produces a wide variety of cells. The ones we will be most concerned about are the fibroblast, osteoblast, osteocyte and chondrocyte.

In many minds, the most important component of the extracellular matrix is collagen. The typical pattern array of collagen fibers, exemplified by type I collagen (Fig. 1) is due to the domain organization of the molecule, where the triple helix is the major element. This molecule begins life as procollagen, and most of the globular ends are cleaved during post-translational modification. More than a dozen different enzymes are responsible for modifying procollagen after the triple helix has formed. So there are a number of places where this process of modification can go awry for both genetic and environmental reasons. Moreover, there is plenty of opportunity for variation short of overt disease.

I now want to emphasize a point that should permeate everything that I have to say. Those who think at all in genetic terms tend to place great stock in the outliers with rare conditions that might be referred to the genetics clinic, and that are clearly phenotypically extreme. However, outliers are, literally, just the tip of the iceberg. A more appropriate way to view life is in terms of a continuum, where extreme phenotypes merge with the general population. Along this continuum of, for example, joint mobility, it becomes impossible to define a boundary between what is normal and what is abnormal. This creates problems in clinical nosology that is not solved by biochemistry or molecular biology, and is something that we have to grapple with in studying a common phenotype such as glaucoma.

Thus, for type I collagen, there are the two structural genes for mutations for this molecule (Fig. 2), and mutations in the enzymes that catalyze the post-translational modifications that cause overt disease (Fig. 3). But there are also hereditary variations that are not pathologic, but account for the qualities that make humans different from one another. This should be one of the major themes of this symposium: trying to identify which of these subtle variations predispose us to pathological processes such as degenerative arthritis, fractures, or glaucoma.

There are now at least 16 genetically distinct collagen molecules. They have different tissue distribution and different functions within the extracellular matrix. Type I collagen, the most prevalent protein in the human body, is primarily found in bone, ligament, tendon, skin, fascia, and vascular walls, and is responsible for tensile strength. Type II collagen is found primarily in cartilage and the vitreous, and has important roles in terms of the strength and maintaining hydration of those tissues. Type

*Optic Nerve in Glaucoma, pp. 37–56*
*edited by S.M. Drance*

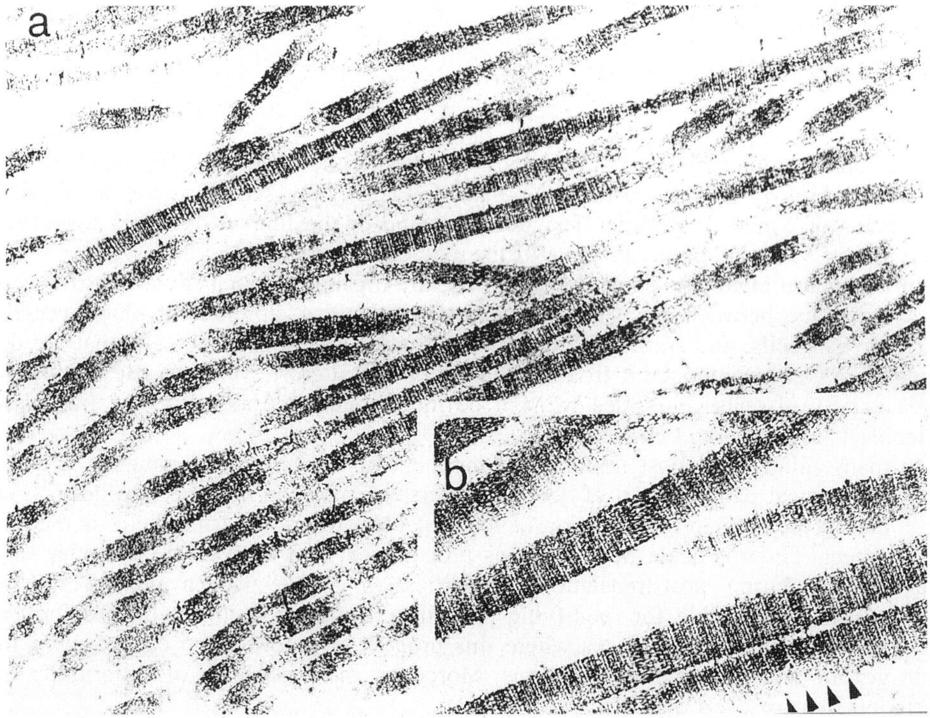


*Fig. 1.* Transmission electron micrographs of collagen fibrils in the intermediate (*a*) and reticular (*b*) dermis fixed in the presence of ruthenium red. The glycosaminoglycan moieties (GAGs) of the proteoglycans associated with the fibrils are retained by binding with ruthenium red. GAGs decorate the surface of collagen fibrils (*a*) and can be seen in periodic association with regular banding patterns (*b*) (arrowheads). (*a*) x 57,000; (*b*) x 66,700.

III collagen is in many respects similar to type I, it is found in the same tissue distribution, but has an important role in the early development of collagen fibers (Table 1).

Most of the other collagens are much less typically triple helical, and have different biophysical properties as a result. Type IV collagen, found virtually everywhere but particularly in basement membranes, does have a role in support, but also in filtration. Type V collagen has a postulated role in adhesiveness. Each of these collagens is encoded by one or more genes, depending on how many procollagen chains comprise these individual collagen types. The genes are scattered throughout the human genome. There are a few clusters that probably arose through gene duplication, and there certainly is homology among some of the genes, but by and large they are distinct and independently regulated.

Type IV collagen will have a prominent role in some of the discussions today. This molecule has some triple helical regions, but aggregates quite differently from the collagens of skin and bone. Figure 4 shows the different types of collagen molecules arrayed with the straight lines indicating the portions of the molecule that are triple helical, and the balls indicating the regions that are globular. There is substantial variation in the amount of triple helical domain in the different collagen molecules, some of them being almost entirely globular.

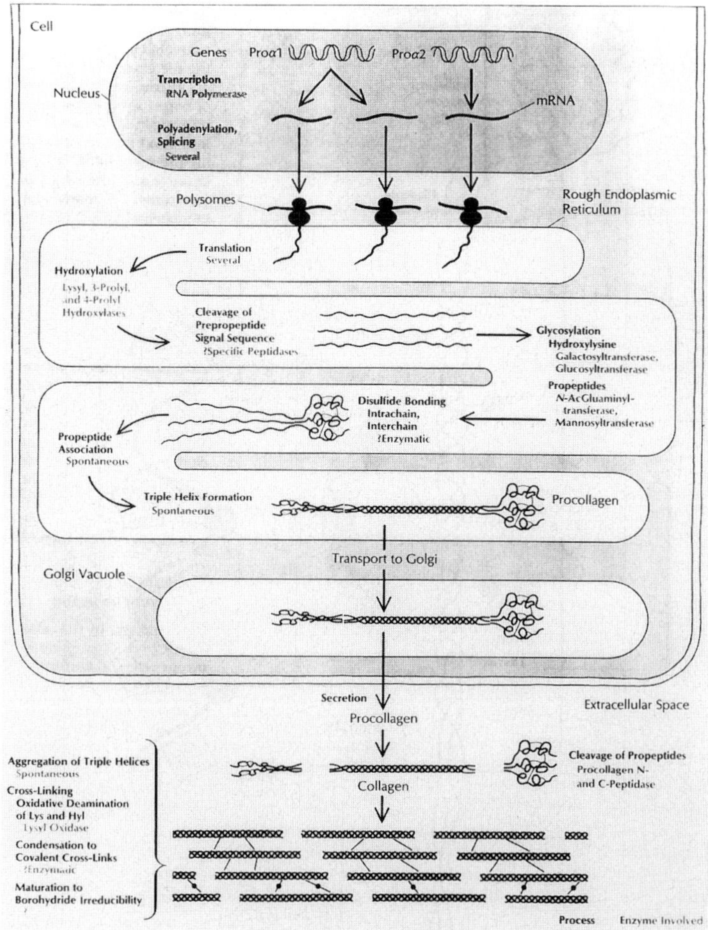


*Fig. 2.* Biosynthesis of type I collagen is traced diagrammatically. The pro-α-chains are synthesized by translation of the appropriate mRNAs on ribosomes attached to the rough endoplasmic reticulum. As the newly assembled chains pass into the cisternae of the RER, a series of post-translational processing steps extend through the Golgi into the extracellular space. Cross-linking provides the collagen fibril with rigidity. Enzymes involved are indicated.

Other fibrous structures occur in extracellular matrices of skin, lung, arteries, ligaments, and any tissue required to stretch reversibility. These are elastic fibers, composed of a rather boring, amorphous core (we are allowed to give biased talks here, are we not?) of mature elastin surrounded by fascinating structures called microfibrils. Microfibrils are laid down first, and tropoelastin is deposited on microfibrils in ways that are still totally unclear. As the elastic fiber is built up on the scaffolding of microfibrils, tropoelastin is post-translationally processed and undergoes intra- and interchain bonding, which is catalyzed primarily by lysyl oxidase, a copper-requiring enzyme.

**Dr. Zeimer**: When you said the fibrils are laid down first, what do you mean first? When does this happen, at what age?

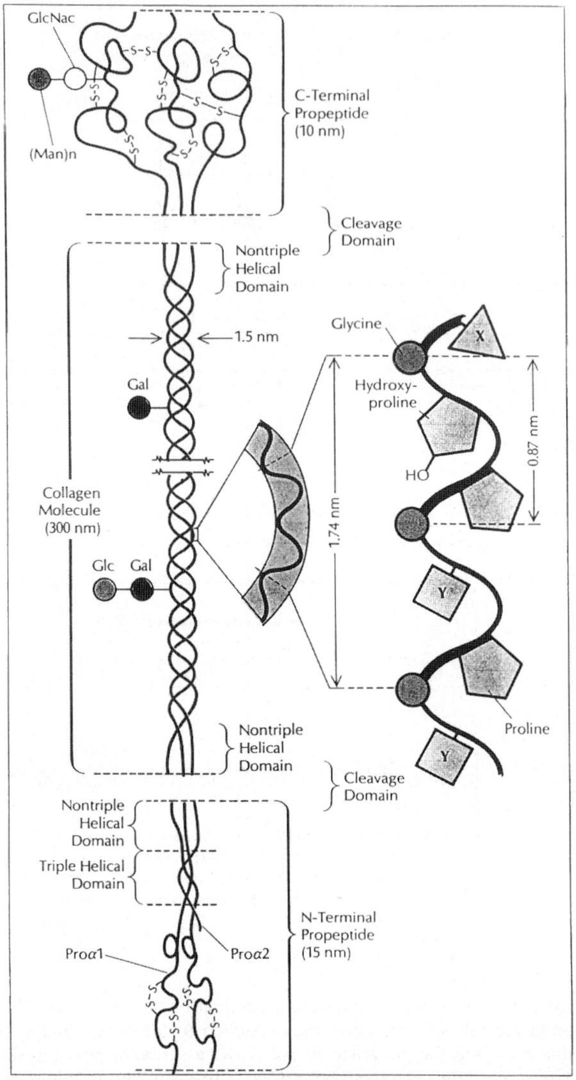


*Fig. 3.* Domains of type I procollagen molecule are defined structurally and functionally. After formation of intra- and interchain disulfide bonds, coiling of triple helix begins near C-terminal peptide cleavage domain. Any alteration in amino acid sequences that slows coiling increases glycosylation and hydroxylation of uncoiled propeptides, adversely affecting cross-linking and exracellular secretion.

**Dr. Pyeritz**: The microfibrils are laid down very early in embryonic life, and they continue to be laid down throughout growth, as far as we know. Elastin deposition begins in fetal life and proceeds during growth and development, and then is markedly reduced in adult life, so that in the adult, in virtually all tissues in which we find elastic fibers, there is extremely low turnover of elastin. What controls the tropoelastin gene on chromosome 7q11 is not known yet. But the characteristic of mature elastin is the formation of isodesmosine and desmosine cross-links, which

*Table 1.* The major collagen molecules

| | *Structure* | *Tissue distribution* | *Function* |
|---|---|---|---|
| Type I | $\alpha1(I)_2\alpha2(I)$<br>$\alpha1(I)_3$ | Major in bone, tendon, ligament, fascia, skin<br>Fetal tissues, inflammatory and neoplastic conditions | Tensile strength |
| Type II | $\alpha1(II)_3$ | Cartilage, vitreous, nucleus pulposus | Strength, hydration |
| Type III | $\alpha1(III)_3$ | Same as type I, but only in bone and tendon, and in distensible tissues (*e.g.*, gut and arteries) | Fibrillogenesis, strength, elasticity |
| Type IV | $\alpha1(IV)\alpha2(IV)$ dimer | Ubiquitous, prominent in lens capsule, glomerular and other basement membranes | Support, filtration |
| Type V | $\alpha1(V)_2\alpha2(V)$<br>$\alpha1(V)_3$ | Cornea, heart valve, fetal membranes<br>Cartilage | ?Adhesiveness |
| Type VI | $\alpha1(VI)\alpha2(VI)\alpha3(VI)$ | ?Ubiquitous | Microfibril constituent |
| Type VII | $\alpha1(VII)$ dimer | Skin, fetal membranes | Anchoring-fibril constituent |
| Type VIII | $\alpha1(VIII)_3$ | Endothelium | Unknown |
| Type IX | $\alpha1(IX)\alpha2(IX)\alpha3(IX)$ | Hyaline cartilage | Unknown |
| Type X | ?$\alpha1(X)$ | Cartilage | Calcification |

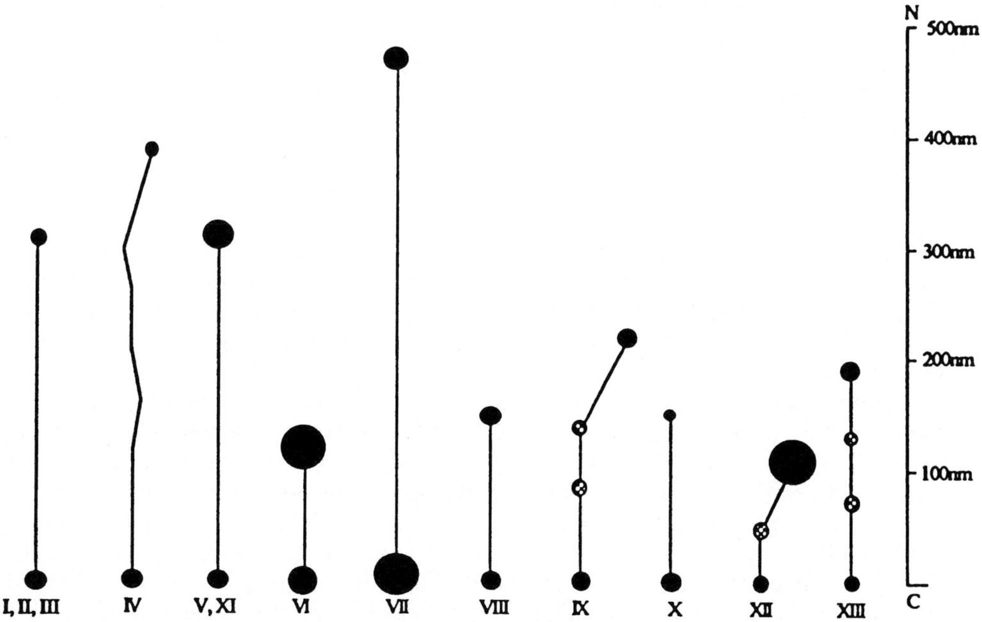


*Fig. 4.* Diagrammatic representation of the molecular morphology of individual collagen molecules and their macromolecular architecture. The line diagram illustrates the extent of the variations in domain structure within the molecules of the collagen family (types I to XIII). The relative dimension of the triple helical and non-collagenous domains are based largely on data accumulated from rotary shadowing images, but also rely where appropriate on predicted amino acid sequences obtained from cDNA sequence analysis.

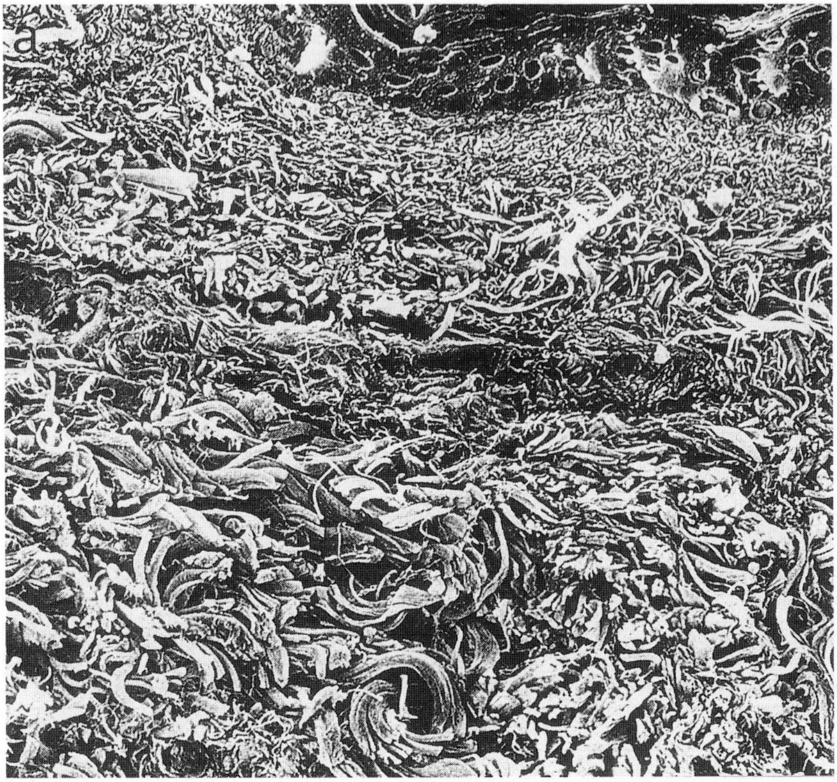

*Fig. 5.* Scanning electron micrograph of a portion of the epidermis (top), papillary dermis and intermediate dermis (bottom). The vessel (V) demonstrates the approximate boundary between the papillary and upper reticular (intermediate) dermis. Note the very fine bundles of collagen fibrils immediately beneath the epidermis and the increasing larger collagen bundles (C) deeper in the dermis. x 500.

can be isolated by degrading elastic tissue. These can be actually assayed from urine to give a rough estimate of elastic tissue turnover.

A scanning electron micrograph of skin, shows collagen bundles and the somewhat thinner elastic fibers (Fig. 5). The primary protein constituent of the microfibril, called fibrillin, is a 350 kilodalton glycoprotein. Fibrillin resides on the surface only of the elastic fibers and not on any of the other structures of the deep, reticular dermis.

Microfibrils can be isolated from a number of tissues, but importantly, from tissues in which there is no elastin (Fig. 6). So microfibrils are ubiquitous. From the perspective of my clinical interest and perhaps some of yours, microfibrils *are* the ocular zonules (Fig. 7). Dr. Barbara Streeten has been especially interested in the structure and composition of zonules, and I thank her for her excellent figures. Zonular fibers, when purified, are shown in Figure 6 and this is exactly what microfibrils look like isolated from other tissues. There is a regular repetition of beaded structures with an intervening fiber, and if you purify the protein fibrillin into monomers and then allow it to aggregate in vitro, you wind up with structures that look much like this.

There are other proteins in microfibrils besides fibrillin. In fact, at least two

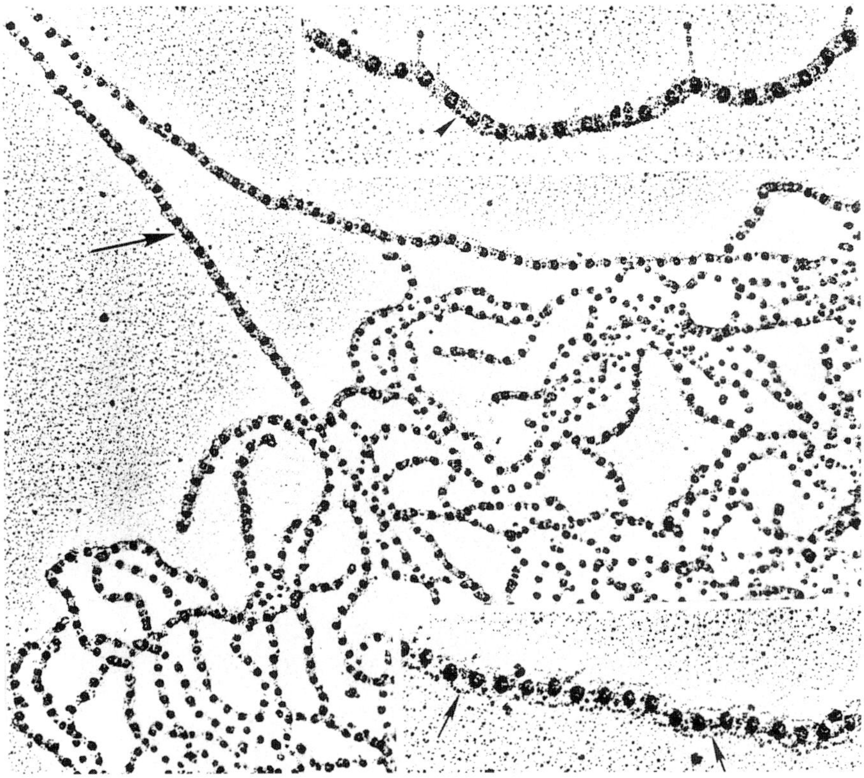

*Fig. 6.* Zonular fibers isolated from a 19-year-old human. Note the beaded repeats, thought to consist of individual monomers of fibrillin-1. Magnification of the large array is 67,800 × and the inset is 107,700 ×. (Reproduced with permission from: Wallace, Streeten and Hanna: *Current Eye Research* 10:99–109, 1991.)

fibrillins, encoded by two different genes on chromosomes 5 and 15 are involved. There is still a lot of active work on the biochemistry of microfibrils.

When I began work on connective tissues with Victor McKusick back in the late '70s, life was simple. The extracellular matrix was divided into the fibrillar portion, *i.e.*, collagen and elastic fibers, and into ground substance, *i.e.*, everything other than the fibrillar portion. Ground substance consisted primarily of glycosaminoglycan. We clinicians could parse the world into these two major camps, and the disorders seemed to follow.

This view of the extracellular matrix, and ground substance in particular, was far too naive. Proteoglycan is extraordinarily complex. A hyaluronic acid backbone has various glycosaminoglycan side chains joined via a link protein. The side chains can be keratan sulfate or chondroitin sulfate, aligned along a core protein (Fig. 8). The genes for the link protein and the core protein have been identified and cloned. Many of the enzymes involved in the catabolism of proteoglycan have been identified. Fewer of the enzymes involved in the synthesis of proteoglycan have been worked out. These are extraordinarily large molecules, many million molecular weight, and the more that they are examined in synthetic terms one finds increasingly complex interactions and tremendous tissue diversity.

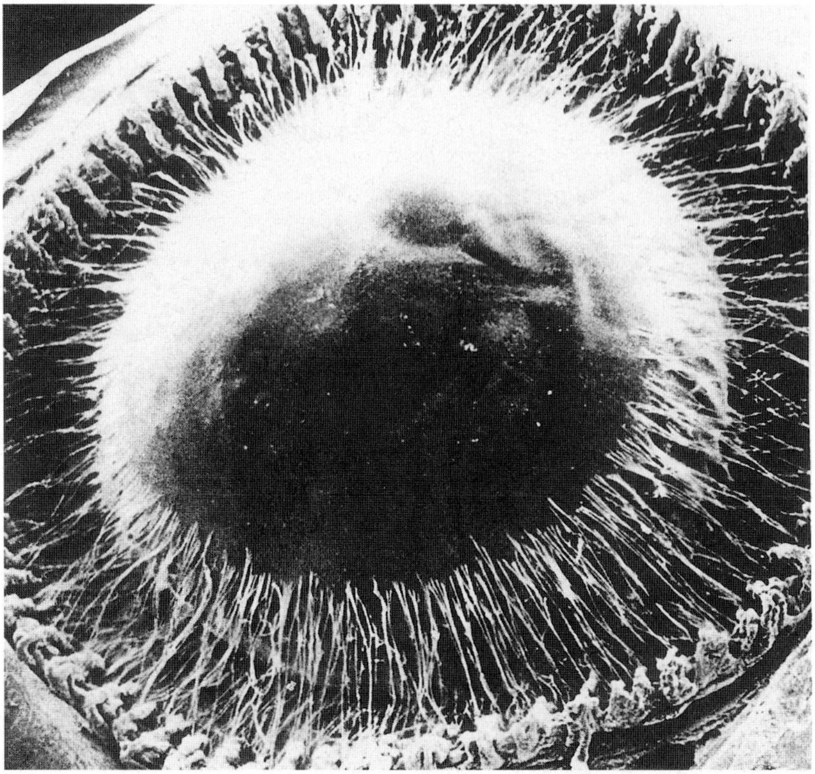

*Fig. 7.* The anterior insertions of the zonules. A scanning electron micrograph after removal of the cornea and iris. (25×) (Reproduced with permission from: Streeten, BW: Anatomy of the zonular apparatus. In: Tasman, W, Jaeger, EA (eds) *Duane's Foundations of Clinical Ophthalmology*, pp. 1–27, 1992.)

Figure 9 shows some potential interactions of these molecules in cartilage, where the primary structural molecule is type II collagen. Other collagens, type IX collagen, for example, interact with both type II collagen and the proteoglycan. There are other components, decorin and fibromodulin, which interact with collagen in highly specific ways, and the charge specificity is crucial to the proper alignment of the individual molecules. But all of these molecules have specific domains that are responsible for these interactions. And again, looking at the kinds of extracellular matrix components produced by a specific cell type, in this case a chondrocyte, a whole array of individual molecules are produced and secreted into the matrix. To some extent, the molecules are processed according to the way they interact with their compatriot components in the matrix.

Each of the molecules that has been identified in the extracellular matrix and cloned is found in Victor McKusick's catalog, which began as a catalog of human mendelian phenotypes, that is, phenotypes that are inherited as Mendel would have predicted, as either autosomal recessive, autosomal dominant, or X-linked. But in the more recent editions of the catalog, and it is now up through the 11th edition, molecules that have been identified but for which there is no known human disease

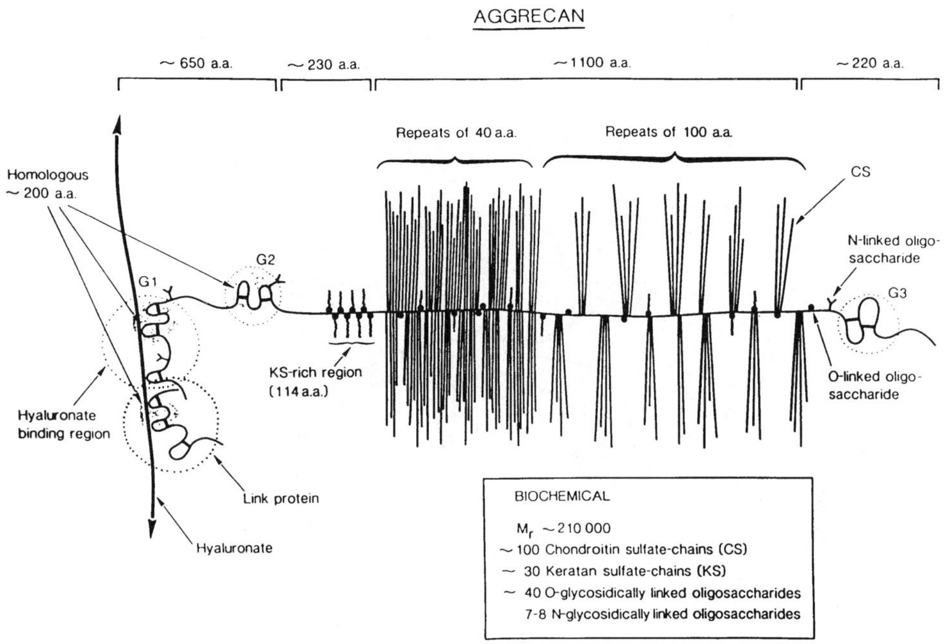


*Fig. 8.* Schematic illustration of aggrecan (the large aggregating proteoglycan from cartilage).

are also listed. This is a catalog that is now on line, called "On-Line Mendelian Inheritance in Man", available to anyone through the Welch Library at Johns Hopkins.

We are used to viewing connective tissue simply as the glue and the scaffolding of the body. However, the extracellular matrix clearly has many other functions. One area of particular interest is the involvement of the extracellular matrix in growth, development, and morphogenesis. An extracellular matrix is laid down extremely early in embryonic life, and is the matrix upon which the various cell types migrate. Thus, the nervous system is formed on an extracellular matrix that contains many of the components that we have been discussing. Moreover, healing and scarring, which unquestionably must be going on in, for example, the eye, as it is subjected to abnormal forces be they traumatic or chronic, is going to be determined by the nature of the connective tissue components that an individual is making. So all of these factors have to be kept in mind as we think about the kinds of variations in tissue biochemistry that can predispose individuals to disease.

In quiet moments of reflection, I am willing to accept that not everything in the world is genetic. There are exogenous factors that affect the extracellular matrix. Some are listed in Table 2; for example, the maturation of collagen fibers is age-dependent. The activities of some of the enzymes that are involved in post-translational modification decrease over time. We know that the number of collagen cross-links of a particular kind increase with age. Collagen turnover decreases as adults age. Inflammation affects the biochemical modification of the extracellular matrix. Many acquired disorders of connective tissue are due to autoimmunity. Vitamin deficiencies, diabetes, sepsis, and steroid therapy are other factors that can all affect the quality of the extracellular matrix.

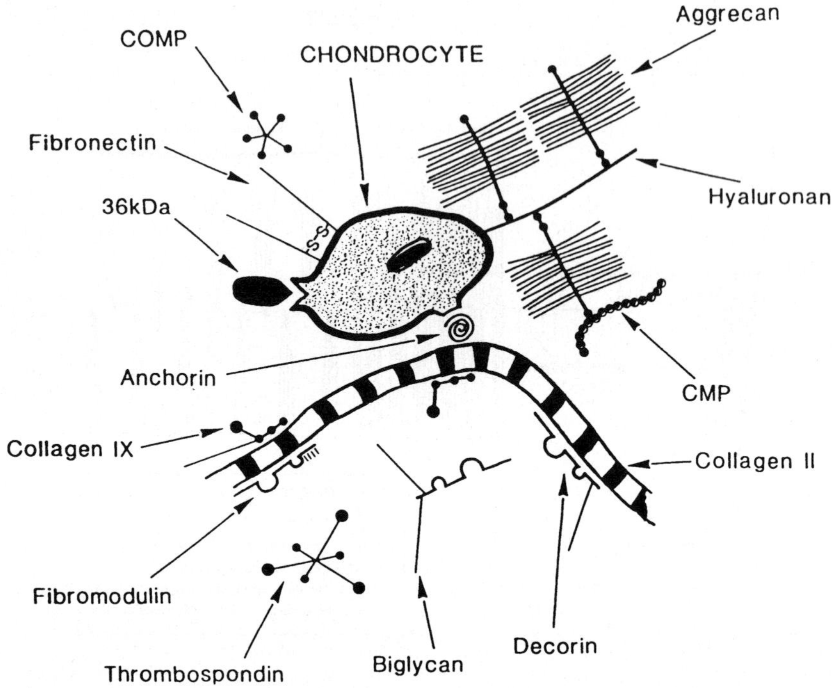


*Fig. 9.* Schematic illustration of cartilage matrix constituents and their proposed interactions. CMP, cartilage matrix (148 kDa) protein; COMP, cartilage oligomeric protein.

The remainder of my remarks will address connective tissue disorders, but we must first define terms. For example, some people have joint laxity clearly out of the normal, but have no intrinsic defect of the extracellular matrix. It is a learned trait. We might describe such people as being abnormal, but double-jointedness is something that they trained themselves to have, not something they were born with. This is one extreme of connective tissue function that is not genetic but is clearly exogenous. Another example is systemic lupus erythematosus, often categorized as a "collagen disorder" or "connective tissue disorder", but not the type that I am going to focus on, because this is due to autoimmunity. Not to say that genetic factors might not be important in autoimmunity, and indeed they are, but this is not due to a primary abnormality of the extracellular matrix.

What I am going to talk about is the group of disorders that was first codified by Victor McKusick in 1955 as the heritable disorders of connective tissue. When he first described Marfan's syndrome in these terms, there were less than a dozen other disorders that he could find that merited description as heritable disorders of connective tissue. I want to emphasize that all of us have a heritable disorder of connective tissue, and that is, we have an inborn error of metabolism that prevents us from synthesizing vitamin C, or ascorbic acid. Now, there are a few mammals, such as the Indian fruit bat, that are like us. Most mammals, however, can make vitamin C, and hence not require a dietary source of the vitamin. But if we lack ascorbic acid then we lack the cofactor for proline hydroxylase, which converts proline in procollagen to hydroxyproline, which is involved in cross-linking. Inability to perform this post-translational modification of collagen results in the disease scurvy.

*Table 2.* Effect of endogenous and exogeneous factors on the extracellular matrix

| *Process* | *Aspects of connective tissue or extracellular matrix affected* | *Alteration* |
|---|---|---|
| Development | Collagen types in skin<br>Collagen fibril diameter | Ratio type III:type I ↓ postnatally<br>↑ During embryogenesis |
| Aging | Maturation of collagen fibrils | ↓ Activities of prolyl and lysyl hydroxylysine<br>↑ Borohydride irreducible cross-links<br>↓ Collagen turnover, ↓ urinary excretion of hydroxylysine |
| Injury | Cartilage<br>Endothelium basement membrane<br>Epidermis<br>Fibrosis<br><br>Angiogenesis | ↑ Proteoglycan turnover and chain length<br>Altered glycosaminoglycan composition<br>↑ Fibronectin<br>↑ Amount of collagen, preferential type III collagen production, mature cross-links<br>Degradation of basement membrane |
| Inflammation | Cartilage | Degradation of proteoglycan and type II collagen |
| Autoimmunity | Basement membrane | ↓ Integrity due to antibody binding to type IV collagen antigen (Goodpasture antigen) |
| Vitamin C deficiency | Collagen cross-linking | ↓ Due to decreased lysyl hydroxylase activity |
| Hypoxemia | Collagen cross-linking | ↓ Due to decreased lysyl and prolyl hydroxylase and lysyl oxidase activities |
| Diabetes | Basement membrane thickness<br>Collagen | ↑ Cause unclear<br>↑ Glycosylation |
| Sepsis | Basement membrane and endothelial integrity | ↓ Serum libronectin |
| Steroid therapy | Fibrosis | ↓ Collagenase; regulation of type I synthesis |

In 1956, McKusick published the first volume of Heritable Disorders of Connective Tissue. By the fourth edition in 1972, there were about 50 disorders included. Last year, a group of McKusick's trainees got together and published the fifth edition of Heritable Disorders of Connective Tissue, and there are now 200 identifiable entries each presumably due to its own specific gene defect. So there has been a tremendous increase in the number of conditions which have been identified as due to a mendelian disorder of connective tissue. And of course, keeping everything categorized properly is quite difficult. For that reason a group of us get together every couple of years somewhere warm by the sea, and talk about nosology, and come up with diagnostic criteria to try to keep the field organized.

In general, the conditions are divided into those which, while mendelian, are not due primarily to abnormalities of the components of the extracellular matrix, versus those that are. An example of the former is one of the first inborn errors of metabolism to be described, by Alexander Garrod in 1903. Alkaptonuria causes deposition of the ochronotic pigment, homogentisic acid, in the vertebral column, with the typical bamboo spine changes on radiography. Ochronotic pigment is deposited in the sclera and in cartilage, leading to arthropathy. But this is a secondary disorder of connective tissue, due to a primary defect in metabolism of the amino acid tyrosine.

Another example of a secondary heritable disorder of connective tissue has a habitus very suggestive of the Marfan's syndrome, with long arms, long legs, long fingers, ocular problems, and vascular problems. This is homocystinuria, another inborn error of metabolism due to a deficiency of the enzyme cystathionine β-synthase, which catalyzes conversion of homocystine to cystathionine. Somehow, elevated homocystine results in dislocation of the lens due to breakage of the ocular zonules.

Most heritable disorders of connective tissue are due to defects in components of the extracellular matrix. One such group of conditions is osteogenesis imperfecta, the ocular hallmark of which is blueness of the sclerae. This breeds true in the family and there are forms of osteogenesis imperfecta in which the sclerae are normal in color, and that breeds true as well. But there is tremendous phenotypic diversity in osteogenesis imperfecta, including patients with a lot of fractures as a child, severe bony deformities and short stature, to infants who have a myriad of intrauterine fractures and who die either at birth or shortly thereafter of profound cardiopulmonary problems, to people with few problems at all. They all have osteogenesis imperfecta and all have one or another defect in exactly the same molecule. Ninety percent plus mutations leading to osteogenesis imperfecta occur in type I collagen, in the gene that encodes either pro-α-1 or pro-α-2. Type I collagen is composed of two pro-α-1 chains and one pro-α-2 chain. One particular mutation leading to osteogenesis imperfecta results in a shortened pro-α-1 chain. The other allele is normal, because this is an autosomal dominant condition, so there are two populations of pro-α-1 chains and a normal population of pro-α-2 chains. Given the stoichiometry of formation of the type I procollagen heterotripolymer, there is a three in four chance that any triple helical molecule will contain at least one of the mutant pro-α-1 chains. In this situation, the patient is heterozygous (has one mutant allele and one normal allele) and you might expect they would be producing half normal amounts of a normal protein. In fact, because of heteropolymer formation, the patient has three-quarters abnormal product. The situation is worse than you would expect based on a 50-50 combination of the precursors. This has been called protein suicide, a term I detest. It is better called a dominant negative effect, where a dominant condition has a worse phenotype because of the molecular pathophysiology.

Other defects of connective tissue are quite distinct from osteogenesis imperfecta, and the Ehlers-Danlos syndromes are illustrative. The hallmarks are marked joint hypermobility, fragility of the skin leading to atrophic scarring and inability to hold standard sutures, and easy bruising. There are about 10 distinct types, separable by relative severity of joint, skin and vascular problems, and by inheritance pattern. One form, type VI, has conspicuous eye pathology, *fragilitis oculi.* The globe tends to rupture with mild trauma. This form, and at least one other, are due to defects in post-translational modification of type I collagen. The most lethal form, type IV, is caused by defects in type III collagen. This collagen plays a crucial role in the integrity of the walls of arteries and the gastrointestinal tract. Patients succumb to rupture in these sites.

An interesting and informative principle – allelic diversity – is illustrated by disorders associated with type II collagen. Recall that this collagen is found in cartilage and vitreous. The most severe condition is achondrogenesis, which is lethal in the neonatal period. There is a virtual lack of cartilage developed, and the biochemists a dozen years ago showed that these patients lack normal type II collagen. A milder condition is spondyloepiphyseal dysplasia congenita, a long name meaning that the growing points of bones in both the axial and appendicular skeleton do not function properly. Patients do not make normal cartilage, but they have cartilage. The result is marked short stature. They are also prone to retinal detachment. At the milder end of the spectrum is the Stickler syndrome, with cleft palate, hearing loss, characteristic midfacial hypoplasia, and mild spondyloepiphyseal dysplasia. This is an autosomal dominant disorder which often comes to medical attention because of the ocular complications of vitreoretinal degeneration, myopia, cataracts, and retinal detachment. Clair Francomano in our group showed that Stickler syndrome is linked to type II collagen gene in some families. A number of mutations have been found. At their mildest, defects in type II collagen present as familial early onset osteoarthritis. But not all pedigrees show linkage, so there must be at least one other locus capable of producing the Stickler phenotype.

The concept of unilocus diversity is prevalent in medical genetics, but particularly nicely illustrated in the connective tissue disorders, including mucopolysaccharidoses. Children with the Hurler syndrome are profoundly mentally retarded and will die in early teenage years of cardiopulmonary problems. Hurler's syndrome is due to mutations in the catabolic enzyme α-iduronidase. Some patients with this same enzyme deficit present in adulthood with hip disease and clouding of the corneas. This same phenotypic spectrum is illustrated by the Hunter syndrome which is much like the Hurler syndrome, but only affects males and not the corneae. This is the form of mucopolysaccharidosis that is X-linked, and for unclear reasons the corneae are spared.

Pseudoxanthoma elasticum is characterized by abnormal skin, angioid streaks, and calcification of Bruch's membrane. The elastic fibers are calcified but the basic defect is unknown.

**Dr. Quigley**: Interestingly, not too long ago somebody said, You know, I have seen a lot of disc drusen in patients with pseudoexfoliation, do you know any reason why that may be the cause? And I said, well, it calcifies elastin in other parts of the body. He said, Is there any elastin in the lamina cribrosa? And John Morrison is going to show you in a few minutes that elastin is in the lamina.

**Speaker**: The Marfan's syndrome is often thought of as a disorder that affects only three organ systems including the eye with ectopia lentis present in about 50-60%. The skeleton shows long arms and legs, long fingers, and chest deformity. The cardiovascular system, with mitral valve disease and dilation of the ascending aorta, causes life-threatening problems. But in fact, virtually every organ system is affected in the Marfan's syndrome. One of the ones that we discovered was the central nervous system, in terms of learning abnormalities, hyperactivity, and attention deficit disorder, but also in terms of stretching of the dura leading to dural ectasia. This latter observation is intriguing in terms of the ocular manifestations. I asked Irene Maumenee whether, in her wide experience with Marfan's syndrome, she thought there was an increased prevalence of glaucoma, and she said most definitely not.

**Dr. Quigley**: She then proceeded to report the fact that there is, and we are trying to find out whether in fact that is true by pursuing a more detailed definitional study of patients with Marfan's syndrome.

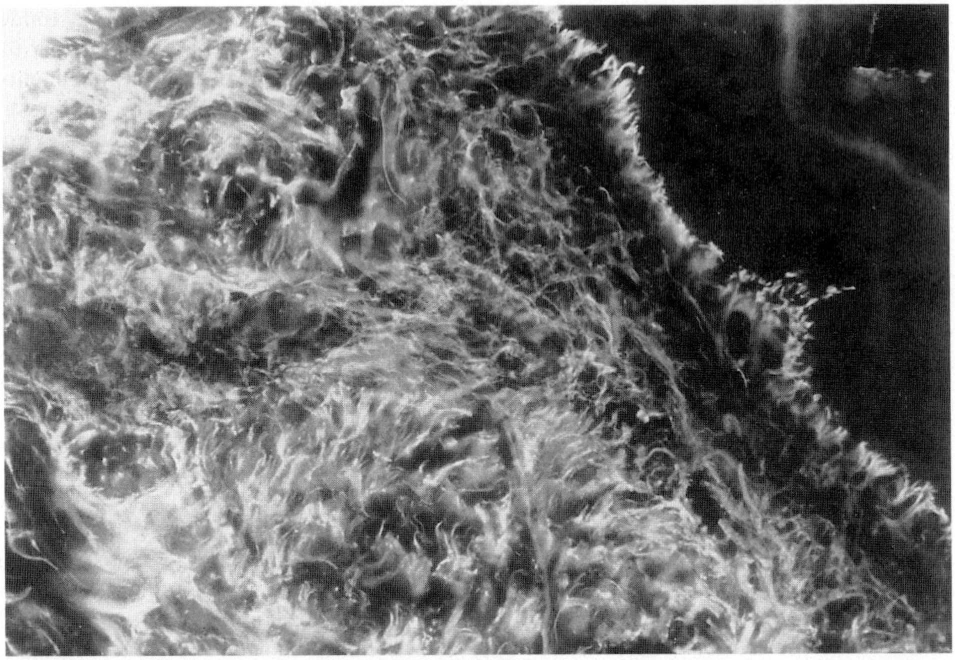

*a.*

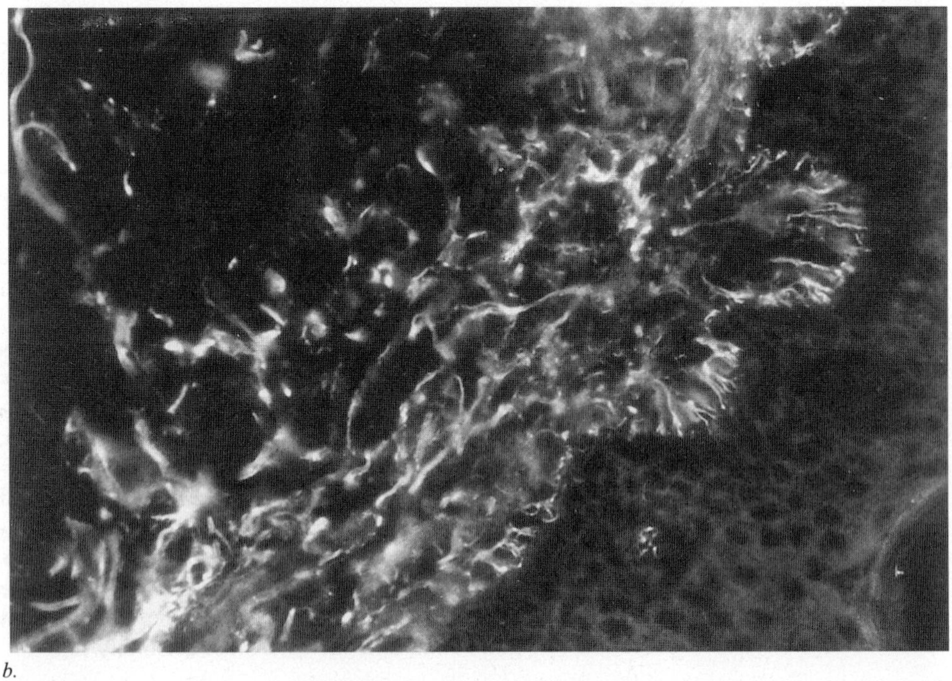

*b.*

*Fig. 10.* Sections of human skin, showing the epidermis to the right and the dermis to the left. The sections were exposed to a monoclonal antibody specific for fibrillin-1, and then to a fluorescein-labeled anti-mouse IgG antibody. In panel *a* from a normal control individual, the bright immunofluorescence identifies microfibrils at the dermal–epidermal junction (oriented perpendicular to the surface) and coating the extensive array of elastic fibers in the papillary and reticular layers of the dermis. In panel *b* from a patient with the Marfan syndrome, immunofluorescence is markedly reduced (100×).

**Speaker**: I do not need to emphasize to this group the ophthalmologic features, but what I always tell our residents is that the lens tends to migrate northward in Marfan's syndrome and southward in homocystinuria. One of the reasons for this is that the zonules break in homocystinuria, so the lens falls because of gravity, whereas in Marfan's syndrome the zonules rarely break. There are families in which they do break, and they are very interesting to us, but by and large the zonules stretch and the lens migrates upward.

What kills people with Marfan's syndrome, on average in their 30s and 40s, is dissection of the aorta or chronic aortic regurgitation. The dilated aorta can be fixed, and patients can live a relatively normal lifespan if the cardiovascular surgeons get to them.

The stretch marks emphasize that other organ systems are affected. Striae atrophicae are extremely common in Marfan's syndrome, and because our Institutional Review Board would not allow us to biopsy the aorta in our patients, we instead decided to biopsy skin in an effort to try to find the basic defect. The normal aorta shows nice contiguous wavy elastic laminae, whereas the aortic media of someone with Marfan's syndrome shows disarray and fragmentation of the elastic fibers. McKusick back in 1956 said, if you can figure out what zonules have in common with the aortic media, you will understand the cause of Marfan's syndrome. And we decided to approach it through the skin by looking at microfibrils, which of course are present everywhere: they are the zonules, they are present in the elastic fibers, and they are even present in bone. Fibrillin was purified first by Lynn Sakai at the Portland Shriners Hospital, and she developed monoclonal antibodies. The late Dave Hollister, in collaboration with me, examined the skin of patients with Marfan's syndrome. Normal skin shows considerable immunofluorescence due to binding of antibody to fibrillin. Patients with Marfan's syndrome had a marked reduction in fibrilin in skin (Fig. 10a and b). Dermal fibroblasts in tissue culture make an extracellular matrix that includes microfibrils. These can be detected with the anti-fibrillin antibody. Cells grown from most patients with Marfan's syndrome do not make these microfibrils. These studies suggested that microfibrils were indeed abnormal in Marfan's syndrome.

Leena Peltonen, in Helsinki, first mapped the gene for Marfan's syndrome to chromosome 15q. Bryan Hall told me about a large pedigree with Marfan's syndrome in Eastern Kentucky. A pediatric cardiologist at Hopkins, Hal Dietz, went with me to Kentucky; we took a slit lamp, we took an echocardiograph machine and we drove to where the road ended. We met this family, worked out the pedigree, drew blood from them and were able to map the gene for Marfan's syndrome to a specific region on chromosome 15. Fortuitously, the gene for fibrillin was mapped to exactly the same region by Lynn Sakai and then by us, so we had these two lines of evidence suggesting that the gene for Marfan's syndrome and the gene for fibrillin occur at the same place on chromosome 15. It then just remained to actually find mutations in the fibrillin gene in a patient with Marfan's syndrome and Hal Dietz did that in a patient with severe, sporadic Marfan's syndrome. This mutation resulted in a change of a single amino acid out of over 3,000 in the fibrillin protein. The patient's parents did not have this mutation. That clinched that this was indeed the cause of Marfan's syndrome in this girl. The gene for fibrillin has now been completely cloned. The coding sequence encompasses 10,000 nucleotides and 65 exons (Fig. 11). More than four dozen mutations have been found in different patients with Marfan's syndrome. Almost every patient has a different mutation. Obviously, patients in the same family share the same mutation, but a great diversity of mutations in fibrillin can all lead to Marfan's syndrome and abnormalities of microfibrils.

An extremely important point I would make is that, having discovered the cause, we really do not understand how Marfan's syndrome arises. This is the distinction between etiology and pathogenesis. A pathogenetic "three" attempts to express how the different phenotypic features out at the leaves arise from a single root cause. We now know that the root cause is an elastic fiber abnormality, or a microfibril abnormality. But even knowing that, we can only speculate how all of the different phenotypic features arise, and that is the challenge for the future. Part of the explanation will involve the many epidermal growth factor (EGF) repeats that occur throughout the fibrillin molecule. Most bind calcium and we know that in patients who have mutations affecting one or more of the amino acids in these regions, that particular EGF motif does not bind calcium properly. What that means in terms of cross-linking, in terms of polymerization, in terms of interaction with tropoelastin or other constituents of the extracellular matrix is just not known.

We are trying to understand what causes the wide phenotypic diversity in Marfan's syndrome. Some patients die in the first weeks of life, because they are so severely affected; other patients are not diagnosed until their 30s or their 40s because they are relatively mildly affected. This variability might be explained, in part, according to the following model (Fig. 12). Two alleles make fibrillin. All of us are making normal amounts of normal monomers, this huge 350 kDa protein. These combine with each other to form microfibrils that give you a normal phenotype, shown in the figure by a normal aortic root and normal mitral valve. The patients with severe Marfan's syndrome have a point mutation or a small defect in one allele of the fibrillin gene. They make 50% normal fibrillin and 50% abnormal fibrillin. When you mix and match to form these large aggregates called microfibrils, every microfibril winds up being abnormal, and you wind up with a severe phenotype with an aortic aneurysm and severe mitral regurgitation, for example. On the other hand, there are patients in whom the defect, at the molecular level, is much more severe; the whole protein is truncated for example, because of a frame shift in the gene. Here you wind up with 50% normal and 50% extremely abnormal monomers that cannot combine with the normal ones, so you wind up with normal microfibrils, but in reduced quantities, and this gives rise to a milder phenotype. Likewise, there are mutations now that result in decreased synthesis of an abnormal protein, so that the stoichiometry predicts that there will be relatively few abnormal microfibrils, a lot of normal ones, and again, a milder phenotype.

One important goal is to construct these genotype-phenotype correlations, looking at how mutations give rise to different levels of severity. We would predict that

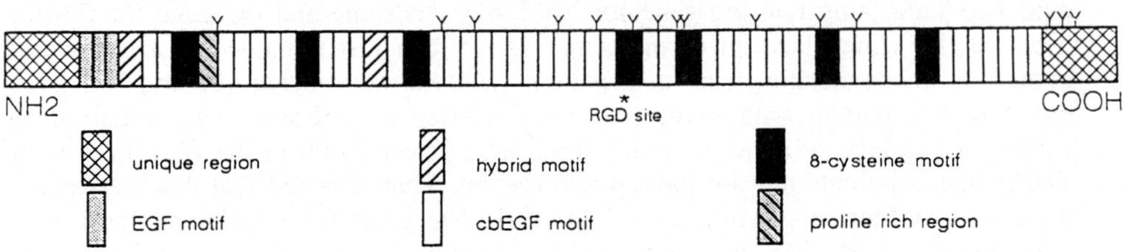


*Fig. 11.* Schematic of the gene for fibrillin-1 (FBN-1). The individual motifs are identified in the key. EGF: epidermal growth factor-like motif; cbEGF: calcium-binding epidermal growth factor-like motif. (Modified after a drawing by Lynn Sakai, PhD, with permission.)

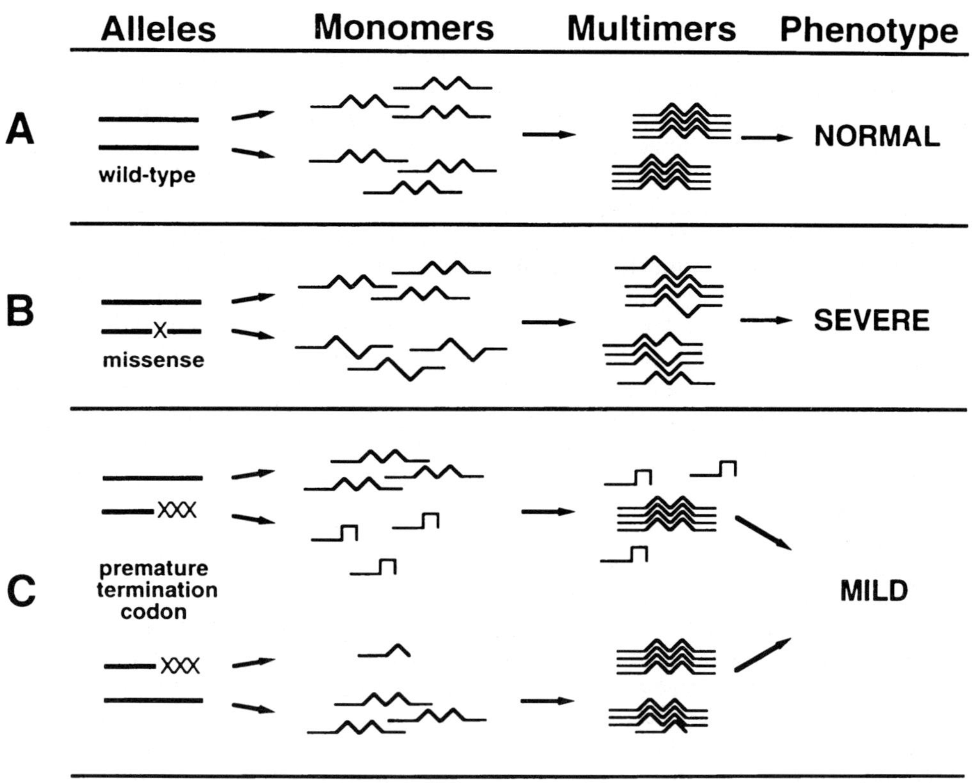


*Fig. 12.* A dominant-negative model for Marfan's syndrome. (A) Two wild-type alleles produce a homogeneous population of normal momomers, which form normal multimers (microfibrils), and the phenotype is normal. (B) Heterozygosity for a missense mutation (X) produces equal amounts of normal and mutant momoners. Because all multimers will contain some mutant monomers, all microfibrils will be defective, and the phenotype will be severe (indicated by aortic root dilation and atrioventricular valve redundancy. (C) A mutation that causes a premature signal for termination of translation (XXX) might produce a truncated monomer incapable of multimer formation (upper panel). Alternatively, a reduction in mutant allele transcripts might produce few defective monomers capable of forming multimers (lower panel). Both situations predict a relative preponderance of normal microfibrils, and the phenotype will be mild (shown by isolated atriventricular valve redundancy).

some defects in this gene will result in very subtle clinical disorders, such as late onset aortic aneurysms, isolated mitral valve prolapse, or ectopia lentis, but not Marfan's syndrome. So I think this is a model of pathogenesis with which to end and stimulate you to think about what other defects in the extracellular matrix will predispose some people to glaucoma. I would urge you to look carefully at some families which develop glaucoma despite normal pressures. They well may have an abnormal extracellular matrix.

**Dr. Drance**: I would like to ask whether the elastin determination from the urine, whether in fact the elastin is controlling the whole body at the same time, or are there variations in the organs. If an organ like the eye, for instance, behaved differently from the joints that would not be picked up by urinary sampling.

**Dr. Pyeritz**: The amount of desmosine and isodesmosine found in the urine is a very crude measure for elastin turnover. As you can imagine, any turnover that is occurring in the eye would account for a minute fraction of what you would pick up in the urine. Primarily you are dealing with skin and lung elastin turnover and to a certain extent vascular, primarily aortic, turnover, so that I do not see that as a way of assaying it. One point that I think is worth making, to perhaps illustrate the kind of regulation that occurs within a single organ, is illustrated by the aorta. The amount of elastin tissue in the proximal aorta, in the region where the aneurysm forms in Marfan's syndrome, is much higher than the amount of elastic tissue found in the distal aorta, say, in the abdomen, where some of us will get aneurysms. The amount of type I and type III collagen in the aorta shows the reverse pattern, with less in the proximal aorta and more in the distal aorta. This accounts for the difference in the elastic and tensile strength properties of the aorta, the proximal being much more elastic, the distal being much stronger. So, using that as a model for the eye, it is quite possible that the time of maturation and deposition of, say, elastin in the lamina cribrosa is different from the timing of deposition and maturation of elastin in the sclera.

**Dr. Anderson**: I wonder if I could ask a few questions which perhaps I will pose simultaneously and then you can deal with any of them or all of them as you like. I will put them more in the way of comments, to see whether I have correctly perceived what you have taught us today about connective tissue. I am thinking, first of all, that there is a tendency in thinking in terms of disease genetics to talk in terms of a defect, and as you point out, we all have a defect in a sense, in at least one enzyme, for vitamin C. Is it not true also that there is such a thing as simply physiologic variation that might be inconsequential, represented by blood types. There is type A, and type B, and there are other biochemical differences among us that are not of much consequence, really, physiologically. We may have collagen I, for example, there may be, I do not know, 50 or however many different kinds you could describe, and you might know exactly how many kinds there are, each one having some slight different amino configuration which may or may not be of particular consequence. But a few of them may give a little less tensile strength, or a little bit more, or something like that.

We are looking now at glaucoma, where we see a variation in the ability of the optic nerve head to withstand whatever pressure the eye carries without having something bad happen to it. There may be a number of different alleles that make up each particular connective tissue component. We do not know whether it is collagen I, II, IV, V or whether it is one of the polysaccharides, or mucopolysaccharides, or whether it is something else that is relevant for the reaction of the lamina cribrosa to pressure. Some of these things determine what shape our ears will be and inconsequential things like that, but others may have something to do with the disease.

So I wonder to what degree we should think in terms of a continuum of variation as opposed to presence or absence of a disease and defect. Continuous variations may become crucial when some other factor comes into play, such as the level of intraocular pressure (also a continuous rather than discreet variable) which is separately determined by a different set of genes, and so on.

Secondly, is it really the variation in the type of connective tissue we have, or is there something that may be different in how the connective tissue responds to a circumstance. There was the person you illustrated, who was very flexible and had taught herself to become quite flexible. Now, some of us could never do that, presumably because no matter how many times we stretch ourselves, our connective tissues would not remould themselves as a gradual response to this chronic or repeated stretch such that it then makes a change in its connective tissue structure. Might that also be true in the lamina cribrosa, where some people have the same kind of collagen, same kind of elastin make up as everybody else, but is there something different in the post-translational changes that occur physiologically following whatever physiologic stretch, or I am talking about stretch because we think of pressure and stretch, but it could be something else. And I am talking about the response in terms of remoulding and restructuring that being a new configuration, has some effect on the axons.

So I have made this as a comment, but I really mean it as a question, that is to say, is this the proper way that we should be looking at glaucoma? And if so, would there be tests, even by skin biopsy, that might be done to discover how glaucoma patients differ either in (1) their connective tissue component nature, or (2) could there be a stretch test, that is to say, to put some sort of stretching device on the skin for a week and look at what that skin did over the course of a week, and compare that to whether the patient is or is not harmed by elevated intraocular pressure.

**Dr. Pyeritz**: I certainly agree with all of the points you raise, and think that life is a continuum, and what we choose to call a defect is purely arbitrary and a figment of our own biases and experiences. And we need to look at health and disease as a continuum, both in terms of the underlying composition of the patient but as well to that patient's response or ability to respond to exogenous forces. I could not agree more. Let me just emphasize that each of us differs from the other in our DNA once every 400 nucleotides, on average, and we have 3 billion nucleotides in our genome. So once every 400 bases there is a change in the sequence, on average, between any two of us. Now, some of these changes mean absolutely nothing because they occur in junk DNA, or spacer DNA. Some result in a change in the coding sequence but not a change in amino acid, because of the degeneracy of the code. Some result in a change of an amino acid in a protein, but the change is between amino acids that look enough alike that you do not change the function of the protein, probably, or at least we do not have a good way of assaying it. And then, of course, some of the changes are flagrant enough to be termed mutations, and you do have a phenotype that results from that change. This gives an idea of the amount of genetic variation that is out there and its possible consequences. This is currently being studied extensively in other common disorders, aside from glaucoma, and I think there are probably some general lessons that we all could take from the study of hypertension, for example, where there is much interest in looking at the individual components of the homeostatic system controlling blood pressure. Looking at, for example, subtle variations among us in angiotensin converting enzyme, where some of us do not have an abnormality that is a true defect, but do have less of an ability to regulate our production and modification of angiotensin compared to others, might be instructive. Similarly, atherosclerosis: subtle variations in apolipoproteins that make up low density lipoprotein or high density lipoprotein, likely make subtle differences in our ability to manage cholesterol, and render some of us slightly more susceptible to that extra pat of butter in the morning compared to others.

And the final point I would emphasize is that you all have available to you a very strong and powerful means of looking at the variation you might detect, and that is, the family study. Find individuals who have a predisposition to glaucoma, and here I would urge you to begin with the young patients who develop glaucoma, because they will be the entrée to these hereditary variations. Then use the family of those individuals to define the phenotype and begin looking for the subtle hereditary variations that would be predisposing others. Where you would find the surrogate marker for what you are looking for depends on the development of techniques for looking at components of the extracellular matrix. The most refined way would be to look at the genes themselves, and here all you need is blood specimens, because you can get the DNA from lymphocytes. But I would caution you that that may not be the best way to approach it, because as we learn from Marfan's syndrome, much to our chagrin, once we knew the defect and once we could identify mutations at the highest level of resolution possible, we were no closer to a laboratory test for the diagnosis. First of all, the gene is too big to screen routinely, and second, we have found mutations that probably do not cause Marfan's syndrome. And the same is going to happen repeatedly when you start looking at these individual extracellular matrix molecules. But I would urge those of you who have the capability to look at families, to save at least blood in purple-topped tubes, EDTA preservative, so that you can go back to those patients and those families at some time in the future to look at them.

**Dr. Quigley**: Reed. Thanks. One of the lessons so far this morning and one that I found in beginning to work in molecular biology related to glaucoma, is illustrated by one of my students who about 3 months ago, when an article appeared dealing with the Iowa family that has very strongly inherited very high pressure that develops at an early age, he said, Dr. Quigley, is not it wonderful, we found the gene for glaucoma. And I think, as Reed has just illustrated, when you know which molecule happens to be abnormal in a clearly genetically inherited disease, Marfan's syndrome, you learn to your chagrin, as he said, that every patient with this disease has a different gene defect, that is, that there is quite a variety of gene defects. And we are seeing the same in retinal degenerations, that some of them are due to defects in rhodopsin and some in peripherin, and some in other things, and in fact, there are hundreds of different rhodopsin mutations now known, some of them trivial, some that lead to disease. So there are some powerful tools at hand, I do not want to sound pessimistic, but there will be multiple genetic factors that are found in glaucoma, and not a single one.

# 4. THE MICROANATOMY OF THE OPTIC NERVE

JOHN C. MORRISON, M.D.

**Dr. Quigley:** John Morrison produced one of the most productive times in the laboratory in which I worked in the mid 1980s, and is now an Associate Professor at the Oregon Health Sciences University. John is now going to talk about what glaucoma does at a level much finer than what my talk included.

**Dr. Morrison:** Thank you, Harry. I first began looking at the extracellular matrix (ECM) of the lamina cribrosa in 1986, when I came to work with Harry for my fellowship. What spurred that work was a description by Tengroth[1], who, using a non-histologic technique, looked at collagen amino acid profiles in glaucomatous optic nerve heads compared with normals. He found a difference in the glaucomatous patients versus the normals, and hypothesized that there is something abnormal about the connective tissue biochemistry of patients with glaucoma, presumably in the lamina cribrosa, that may influence glaucomatous optic nerve damage.

I am going to summarize some of the work done in this area over the years and a few things that I am working on now. I am afraid, though, that I am going to ask more questions in the end than I succeed in answering.

Harry wanted me to talk first a little bit about fine structure. While I am going to spend the majority of my time discussing the composition of the lamina cribrosa, I will occasionally drift anterior and posterior to it, because there are some very interesting things to be seen in those regions as well. After that, I will concentrate on several specific extracellular matrix proteins, looking not only at normal and glaucomatous human specimens but also animal model results, both in monkey as well as some rat model work that we have been doing lately.

Initially we will be covering what I call stable connective tissue proteins, such as collagens, basement membrane components, and so forth. I will then present recent information we have discovered about the more labile proteins that are really cell-associated. At that point, because each topic is really an hour talk in itself, I will be very brief. Hopefully, it will give you an idea of the range of things that we will need to be thinking about when we talk about the extracellular matrix of the optic nerve head. I wanted to present some transmission electron microscopy initially. I am concentrating really in the prelaminar region as well as the lamina, pointing out a couple of features that I think are useful to keep in mind as we think about this question of what it is about the structure of the optic nerve head that either protects optic nerve fibers or in some other way modifies the glaucomatous process.

In the prelaminar region there are two predominant cell types. Glia appear darker due to the very dense fibrillar content of their cytoskeleton. Axons, which appear lighter, are at this point not myelinated, and they do not become myelinated until the posterior edge of the lamina cribrosa (Fig. 1a). Glial cells often appear stacked upon each other, extending up from the laminar beams, which also appear aligned at the light microscopic level. You can see how complicated these are, ultrastructurally, with the axons moving along beside them (Fig. 1b). In longitudinal section, you also get a feel for just how variable the orientation of nerve fiver bundles can be as they course through the optic nerve head. Membranous junctions between astrocytes have

*Optic Nerve in Glaucoma, pp. 57–78*
*edited by S.M. Drance*

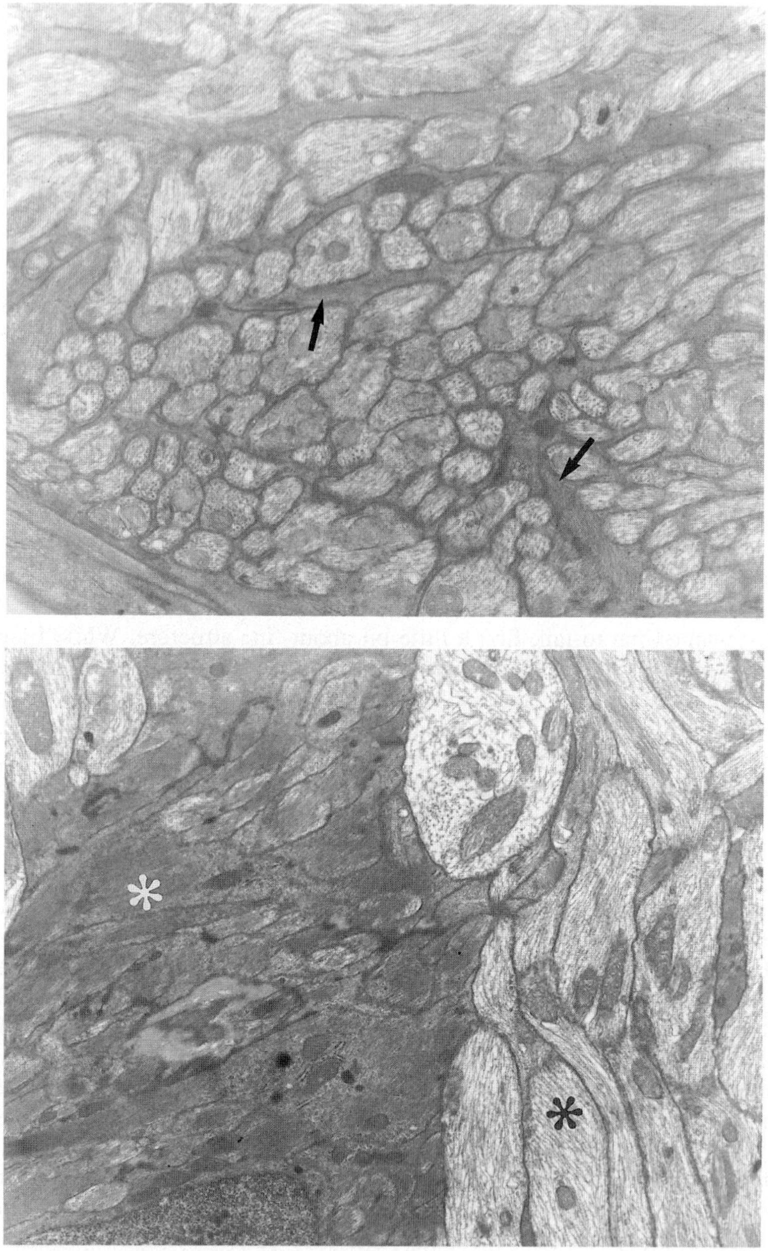

a.

b.

*Fig. 1. a.* Prelaminar optic nerve head showing unmyelinated optic nerve fibers (lighter cells) with associated glial cells (darker cells, arrows). Note variable orientation of nerve fibers within relatively small area (8,100×). *b.* Column of glial cells (white asterisk) with adjacent unmyelinated optic nerve fibers (black asterisk) (5,600×).

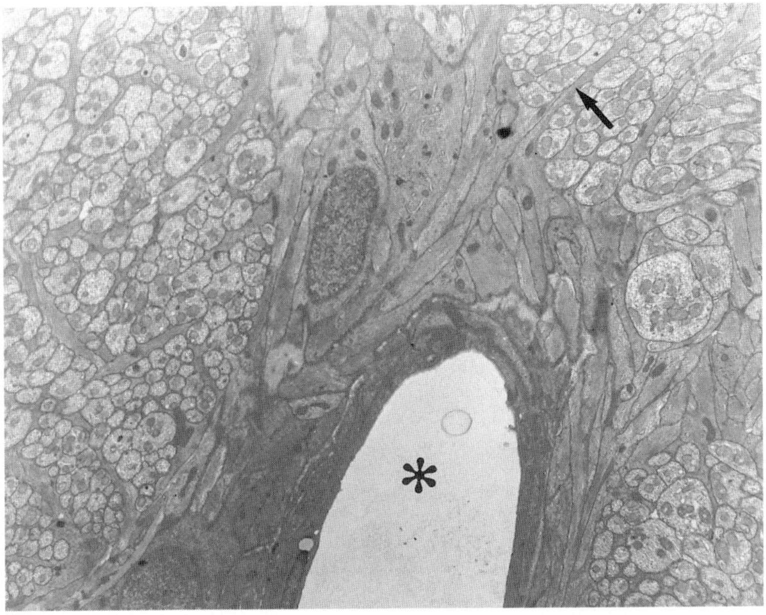

*Fig. 2.* Capillary (asterisk) in anterior optic nerve head with surrounding, complex arrangement of glial cells and processes (arrows) extending into the axon bundles (3,200×).

been described in normal eyes and in those with experimental optic atrophy.

Blood vessels, capillaries mostly, anterior to the lamina cribrosa, are easily identified, with surrounding astrocytes and their processes that extend out into the adjacent nerve fiber bundles (Fig. 2). Approximately 20–30% of nerve fiber bundle tissue in this region is astrocytes and their processes, and they are very prominent in the anatomy of the optic nerve head.

At the lamina cribrosa, individual beams can contain fibroblasts as well as astrocytes (Fig. 3). In addition, the collagen fiber bundles of laminar beams are not all oriented in the same direction. In any one plane of section you will see fibers cut in cross-section while in another area they will be longitudinally cut, and tangential elsewhere. I think this has implications in terms of the physical behavior of these beams. Perhaps Ran Zeimer can speak to that later on.

**Dr. Quigley:** I wanted to say that while there is variation in how the beams have their collagen arranged, the predominant orientation is side to side across the scleral opening. Therefore, when you cut a section of laminar beam, as John is doing here, you will be cutting many more collagen bundles oriented across the opening than anteroposterior. Elastin fibers, in fact, all run side to side, as we are talking about the bundles doing here.

**Dr. Morrison:** Yes, I think that is right. And the other thing to point out, in both the human and monkey, is that each individual laminar beam is not an isolated structure unto itself. That is, it is connected with the other adjacent laminar beams. It is very hard to actually prove this because of the complexity of the structure, but you will often see basement membrane components within a laminar beam, and I think a lot

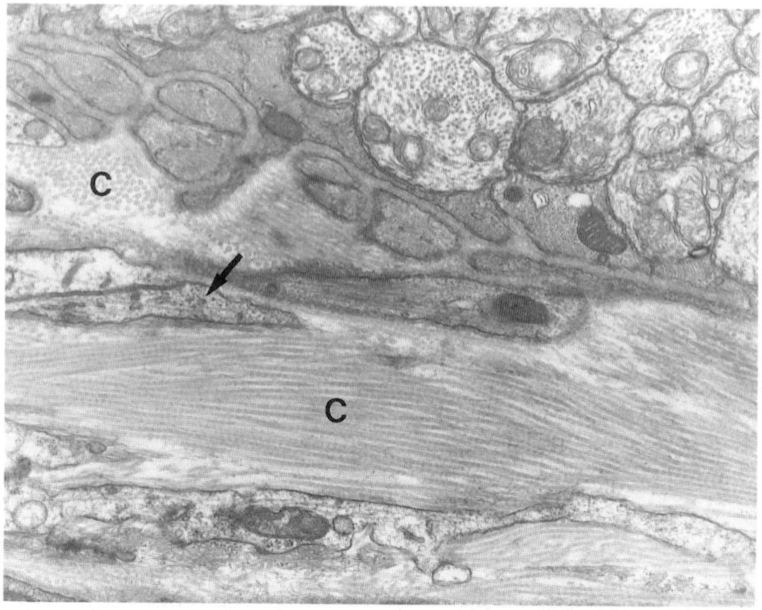


*Fig. 3.* Detail of laminar beam showing collagen bundles (C) cut both longitudinally and in cross-section with apparent fusion of adjacent beams. Note dark glial cells between collagenous beam and nerve fiber bundles. Arrow indicates probable fibroblast (13,000×).

of this is because the adjacent laminar beams are fusing into each other at various points.

When I started working with Harry, we were concentrating primarily on the lamina cribrosa, and we just looked at collagen type I, III and IV, basement membranes and elastin. Since then, my own laboratory has become more interested in a large variety of extracellular matrix molecules. Some of these are structural, but many are not. These latter molecules have functional relationships to cells, involved in both normal and abnormal function of the extracellular matrix. Examples include the metalloprotease enzymes, which are intimately involved in the tissue remodeling seen with wound healing. There is pretty good evidence to indicate that such phenomena are also occurring in the lamina with elevated eye pressure.

The majority of the work I am going to show you is based upon immunohistochemistry, where tissue sections are exposed to primary antibodies directed against the protein of interest, followed by a secondary antibody tagged with a marker which is visible by light microscopy, to show where in the section the primary antibody sticks. Although we have used other methods as well, we have chosen to stay with immunohistochemistry because it has been particularly productive for us. It preserves the complicated histology of the lamina cribrosa and allows us to see the distribution of its different components. A weakness of this technique is that it is hard to quantitate. However, this disadvantage is outweighed by its ability to rapidly evaluate the broad range of molecules that concern us here.

**Dr. Quigley:** The original observation of Tengroth, which was a brilliant approach, to grind up the nerve head and see what the amino acid composition was, suffers unfortunately from precisely that problem. You do not know whether the collagen that

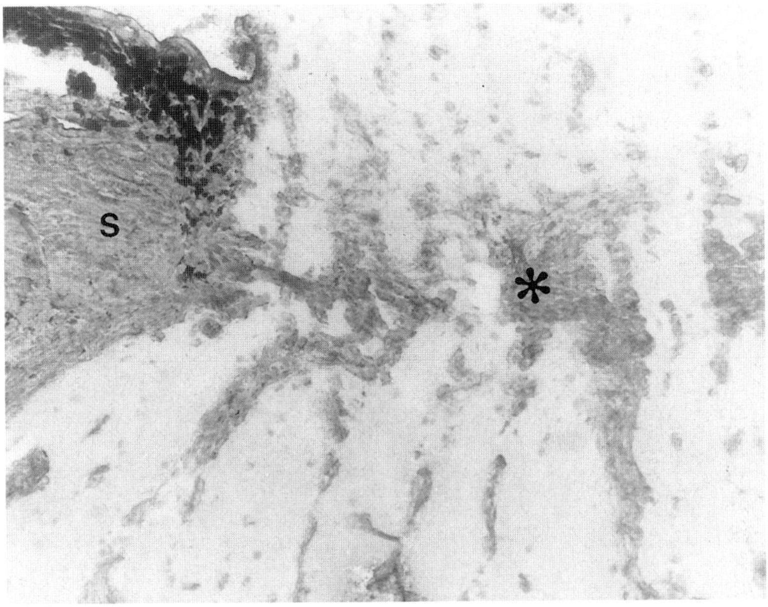


*Fig. 4.* Collagen type I distribution in the monkey optic nerve head. Heavy label is seen over the sclera (S) and the lamina cribrosa (asterisk) (125×). (Reprinted with permission from *Invest Ophthalmol Vis Sci* 1988;29:1141-1150.)

was ground into the amino acid analysis was from the central retinal artery, from the anterior part of the lamina, or the posterior part. So, immunohistochemistry has that as its strong point.

**Dr. Morrison:** What I want to do is review some of the normal composition of the lamina. We will cover both light microscopy observations, and some of the EM correlates to that. Then I will get into some of our observations in the monkey model, and finish up with some newer information on several functional proteins, both in normal and glaucomatous tissue.

We initially found that both collagen I and collagen III are present abundantly within the laminar beams (Fig. 4). There really is not a whole lot of difference in the qualitative distribution and density of either component as you see it in longitudinal section[2,3]. Similar distributions were seen with other types of collagen as well, such as collagen type VI, which tends to be more fibrillar in nature.

Using a pre-imbedding technique, where you expose the antibodies to tissue before the tissue is embedded and sectioned, allows you to cut one micron sections in which it is possible to see the fine distribution of certain basement membrane materials. A collagen type IV antibody shows labeling around margins of the beams of the lamina cribrosa, presumably deposited by astrocytes that line the beams (Fig. 5). Anterior to the lamina cribrosa, we often see basement membrane labeling tailing into the glial columns and the cellular elements that exist between the neural bundles as they are turning to enter the optic nerve head itself. We have seen this with a number of different basement membrane compounds.

At the ultrastructural level, using colloidal gold to visualize antibody location, we also see deposition of type IV collagen at the edges of laminar beams[4], confirming

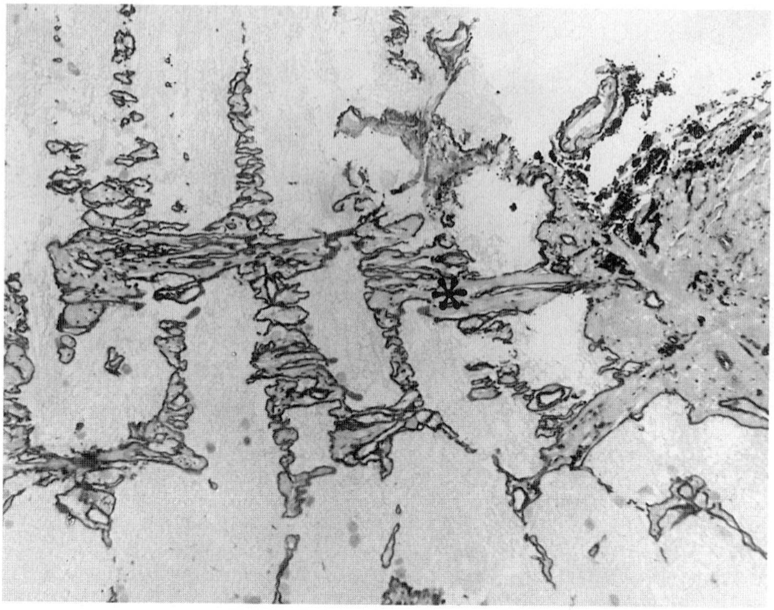

*Fig. 5.* Label with antibodies to collagen type IV is present around the margins of the laminar beams (asterisk), consistent with glial cell basement membranes (340×). (Reprinted with permission from *Invest Ophthalmol Vis Sci* 1988;29:1141-1150.)

its astrocytic basement membrane location (Fig. 6). You can also see focal depositions of basement membrane materials within these laminar beams between bundles of collagen (Fig. 7). Exactly what this is doing here, I do not know. But the point is, even within individual beams, the structure is very complicated.

**Dr. Anderson:** I was going to comment that your finding of this type of collagen type IV going up into the glial columns and forward, if this is equivalent of the electron microscopic basal lamina, would not be surprising, since the basal lamina always separates astrocytes from the capillaries which run in those glial columns. It seems to be an identical distribution. In your last picture, though, how can one be certain that you were not just grazing the surface of a capillary that was embedded within the block, and the label identified only its basal lamina?

**Dr. Morrison:** This could be the case. However, we have seen focal depositions in frozen sections, even 5 and 6 microns thick. In those instances when we see even heavy depositions there is really no evidence of a capillary or any other associated structure. So, while I am sure it is possible, I think it is unlikely in every instance that such depositions are associated with some other structure.

**Dr. Zeimer:** There is a periodicity in the collagen fibers. Could you, when you get to glaucoma, could you show us the periodicity and try to compare it to the normal and abnormal?

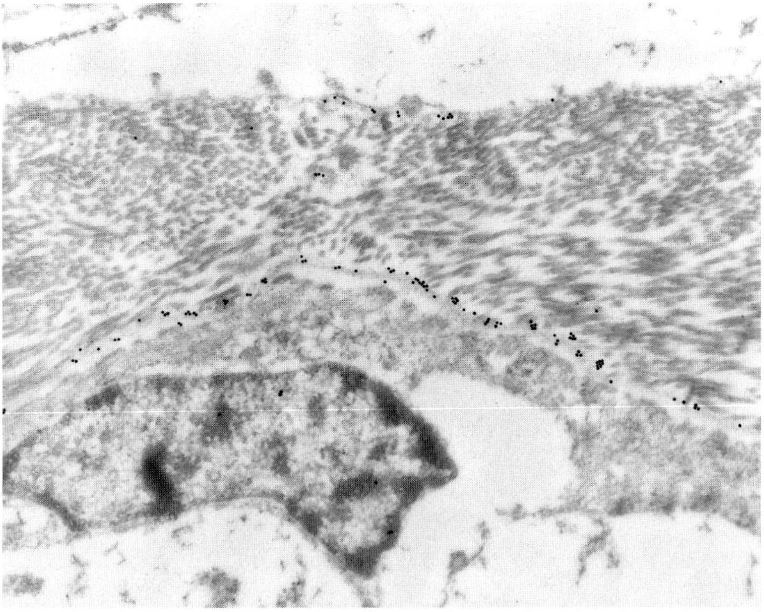

*Fig. 6.* On-grid labeling of type IV collagen with colloidal gold-conjugated secondary antibodies confirms the label of astrocyte basement membranes (22,100×). (Reprinted with permission from *Arch Ophthalmol* 1989;107:123-129.)

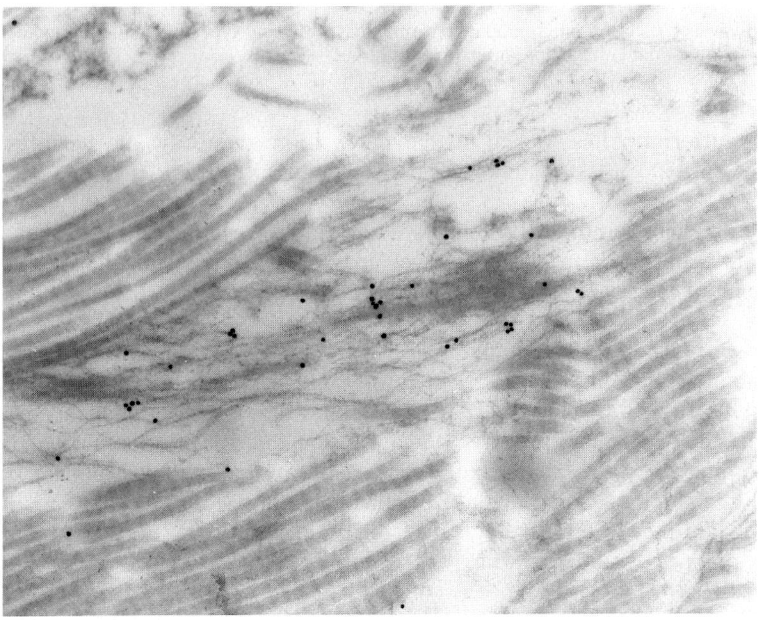

*Fig. 7.* Apparently isolated patch of fibrillar material labeling with antibodies to collagen type IV between bundles of cross-banded collagen fibrils (27,000×).

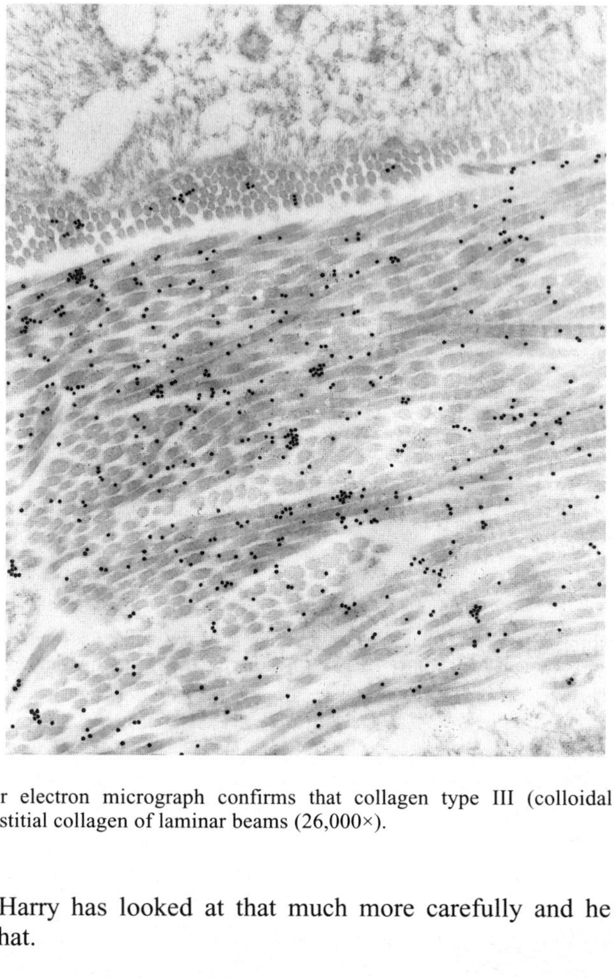

*Fig. 8.* High power electron micrograph confirms that collagen type III (colloidal gold) contributes substantially to interstitial collagen of laminar beams (26,000×).

**Dr. Morrison:** Harry has looked at that much more carefully and he might want to comment on that.

**Dr. Quigley:** There is not a difference we can find. Nor is there a difference in diameter of collagen fibrils in glaucoma eyes compared to non-glaucoma eyes, if you accept the monkey model as glaucoma.

**Dr. Morrison:** Using the immunogold technique, you can also illustrate at the ultrastructural level that the collagen throughout the laminar beams is composed of collagen I, III, and V (Fig. 8). Anterior to the lamina, the collagen and basement membrane components taper off, indicating that there is no distinct anterior border to the lamina cribrosa. Finally, an alpha elastin antibody shows that the amorphous deposits that look like they should be elastin among collagen fiber bundles within the beams are indeed immunologically consistent with that[5] (Fig. 9).

At this point, I would like Harry to comment about the appearance of elastin in glaucoma.

**Dr. Quigley:** I first want to comment on the uniform collagen fibril diameter in the lamina cribrosa. In monkey and in human, if you had all the fibrils cut in exact cross-section you would find that their diameter in the lamina is absolutely dead

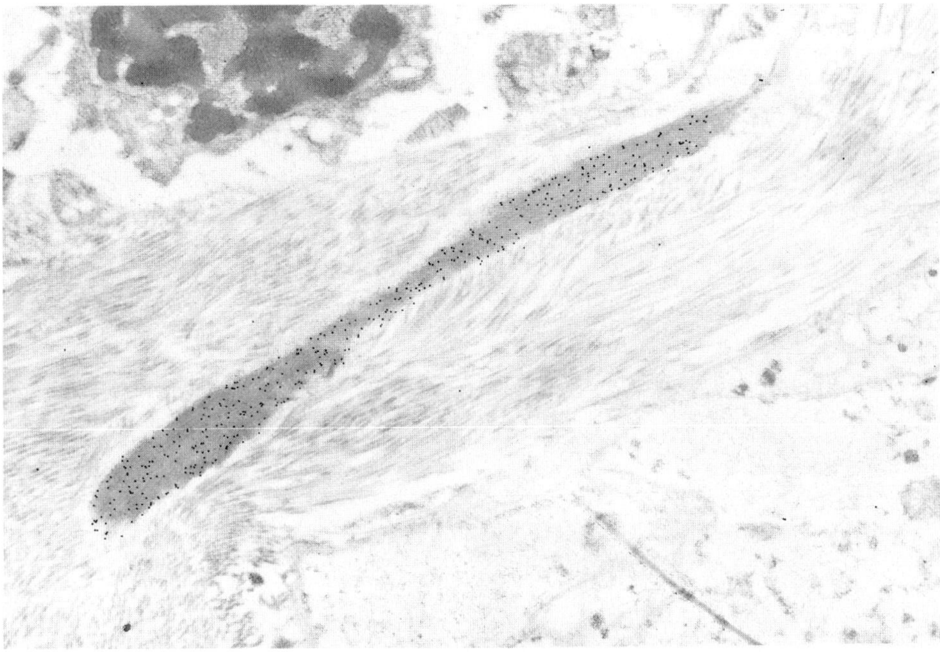

*Fig. 9.* Electron micrograph of amorphous material within a human laminar beam labeled with elastin antibodies and secondary antibodies conjugated to colloidal gold (13,000×).

uniform; 50 nm. Why would it be that the fibrils are all the same size in the lamina? What does that do for you in terms of structure?

Figure 10a shows human laminar beams stained with Luna's technique. They are cut in longitudinal section, so the bundles of nerve fibers are going vertically out of the eye. This is the normal human appearance, and you can see how much elastin there is in each beam. John showed you how hard to find it is in transmission electron microscopy, but when you stain it specifically at the light level it looks sort of like the Eiffel tower. And it is straight. In other words, no matter whether you fix this tissue at atmospheric pressure or fix it at various "elevated" pressures, it has the same appearance.

The next two pictures are from glaucoma eyes with mild (Fig. 10b) and severe (Fig. 10c) optic nerve damage. We have done a masked examination of a series of glaucoma eyes and normal eyes to prove that this appearance is typical in glaucoma. While it may look as if there are fewer elastin fibers total, we cannot prove this. But the appearance in glaucoma is quite different in that they look wavy[6]. They almost never look wavy in the normal eye. Why is it that the elastin fibers look wavy in a glaucoma eye? Is it a fundamental change in the elastin molecule, what you call alpha elastin, or is it the way in which alpha elastin molecules, these black fibers, are connected to the rest of the matrix? This is one of the changes that we now think worth chasing.

**Dr. Zeimer:** Harry, is it your impression that the elastin fibers run more straight than the collagen fibrils?

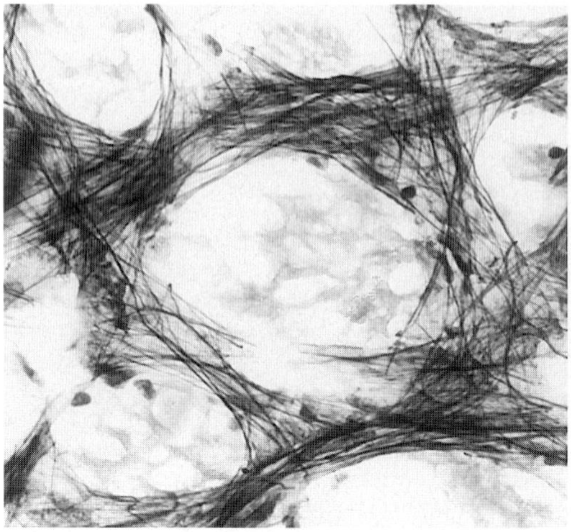

a.

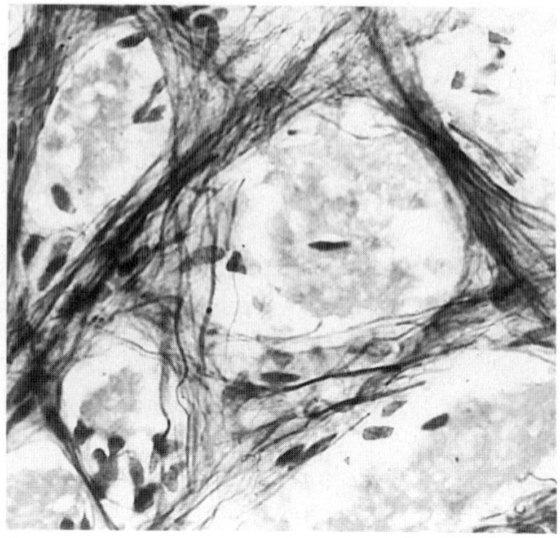

b.

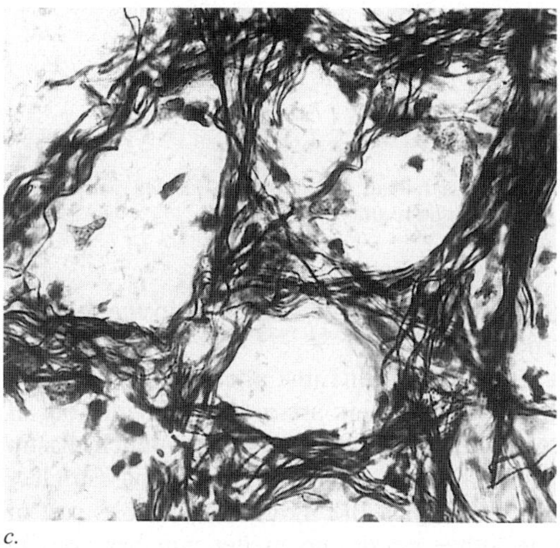

c.

*Fig. 10.* Normal human optic nerve head stained for elastin shows straight elastin bands appear straight (*a*). In glaucoma eyes with mild (*b*) and severe (*c*) glaucomatous nerve damage elastin fibers are more curved and less straight. (490X).

**Dr. Quigley:** I do not know how I can tell, I do not know how we would know that. They are all pretty straight looking, normally.

**Dr. Kaufman:** Harry, in the slide that you have just showed us, how can you be sure that the difference from the glaucomatous to the normal eye is not a secondary one because you have either a skinnier axon, or you do not have an axon, or there is some change in the axon? In other words, rather than a primary change in the support system of the axon, could not this be a secondary change in the surround because the axons are not there to fill out the space?

**Dr. Quigley:** By axon, do you mean fibers of elastin, or do you mean axon bundles?

**Dr. Kaufman:** No, I mean neural fibers.

**Dr. Quigley:** What I was showing you there was elastin, it was not an axon in the picture.

**Dr. Kaufman:** I understand that, but what I am saying is, in the glaucomatous eye, where there may be a change in the neural elements, the changes in the elastin could be secondary to the fact that the whole configuration is different because you do not have the neural tissue there to begin with? In other words, is it the chicken or the egg?

**Dr. Quigley:** Point well taken.

**Dr. Morrison:** Actually, I will speak on that a little later on. In fact, it does seem to be the case, for some things.

At the electron microscopic level, type IV collagen tends to be seen in the basement membranes. Laminin has a similar distribution, but at the ultrastructural level it tends to be located more in the lamina lucida, which is where it promotes attachment between the lamina densa and the cell membrane. Frequently, two laminar beams with astrocyte processes in between them demonstrate a fairly intricate basement membrane pattern, producing a chicken-wire type of connection between the laminar beams. This raises the question of whether or not adjacent beams are really capable of sliding across each other or whether they move together as a unit.

We have also looked at how laminar composition is changed with experimentally elevated eye pressure and damage to the optic nerve in the monkey eye using the laser technique Harry has already described. As Harry has implied, we do not really know whether this is glaucoma or not, but its pathology correlates quite well with what we know of the human situation. Here, we are simply raising the eye pressure to varying degrees for variable periods of time in one eye only, and then looking at the pathology of that eye, comparing it to the fellow eye.

While normal eyes demonstrate linear label with antibodies to type IV collagen around the laminar beams themselves, eyes with moderate to severe cupping show labeling with this same antibody in spaces between the laminar beams, which normally should be occupied by axon bundles alone (Fig. 11). A similar deposition was seen when we looked with antibodies to either collagen I or III[7]. In addition to the extracellular matrix deposition of collagen IV within laminar pores, we noted that the margins of both the laminar beams and the optic nerve septa were more heavily stained than normal in eyes with pressure-induced cupping. Hernandez has also described depositions of collagen type IV within laminar pores in eyes with primary open angle glaucoma[8].

We have confirmed the deposition of extracellular matrix materials within laminar pores using ultrastructural immunohistochemistry. At this level, we also found that the thick appearance of labeling of laminar beam margins was due to thickening of the basement membranes, possibly a reaction by astrocytes to either the increased pressure or the loss of axons.

To differentiate these two possibilities, we transected the optic nerves of several other animals, let the nerves atrophy completely, and processed the tissue for light and electron microscopic immunohistochemistry. We found intense labeling of laminar beam margins with antibodies to collagen IV, and similarly intense label of the retrobulbar septal margins (Fig. 12). However, in contrast to the experimental glaucoma eyes, we did not see any deposition within laminar pores using either antibodies to collagen I, III, or IV. At the electron microscopic level, the increased label

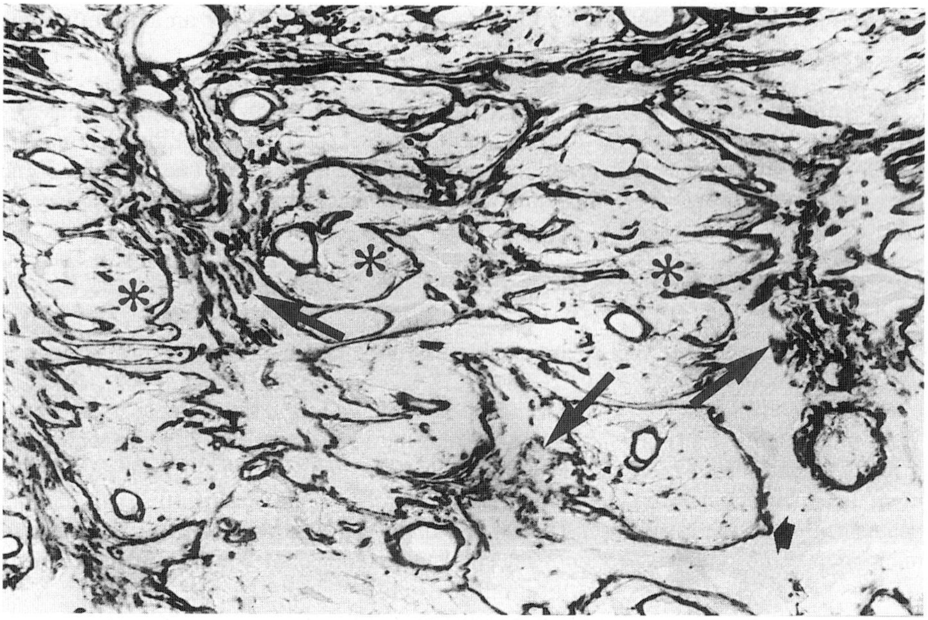

*Fig. 11.* Monkey eye with experimental glaucomatous optic nerve damage shows abnormal deposition of type IV collagen (arrows) between the laminar beams (asterisks), which also have heavier than normal label along their margins (small arrow) (1250×). (Reprinted with permission from *Arch Ophthalmol* 1990;108:1020-1024.)

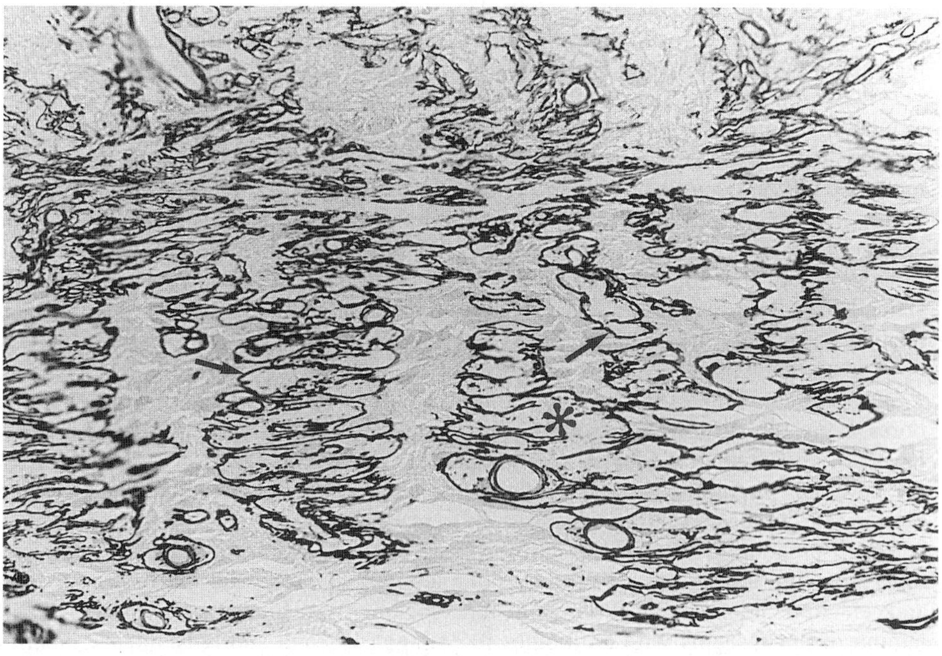

*Fig. 12.* Monkey eye after optic nerve transection showing prominent collagen type IV label of laminar beam margins (arrows) but no significant deposition between the beams themselves (asterisks) (700×). (Reprinted with permission from *Arch Ophthalmol* 1990;108:1020-1024.)

of basement membranes in both the lamina cribrosa and optic nerve appears to be due to a ruffling up of the membrane. This is probably not a reduplication, but a folding up of redundant basement membranes as the axonal bundles shrivel and die. Joe?

**Dr. Caprioli:** Do you think the change that you see with a transection of the optic nerve, I mean change relative to the glaucomatous process with the elevated pressure, may have something to do with rates rather than mechanism *per se*? In other words, the rate at which the axon will be lost, when you transect the nerve, is undoubtedly a lot faster than the glaucomatous process, I would guess. Would you comment on that.

**Dr. Morrison:** I think that is possible. However, with these particular models, the time period over which we let these animals go was about the same. It is just that in the glaucomatous animal the pressure was up around 35 mm Hg for the entire time. However, rates of axonal loss could still be an important factor.

We have started looking at a wide variety of proteins that have various roles in the extracellular matrix. Certainly the proteoglycans are a very large part of this, and Reid covered their general structure very nicely. Their range of potential interactions appears very broad. They have effects on the extracellular matrix itself, and they have cell–cell interactions. They modulate the reaction of cells to the extracellular matrix, and they bind growth factors. The entire range of responses that the extracellular matrix is capable of is probably due in large part to proteoglycans.

We have started looking at proteoglycans using a set of antibodies directed against the stub of either chondroitin or dermatan sulfate on the core protein that is left over after you use enzymes to digest away their glycosaminoglycans[9]. These antibodies are specific for chondroitin sulfate in either the 4 position or the 6 position.

When we looked at optic nerve sections exposed to chondroitin-4 sulfate following predigestion with chondroitinase ABC, which degrades both the dermatan and chondroitin sulfate glycosaminoglycans, you see heavy and confluent labeling of the laminar beams themselves, with some in the anterior part of the nerve (Fig. 13). This would indicate that a chondroitin sulfate/dermatan sulfate-containing type proteoglycan is present in these areas. Probably more that just one type of proteoglycan is responsible for this.

The chondroitin-6 sulfate antibodies produced a very different picture. At high magnification you can see that labeling with these antibodies is more fibrillar within the beams and along their margins (Fig. 14). Exactly what all of this means, we do not really know for sure because a wide variety of core proteins can produce this kind of picture.

Now, if you substitute chondroitinase ACII, which degrades only chondroitin sulfate side chains, for chondroitin ABC, you will only be exposing the chondroitin sulfate stub. If you stain that tissue with the chondroitin-4 sulfate antibody you will be able to estimate how much label is due to chondroitin-4 sulfate versus dermatan sulfate. This changes the labeling pattern dramatically (Fig. 15). Instead of labeling all connective tissue structures, the chondroitin-4 sulfate antibody now labels only connective tissue at the level of the lamina cribrosa. We have seen this in both the human and the monkey, and, just recently, in the rat as well. This is the only example I can think of where extracellular matrix proteins appear to be localized to laminar beams but not in the optic nerve septa and sheath as well.

Aggrecan was mentioned earlier by Dr. Pyeritz. This is the large chondroitin

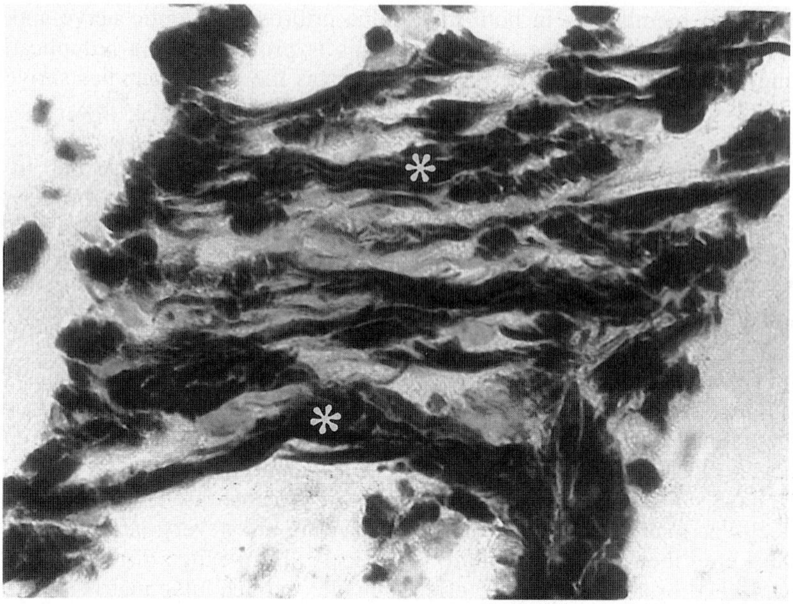

*Fig. 13.* High power appearance of labeling of monkey lamina cribrosa beams (asterisk) with antibodies to chondroitin-4 sulfate stubs after chondroitinase ABC predigestion (1100×).

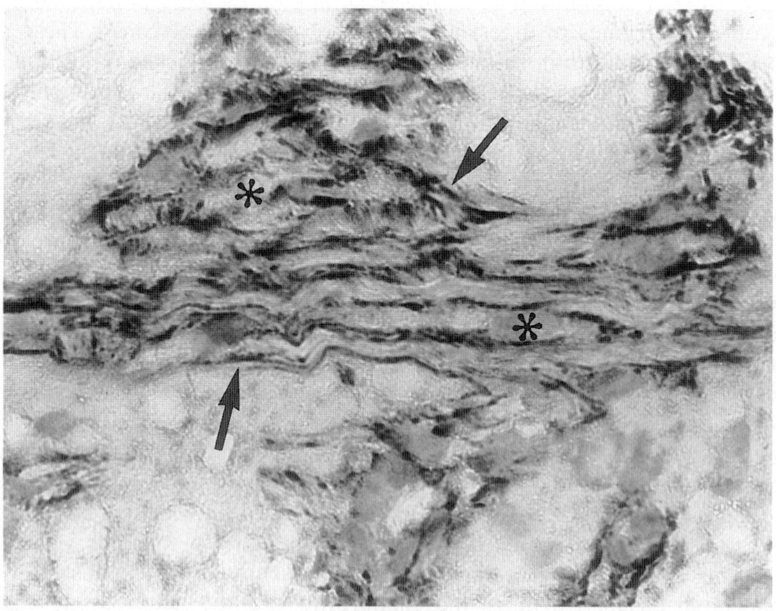

*Fig. 14.* Labeling of laminar beams (asterisk) with antibodies to chondroitin-6 sulfate after chondroitinase ABC appears fibrillar and along the beam margins (arrows) (1100×).

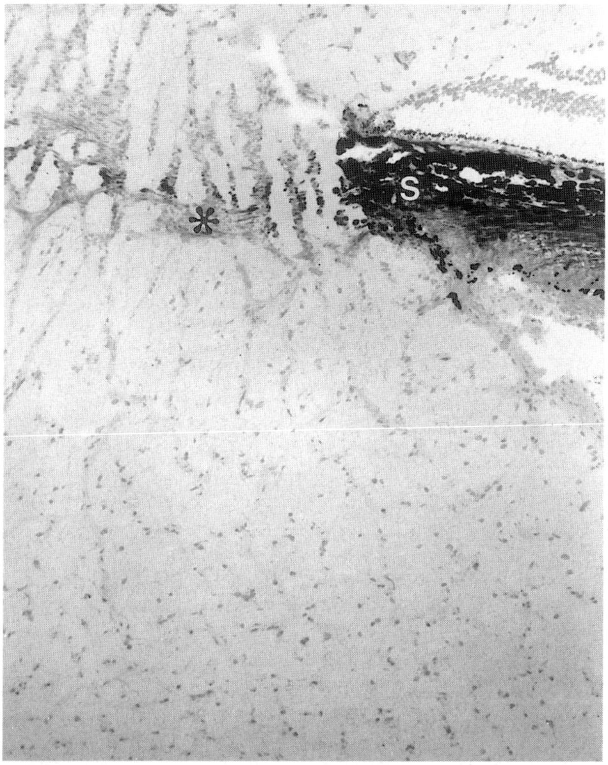


*Fig. 15.* Monkey optic nerve head exposed to chondroitin-4 sulfate antibodies after chondroitinase ACII digestion limits label to the lamina cribrosa (asterisk) and sclera (S), with disappearance of optic nerve septa and pia label (120×).

sulfate proteoglycan of cartilage. It produces the bottle brush appearance of the proteoglycan diagram that you are used to seeing, and it is responsible for the resilient, cushioning physical properties of cartilage in large, weight-bearing joints. This picture is a normal human specimen labeled with aggrecan antibodies obtained from Dr. Kurt Doege, from the Portland Shriner's hospital. In both normal human and monkey, labeling with this antibody is limited to the posterior sclera, with variable label of the laminar beams, but never of the optic nerve connective tissues (Fig. 16a). This is very similar to the antibody labeling that we saw with chondroitin-4 sulfate after chondroitinase ACII digestion. Interestingly, this same antibody used on human glaucoma specimens with moderate to severe damage showed greater labeling intensity within the lamina cribrosa (Fig. 16b). Is this a primary abnormality for people with glaucoma, or only secondary to injury? We do not know for sure, but we have seen this in both primary and secondary glaucoma specimens.

Decorin and biglycan are two other proteoglycans we have found in the lamina cribrosa. These are small proteoglycans with one or two attached chondroitin or dermatan sulfate side chains. They have a wide variety of functions. Decorin interacts with collagen fibrils and governs fibrillogenesis, and spacing among other things. Biglycan is less well understood. It tends to be more associated with cells and with tissues that are under stress. We now have evidence that both proteins are

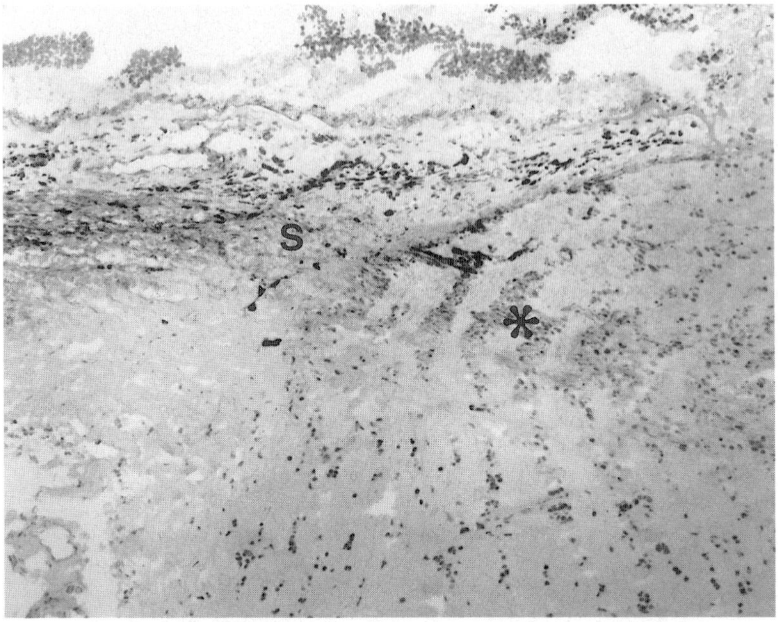


a.

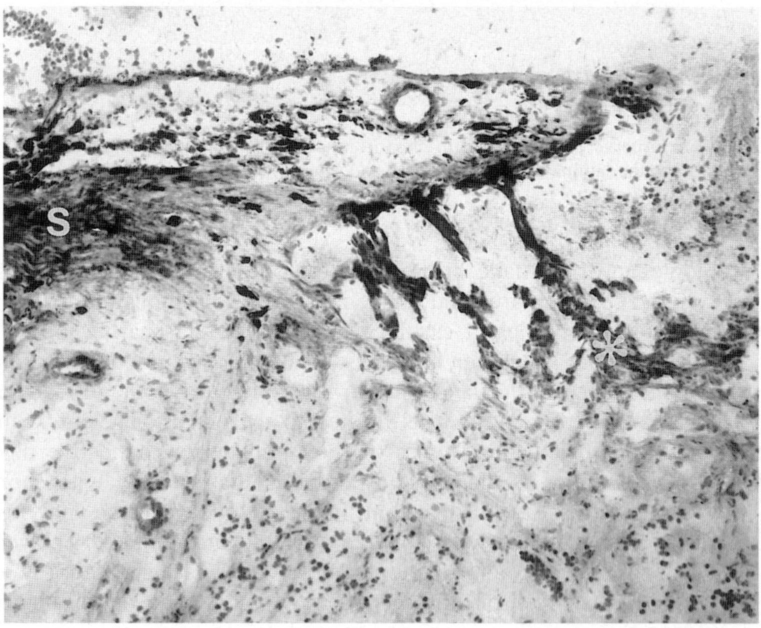


b.

*Fig. 16.* Human optic nerve heads labeled with antibodies to aggrecan. Normal specimen (*a*) shows label of portions of the lamina cribrosa (asterisk) and sclera (S). Glaucomatous specimen (*b*) has more intense label of distorted laminar beams (asterisk) (220×).

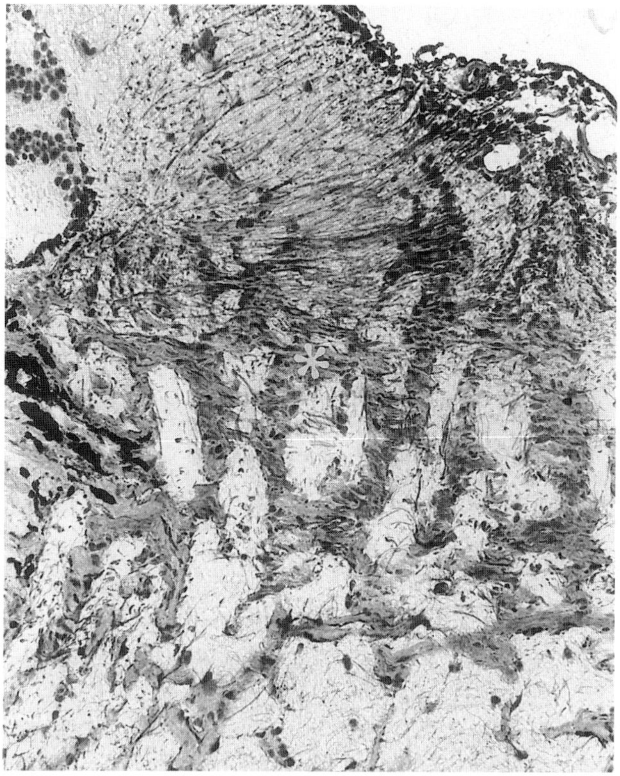

*Fig. 17.* Normal monkey optic nerve head labeled with antibodies to a propeptide fragment of biglycan. Note primarily cellular label with transversely oriented processes, presumably glial, concentrated mostly within the prelaminar and laminar axon bundles. Asterisk indicates laminar beams (110×).

present within all collagen-containing structures in both normal human and monkey tissues. Staining with antibodies to both is nearly identical to that seen with antibodies to the interstitial collagens. Preliminary work also shows that decorin, but not biglycan, may be deposited within laminar pores in eyes with glaucomatous optic nerve damage.

We have also been looking at the distribution of a precursor for biglycan, using an antibody to a propeptide portion of the biglycan molecule. A monkey specimen shows labeling in both the prelaminar and the laminar area, much of it extending transversely into the nerve bundles (Fig. 17). We have seen this same pattern in a number of different tissues, including the rat. At higher power much of this label appears to be associated with astrocyte processes. Obviously, ultrastructural studies are required to understand this distribution fully. As a propeptide, this molecule may regulate cellular processing, possibly through controlling endocytosis. I want to show this mainly to emphasize that studying the extracellular matrix of the optic nerve head is now requiring us to expand our thinking beyond just the lamina cribrosa.

Vitronectin is another cell-associated protein. In normal tissue, antibodies to vitronectin label the lamina cribrosa fairly heavily (Fig. 18a). However, in glaucoma specimens, much of this label is lost (Fig. 18b). Vitronectin bears some re-

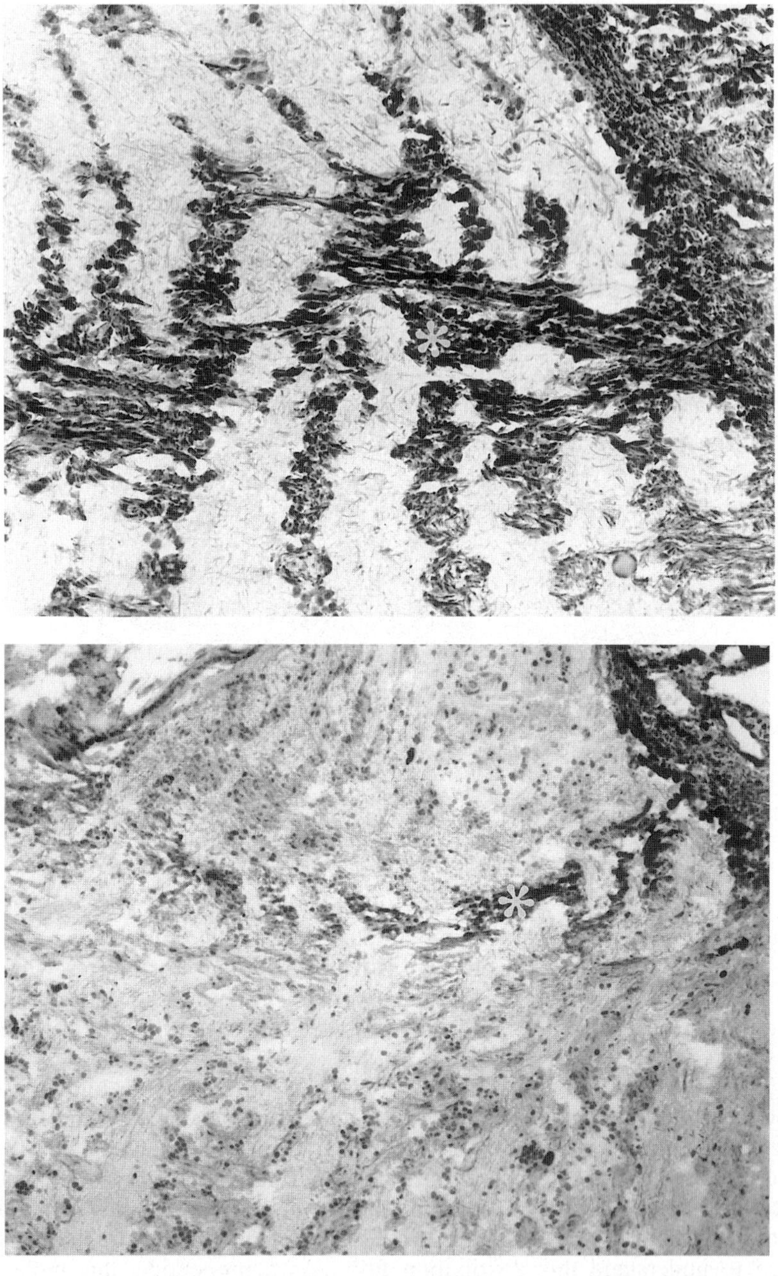

a.

b.

*Fig. 18.* Human optic nerve heads labeled with antibodies to vitronectin. Label of the laminar beams (asterisk), heavy in normal tissues (*a*), appears much less intense in glaucomatous specimen (*b*) (220×).

sponsibility for activating the complement system. It also binds to plasminogen activator inhibitor, possibly to stabilize this inhibitor of plasminogen activator in tissues. A decrease in quantity of vitronectin might release plasminogen to convert to plasmin, which could be an initial event in degrading the lamina cribrosa and surrounding regions in the early stages of glaucomatous nerve head remodeling.

Finally, the integrins, which are important for cell signalling phenomena, are also intimately involved in this whole process. We have now looked at human optic nerve head labeling with a battery of 16 antibodies to the different integrins. This is just one example, using antibodies to the $\beta_1$ subunit (Fig. 19a). Labeling of a human primary open-angle glaucoma specimen shows an overall loss of connective tissue organization and label throughout the nerve head (Fig. 19b).

I would like to make one point about using human tissue to look for these cell-associated antigens. Because these proteins are attached to cells, they tend to be lost fairly early after enucleation and they are often not as easy to find as when you are looking at structural proteins like collagen and basement membranes. This is why, although it is important to look at human glaucomatous tissue, it is important to also use an animal model so that you can have very strict control over how quickly the tissue is obtained and processed. This will allow detailed understanding of the behavior of these important cell-associated constituents.

**Dr. Zeimer:** You mentioned, by the way, that you have a rat model. What is the difference as far as the morphology between the rat intraocular pressure damage and the monkey intraocular pressure damage and the human? Do you see excavation? Do you see enlargement of the scleral canal?

**Dr. Morrison:** We are developing a system where we are getting moderate elevations in pressure, but the ones we have followed through their whole pressure course will elevate after about one to two weeks following the episcleral vein injection of hypertonic saline. If the pressure is very high, I am talking in the 30's and 40's, you will get a rapid loss of nerve fibers. It is my impression so far that the rat optic nerve is more susceptible to elevated eye pressure than the human. The quantity and arrangement of the laminar beams may have something to do with that, although vascular considerations may also be important. As yet, details of rat optic nerve head vasculature have not been worked out. We have indeed seen cupping in many of our specimens. I can not tell you for sure whether we are getting any actual enlargement of the scleral canal or not. There is no question that we see nerve fiber damage. When you look at a section through the retina, the outer retinal layers look pretty normal. However, the ganglion cell and the nerve fiber layer are markedly diminished.

**Dr. Anderson:** I have a comment and a question. The comment is that it is certainly important that all of these various compounds be looked at to see where they are in the lamina cribrosa and what the structure is so that we may then begin to understand what might be abnormal, either primarily or secondarily, as it happens in glaucoma. The question I have relates to your finding of certain of these substances, seemingly in association with a morphology that suggests astrocyte processes and astrocyte cells. Is it possible that some of the antibody staining is to intracellular polypeptide precursors of the substance, rather than the substance itself, reflecting the fact that the astrocytes are responsible for producing some of these extracellular components?

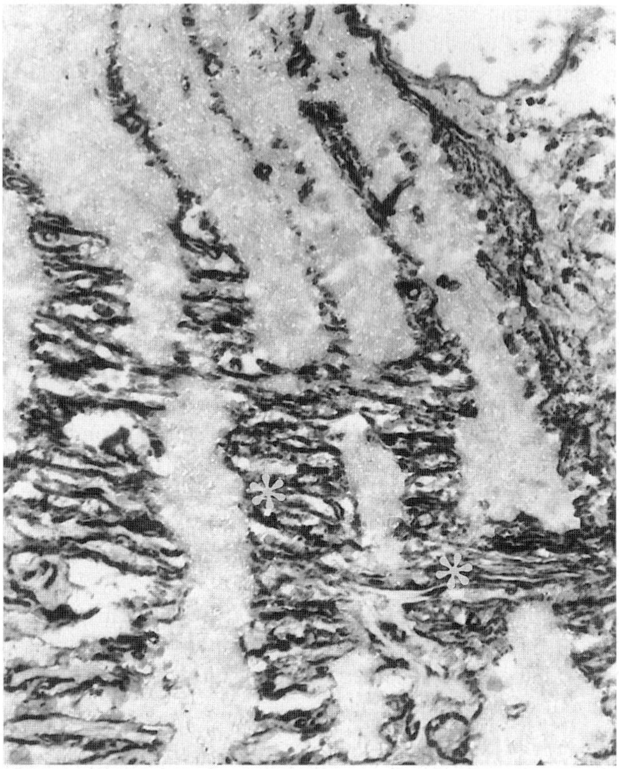

a.

*Fig. 19.* Human optic nerve heads labeled with antibodies to $\beta_1$ integrin. Highly ordered arrangement of label around laminar beams (asterisks) and within glial columns in a normal specimen (*a*) is lost in the nerve head with primary open-angle glaucoma (*b*), which also shows label within optic nerve fiber bundles (arrows) (220×).

**Dr. Morrison:** Yes, I think that is certainly possible. We think there is a very high likelihood of that with the biglycan propeptide antibody that I showed you. There is no question about the intracellular labeling of that, or at least cell surface associated labeling. In the future, it will be very important to identify the cells of origin for these proteins, in both normal and glaucomatous tissues. This will be essential in defining the pathology of glaucomatous optic nerve damage.

**Dr. Quigley:** I want to make a comment that you have stressed already, and that is that the immunoperoxidase method that John showed you, that is, sending an antibody in to try to find the molecule, is something which is difficult to quantitate. When the entire tissue is changing, and when you are using an inherently non-quantitative method, it becomes very hard, unless there is something quite dramatic, to say there is more elastin, or there is less elastin, or there is more biglycan than there was before. So while the work certainly deserves to be followed up, it certainly is controversial at the moment whether there is any more or less of something there than we think is present in normals.

**Dr. Morrison:** One approach to achieving quantification is with methods that look

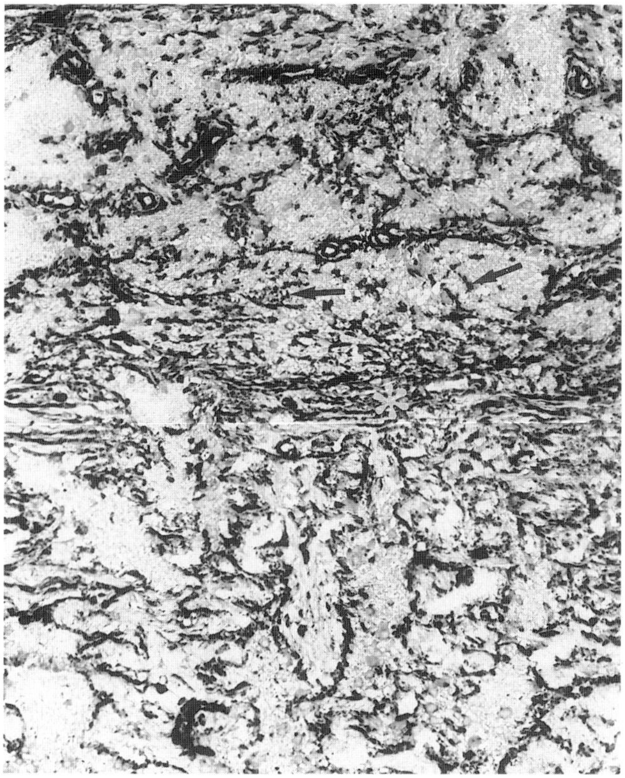

*Fig. 19b.*

specifically at cellular mRNA production. These have been successfully employed by Dr. Rosario Hernandez[10]. She has observed specific changes in cellular production for collagen I, IV, and elastin in many glaucomatous specimens[11]. However, because these methods are very time-consuming, and the range of proteins we are faced with here is very broad, we want to first use immunohistochemistry to get an idea of what specific proteins we need to concentrate on. Then we can use these other methods for more precise, quantitative studies to confirm our initial findings.

## References

1. Tengroth B, Ammitzboll T. A comparative analysis of the collagen type and distribution in the trabecular meshwork, sclera, lamina cribrosa and the optic nerve in the human eye. *Acta Ophthalmol.* 1985;63(suppl):91-93.
2. Morrison JC, Jerdan JA, L'Hernault NL, Quigley HA. The extracellular matrix composition of the monkey optic nerve head. *Invest Ophthalmol Vis Sci.* 1988;29:1141-1150.
3. Hernandez MR, Luo XX, Igoe F, Neufeld AH. Extracellular matrix of the human lamina cribrosa. *Am J Ophthalmol.* 1987;104:567-576.
4. Morrison JC, L'Hernault NL, Jerdan JA, Quigley HA. Ultrastructural location of extracellular matrix components in the optic nerve head. *Arch Ophthalmol.* 1989;107:123-129.
5. Hernandez MR. Ultrastructural immunocytochemical analysis of elastin in the human lamina cribrosa. Changes in elastic fibers in primary open-angle glaucoma. *Invest Ophthalmol Vis Sci.* 1992;10:2891-2902.
6. Quigley HA, Brown A, Dorman-Pease ME. Alterations in elastin of the optic nerve head in human and experimental glaucoma. *Brit J Ophthalmol.* 1991;75:552-557.

7. Morrison JC, Dorman-Pease ME, Dunkelberger GR, Quigley HA. Optic nerve head extracellular matrix in primary optic atrophy and experimental glaucoma. *Arch Ophthalmol.* 1990;108:1020-1024.
8. Hernandez MR, Andrzejewska WM, Neufeld AH. Changes in the extracellular matrix of the human optic nerve head in primary open-angle glaucoma. *Am J Ophthalmol.* 1990;109:180-188.
9. Morrison JC, Rask P, Johnson EC, Deppmeier LMH: Chondroitin sulfate proteoglycan distribution in the primate optic nerve head. *Invest Ophthalmol Vis Sci.* 35:838-845, 1994.
10. Hernandez MR, Wang N, Hanley NM, Neufeld AH. Localization of collagen types I and IV mRNAs in human optic nerve head by in situ hybridization. *Invest Ophthalmol Vis Sci.* 1991;32:2169-2177.
11. Hernandez MR, Yang J, Ye H. Gene expression of collagen types III and IV, and elastin in human glaucomatous optic nerve heads. ARVO Abstracts. *Invest Ophthalmol Vis Sci.* 1992;33(suppl):1091.

# 5. CELL BIOLOGY OF THE HUMAN LAMINA CRIBROSA

ABBOT F. CLARK, Ph.D, SHERRY BROWDER, B.S., H. THOMAS STEELY, Ph.D, KAREN WILSON, B.A., DAVID CANTU-CROUCH, B.S., MITCHELL D. MCCARTNEY, Ph.D

I will briefly review the work that our laboratory has been doing on the culture and characterization of cells isolated from the human lamina cribrosa. All forms of glaucoma are characterized by pathognomonic changes in the optic nerve head (ONH) which involves excavation of the optic cup. The lamina cribrosa (LC) is a complex, reticulated elastic tissue which normally supports the optic nerve head and through which 1-2 million retinal ganglion cell axons leave the eye to form the optic nerve (Fig. 1a). In glaucoma, there is a progressive posterior displacement and compression of the lamina cribrosa as well as a disinsertion of the lamina cribrosa from the scleral rim (Fig. 1b). The size of the lamina cribrosa, approximately 1.5 μm in diameter and 200–400 μm thick, makes this tissue recalcitrant to conventional biochemical analysis. Several years ago, Rosario Hernandez and coworkers reported the successful culturing and characterization of lamina cribrosa cells from the human optic nerve head[1]. This pioneering work has initiated a better understanding of the cell biology and biochemistry of the optic nerve head.

Our technique for culturing cells from the human lamina cribrosa is a slight modification of the technique described by Hernandez and her colleagues[1]. We carefully dissect the lamina cribrosa from the optic nerve head of human donor eyes, place the explant in a single well of a 24-well culture plate in Dulbecco's modified Eagle's medium containing 10% fetal bovine serum. It takes approximately 2-3 months for the cells to reach confluency in a single well. These cells are serially passaged using Cytodex 3 microcarrier beads instead of trypsin passage, so these cells never see trypsin, which appears to be important in allowing us to carry these cells out to about ten passes.

Our work and that of others suggest that there are at least five different cell types that can be potentially grown out of these explants: lamina cribrosa cells, scleral fibroblasts, astroglial cells, vascular endothelial cells, and vascular pericytes. These different cell types can be distinguished morphologically based on their shape in culture (Fig. 2). The lamina cribrosa cells are broad, flat cells with multiple processes and branches. In our hands, they actually grow into a confluent monolayer composed of cells with overlapping cell borders. In contrast, the astroglial cells have large cell bodies with numerous long, thin processes and do not form a confluent monolayer. The scleral fibroblasts are long, thin, spindle-shaped cells that grow in multiple layers. The vascular endothelial cells are polygonal in shape, with smooth borders and a characteristic cobblestone appearance. And finally, vascular pericytes are large dendritic shaped cells with long thin processes. In addition to the different morphological characteristics of these cell types, there are biochemical markers that also allow us to differentiate between the five cell types (Table 1). For example, astroglial cells of the optic nerve head express an intermediate filament protein, glial filament acidic protein (GFAP), whereas the resident cells of the lamina cribrosa do not express glial filament acidic protein. Scleral fibroblasts do not express the basement membrane proteins such as type IV collagen and laminin while lamina cribrosa cells do express these proteins.

*Optic Nerve in Glaucoma, pp. 79–105*
*edited by S.M. Drance*

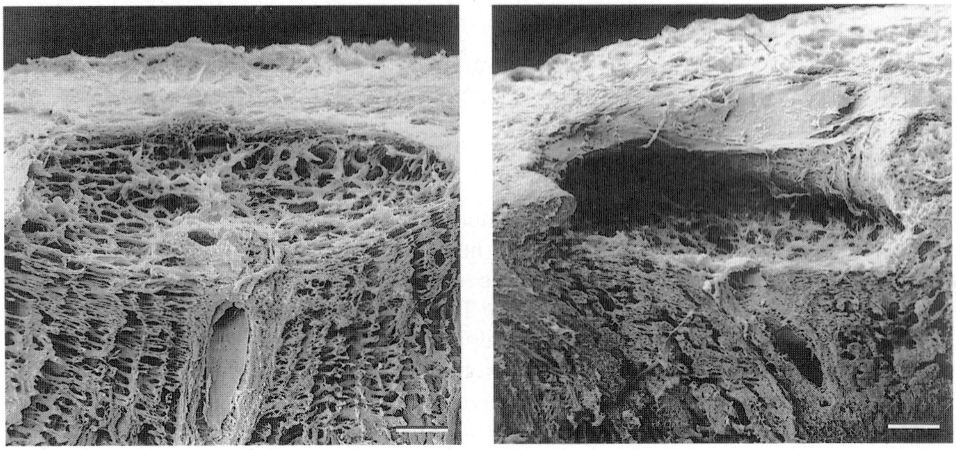

a. b.

*Fig. 1.* Scanning electron micrographs of optic nerve heads from normal (*a*) and glaucomatous (*b*) donor eyes. The optic nerve heads were fixed, digested with trypsin, and prepared for SEM. Bar = 200 μm.

*Table 1.* Biochemical markers for cells cultured from the human lamina cribrosa.

| *Collagen* | *IV* | *LN* | *Factor VIII* | *sm-actin* | *GFAP* | *3G5* |
|---|---|---|---|---|---|---|
| Lamina cribrosa cells | + | + | – | – | – | ? |
| Astroglial cells | + | – | – | + | + | ? |
| Scleral fibroblasts | – | – | – | – | – | ? |
| Vascular endothelial cells | + | + | + | ± | – | – |
| Vascular pericytes | – | – | – | + | (–) | + |

GFAP: glial filament acidic protein

Vascular endothelial cells stain positively for Von Willebrand's factor (Factor VIII) while vascular pericytes do not, but the pericytes do stain with antibody 3G5 which is specific for a ganglioside found in these cells[2].

We find that the vast majority of cells which grow out of the human lamina cribrosa explants are of the cell type which we call lamina cribrosa cells. Indirect immunofluorescent analysis of these lamina cribrosa cells shows that these cells express types I, III (Fig. 3a), and IV (Fig. 3b) collagen, fibronectin (Fig. 3c), laminin (Fig. 3d), and elastin. We are in the process of examining which isoforms of fibronectin are expressed and which extracellular matrix receptors (*i.e.* integrins) are present on these cells. Dr. Morrison has started to characterize a variety of integrins in the optic nerve head, and we are also trying to identify them in our cultured lamina cribrosa cells. We have also been looking at the cytoskeletal components expressed by these cells. We were quite surprised to find that these cells express smooth muscle α-actin (Fig. 3e). The possibility that this cytoskeletal protein may play an important role in cell function is currently only speculative.

It is important to compare the characteristics of the cells from a specific tissue with the characteristics of the tissue from which the cells were isolated because it is possible for cells to change certain features in culture. Our cultured lamina cribrosa cells express the same extracellular matrix molecules that are found in the lamina cribrosa of

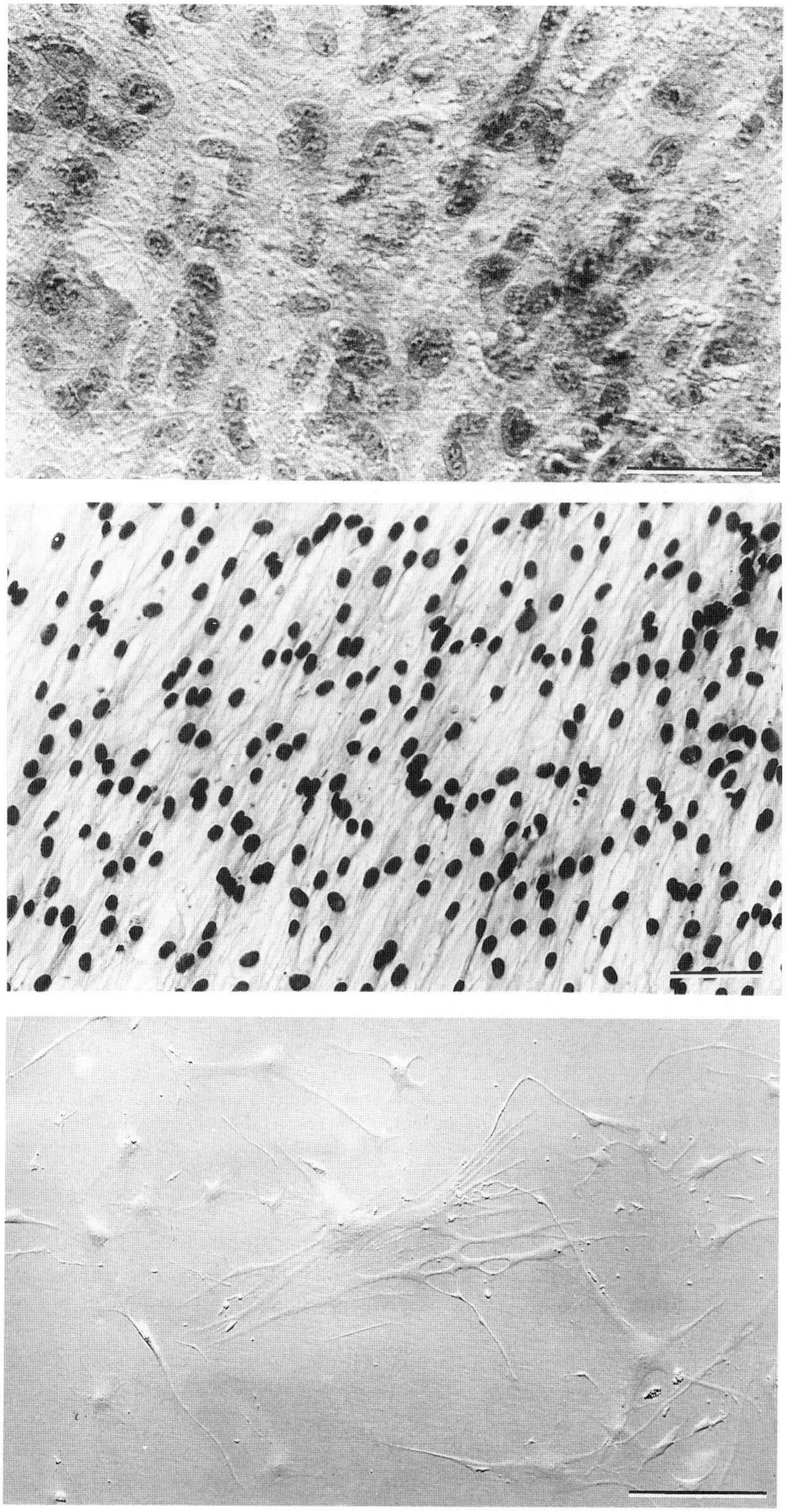

a.

b.

Fig. 2. c.

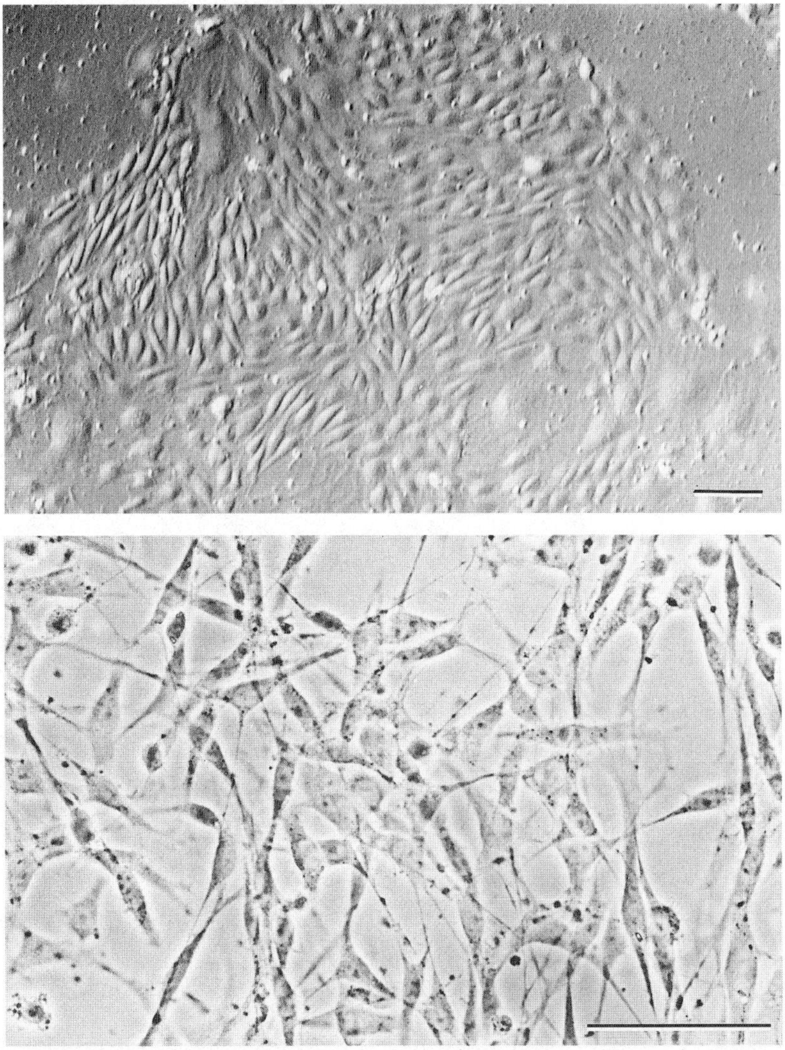

d.

e.

*Fig. 2.* Light photomicrographs showing the characteristic morphology of cells which can be potentially cultured from the lamina cribrosa: (*a*) human lamina cribrosa (LC) cells, (*b*) human scleral fibroblasts, (*c*) human retinal vascular pericytes, (*d*) human vascular endothelial cells, and (*e*) rat astroglial cells. Bar = 150 μm.

the human optic nerve head[3-5]. (Table 2). It is therefore quite likely that the lamina cribrosa cells are responsible for generating and maintaining the unique extracellular matrix of the lamina cribrosa. We do not yet know whether lamina cribrosa tissue has any smooth muscle α-actin staining.

The successful culture of human lamina cribrosa cells allows us to explore a variety of factors that might influence the structure of the lamina cribrosa. For example, studies have suggested that age, genetics, race, intraocular pressure, and optic nerve head ischemia may influence lamina cribrosa structure and thereby predispose an individual to glaucomatous optic neuropathy. The incidence of primary open-angle glaucoma in-

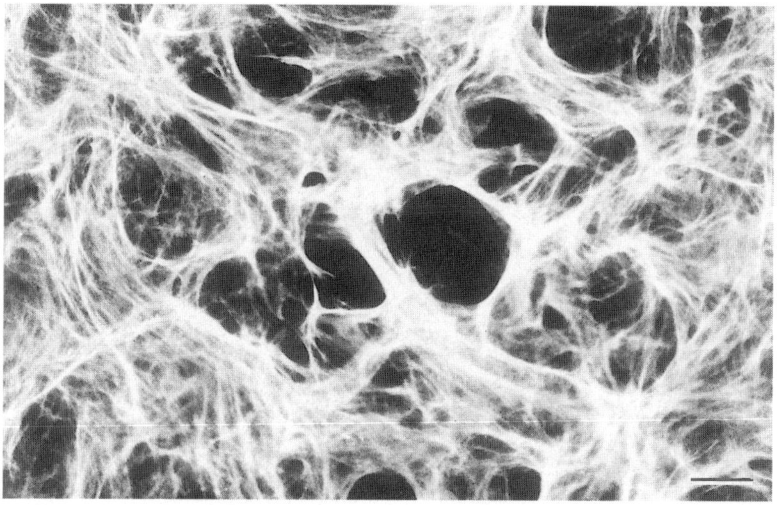

*a.*

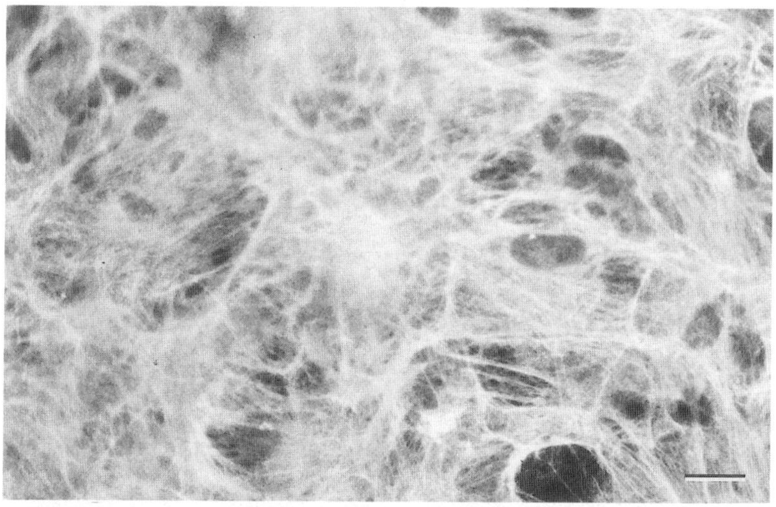

*b.*

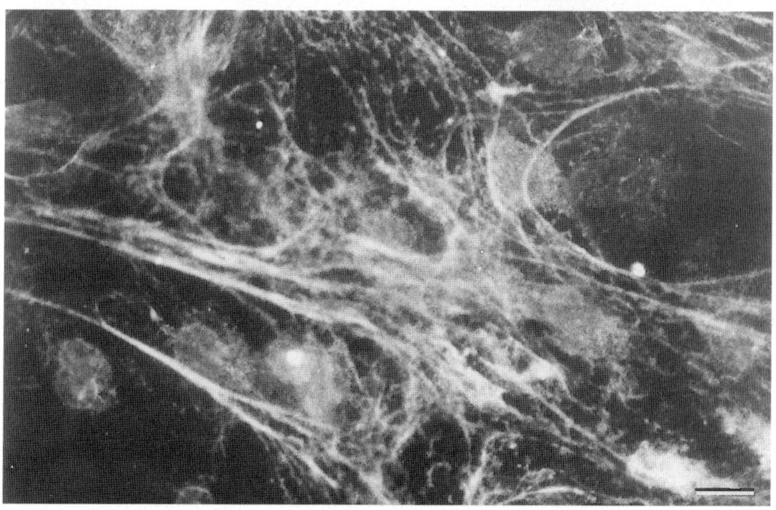

*Fig. 3. c.*

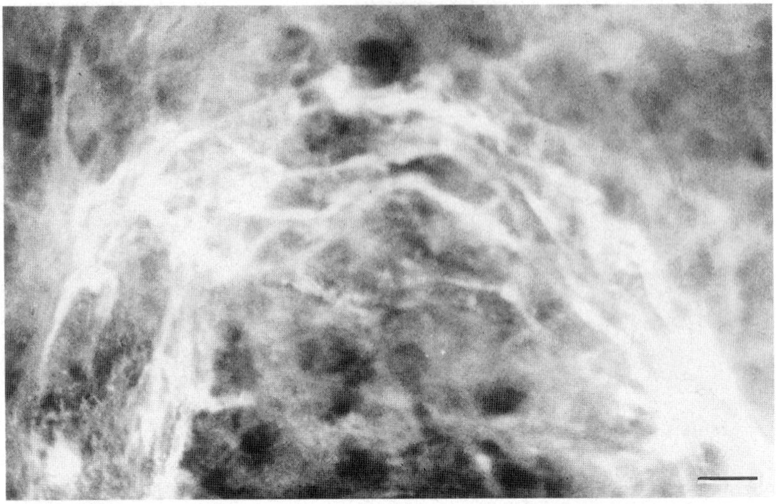

d.

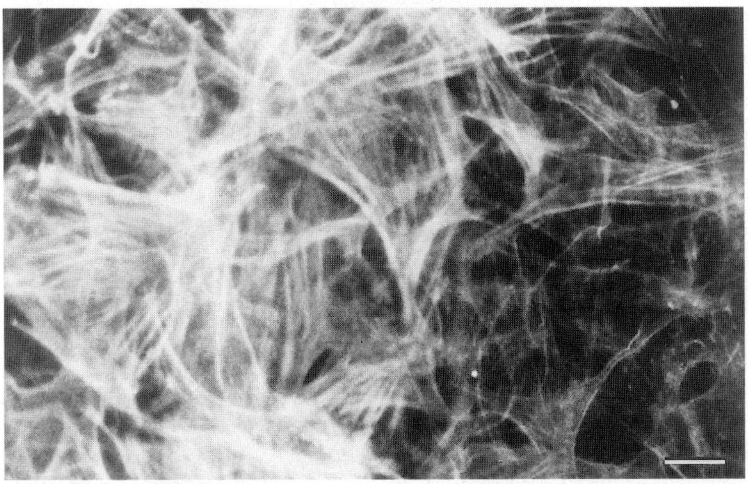

e.

*Fig. 3.* Expression of extracellular matrix and cytoskeletal proteins in cultured human lamina cribrosa cells as determined by indirect immunofluorescence: (*a*) type III collagen, (*b*) type IV collagen, (*c*) fibronectin, (*d*) laminin, and (*e*) smooth muscle α-actin. Bar = 50 μm.

*Table 2.* Comparison of biochemical markers in lamina cribrosa tissue and cultured lamina cribrosa cells.

| *Marker* | *LC tissue* | *Cultured LC cells* |
|---|---|---|
| Collagen type I | + | + |
| type II | + | + |
| type III | + | + |
| Fibronectin | + | + |
| Laminin | + | + |
| Elastin | + | ± |
| Smooth muscle α-actin | ? | + |

LC: lamina cribrosa

creases dramatically after the age of 40[6]; age-related changes in lamina cribrosa structure have been reported[7]. It will be interesting to see if there are any differences in lamina cribrosa cells cultured from young compared to older eyes. Genetics appears to play a role in the development of glaucoma[8-9] particularly as it is related to ocular hypertension[9-10]. Much less is known about how genetics may play a role in susceptibility of the optic nerve head to glaucomatous damage. Several studies have shown that race is a risk factor for the development of primary open-angle glaucoma. African-Americans have a 4-5-fold higher propensity to develop glaucoma[11]. There may be important biochemical differences[12] as well as structural differences[13] in the optic nerve head of blacks which make them more susceptible to glaucomatous damage. Elevated intraocular pressure (ocular hypertension) remains one of the most important risk factors for the development of glaucomatous optic neuropathy[6,14-15]. Experimentally induced ocular hypertension in primates causes progressive optic nerve head damage[16-17] and biochemical changes in the optic nerve head[18-20]. Can elevated pressure be mimicked in any way in cultured lamina cribrosa cells? Rosario Hernandez and colleagues have recently published work describing the effect of elevated hydrostatic pressure on cultured lamina cribrosa cells[21]. Human lamina cribrosa cells were exposed to atmospheric pressure or to an elevated hydrostatic pressure of 50 mm Hg for 7 days. They found a 2-fold increase in the expression of type I collagen mRNA in the pressure-treated lamina cribrosa cells.

**Dr. Quigley**: Can you interpret for us what that experiment might show? What does that mean? Does that mean, for example, that they also showed that other mRNAs also increase, was this a non-specific effect?

**Dr. Clark**: The pressure-induced effect on lamina cribrosa type I collagen mRNA shown by Hernandez and coworkers appears to be specific. They have tested, for example, actin as a control and the actin mRNA did not change with pressure. This effect appeared to be specific for collagen I, as far as the markers they looked at. They have also done earlier immunocytochemical work suggesting that there is an increase in the expression of collagen in the lamina cribrosa of glaucoma eyes[22].

**Dr. Quigley**: Among the things that are important in the measurement of mRNA levels is to know whether it was newly made mRNA or whether the mRNA breakdown rate was changed. It is also important to know whether the increased presence of a specific mRNA results in the increased expression of the specific protein or is the cell just sort of churning out more mRNA but is not really making more protein. But this is an excellent first step for knowing what is going on.

**Dr. Pyeritz**: In very well controlled tissue culture studies, fibroblast monolayers subjected to different tensions and stretch clearly synthesize altered levels of specific components of the extracellular matrix, so that physical forces certainly contribute to the expression, and this is in keeping with these results, if it is real.

**Dr. Clark**: I absolutely agree. One of the things that we would like to try to do is grow these cells on a membrane that is stretchable, and use that model rather than just expose them to pressure. But as Harry has said, the study of Hernandez and colleagues is a really good first start.

**Dr. Zeimer**: In this pressure experiment, were the lamina cribrosa cells grown on a substrate which was put under pressure and therefore the substrate was actually stretching?

**Dr. Clark**: The work of Hernandez and coworkers was done on lamina cribrosa cells that were cultured on a plastic matrix, and therefore the uniform pressure probably did not stretch the substrate.

**Dr. Zeimer**: No, I mean, whether the effect was due to pressure or whether the effect was due to stretching. I think from the literature on fibroblasts that the response of the cells is more to stretching rather than to homogeneous pressure. And I would like to stress that it is not necessarily the direct effect of the intraocular pressure, rather the stretching of the substrate, which could be the lamina cribrosa, on these cells, that caused that change in their expression.

**Dr. Clark**: Very true, and we can experimentally approach this issue by growing the cells on an elastic substrate. That way we can differentiate between pure pressure and stretch.

**Dr. Quigley**: Let us also imagine that we are a native cell in the lamina cribrosa, and 72 times a minute we get stretched. So if you want to duplicate what is going on here, what you want to do is you want to change the natural rhythmic stretching of the extracellular matrix that these cells are normally sitting on. I do not think just pulling on them in a static way is going to tell us very much of anything. Now, it is a very complicated experiment, but it is a good challenge.

**Dr. Clark:** Another risk factor that may play a role in glaucomatous damage to the optic nerve head is ischemia, and this could easily be modeled in lamina cribrosa cultures. We will be hearing a lot more about ischemia later on in the conference. It is also possible that a variety of different biochemical factors, such as hormones and growth factors, can influence the structure of the lamina cribrosa. One very interesting hormone class to consider is the glucocorticoids as these steroids have been suggested to be associated with at least some forms of glaucoma. Most of the evidence that suggests that glucocorticoids are associated with glaucoma has concentrated on their ability to generate ocular hypertension[23], and very little has actually been done on the potential role of glucocorticoids at the back of the eye. A variety of researchers, including work in our own laboratory, have looked at the effects of glucocorticoids on the trabecular meshwork[24-31]. I will not extensively review this literature, but summarize by saying that glucocorticoids change trabecular meshwork cell functions, cytoskeletal organization, extracellular matrix composition, and protease expression. So we asked the question: Do glucocorticoids affect cultured lamina cribrosa cells?

The lamina cribrosa can be visualized as a tissue matrix system, and its detailed structure was described earlier today by Dr. Morrison. There is an extensive connectivity between the laminar beam extracellular matrix and the cells in the lamina cribrosa. This connectivity includes specific molecules in the extracellular matrix, membrane receptors for these extracellular matrix molecules, the cytoskeleton, and the nucleus. Alterations in this connectivity can influence gene expression in these cells. Using the cultured lamina cribrosa cells we can independently test all of these different functions.

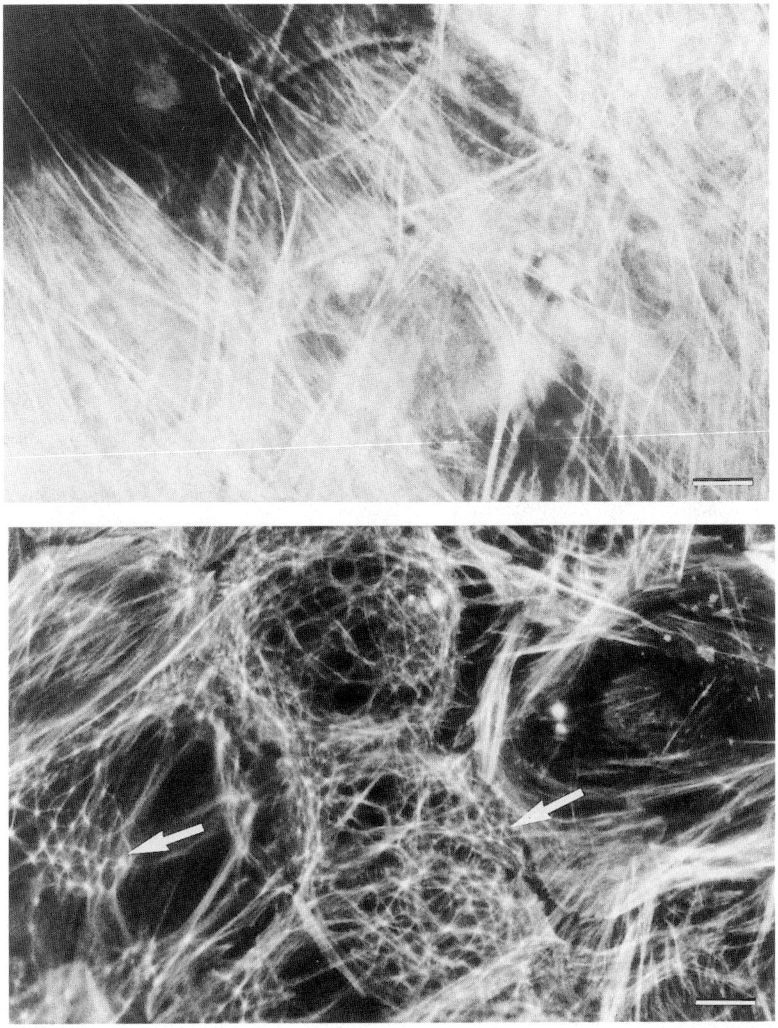

a.

b.

*Fig. 4.* Dexamethasone-induced reorganization of actin microfilament network in cultured human lamina cribrosa cells. Cells were fixed, stained with rhodamine phalloidin, and examined by epifluorescence to visualize microfilaments. *a.* Control LC cells. *b.* LC cells were treated with $10^{-7}$ M dexamethasone for 14 days. The DEX-treated cells form cross-linked actin networks (CLANs) (arrows). Bar = 50 μm.

One of the first things we examined was the effects of glucocorticoids on the cytoskeleton, particularly the microfilaments and microtubules. Cultured human lamina cribrosa cells were fixed in 1% glutaraldehyde buffer containing 0.5% Triton X-100 and stained with rhodamine phalloidin which binds to polymerized f-actin. Control lamina cribrosa cells displayed a linear array of microfilament stress fibers (Fig. 4a). Using whole mount transmission electron microscopy[24-25], you can see the finer details of these stress fibers. These actin microfilament stress fibers are labeled with antibodies against actin and secondary antibodies derivatized with immunogold particles (Fig. 5a). Using this same technique of whole mount transmission immunoelectron microscopy, we can also observe the structure of another cytoskeletal ele-

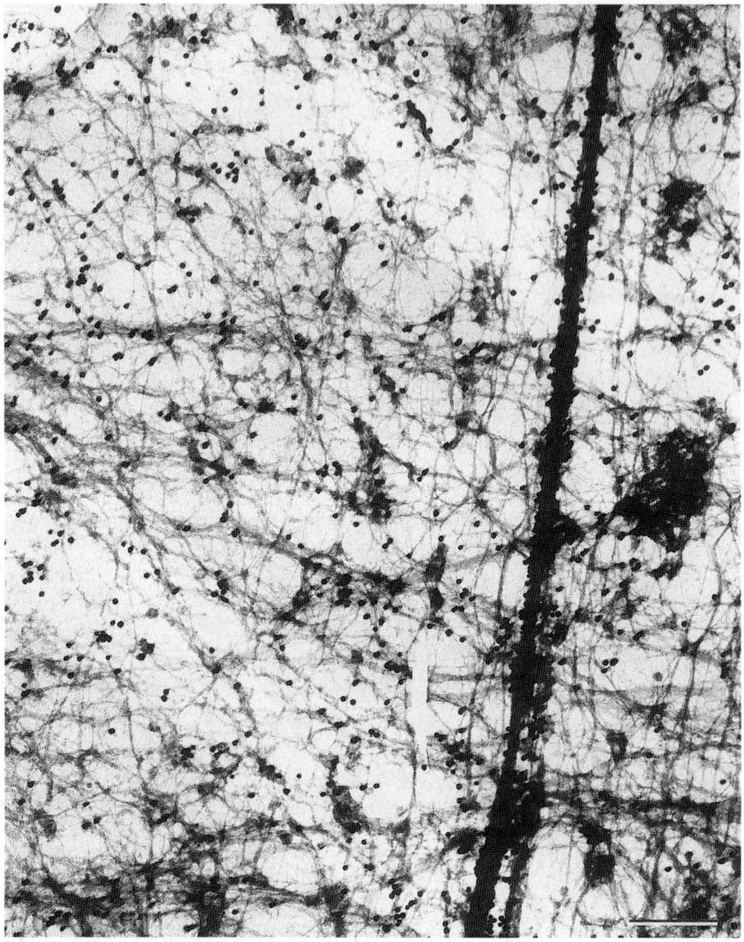

a.

*Fig. 5.* Immunocytochemical analysis of transmission electron micrographs of whole mount cultured human lamina cribrosa cells from control cultures (*a-b*) and cultures treated with $10^{-7}$ M dexamethasone for 14 days (*c-d*). The cells were reacted with antibodies to actin (*a,c*) or tubulin (*b,d*) and labeled with gold-conjugated secondary antibodies. DEX treatment caused the formation of CLANs (*b*) and microtubule tangles (*d*). Bar = 1 µm.

ment, tubulin, which are specifically labeled with anti-tubulin antibodies and secondary antibodies containing immunogold particles (Fig. 5b). The microtubules in these control lamina cribrosa cells form a network of radiating fibers that are decorated with the gold particles.

There is a major reorganization of the cytoskeleton in the cultured lamina cribrosa cells that are exposed to the potent glucocorticoid dexamethasone ($10^{-7}$ M) for 14 days (Fig. 4b). This reorganization of the lamina cribrosa microfilaments involves a transition from linearly arranged stress fibers to a polygonal network of actin which we have previously named cross-linked actin networks or CLANs[24-25]. We have observed the dexamethasone-induced cytoskeletal reorganization in ten independent lamina cribrosa cell cultures. This finding is quite reminiscent of what we have previously shown with trabecular meshwork cells that are exposed to glucocorti-

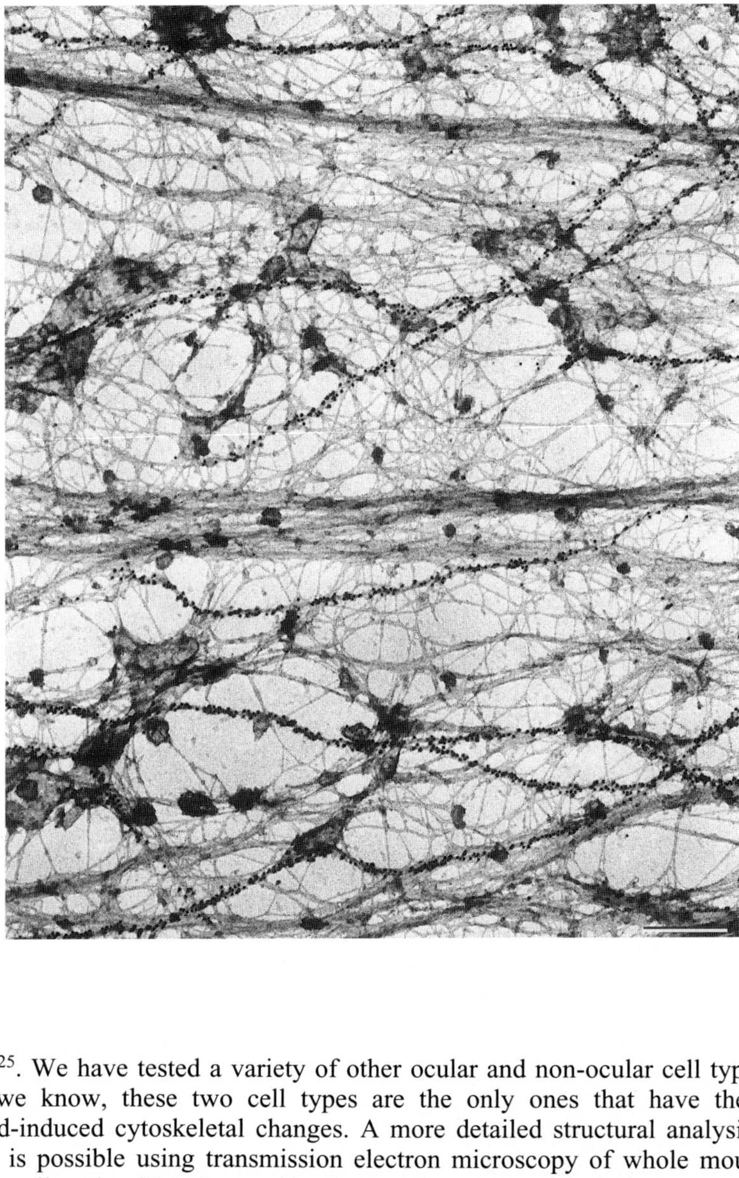

b.

*Fig. 5.*

coids[24-25]. We have tested a variety of other ocular and non-ocular cell types, and as far as we know, these two cell types are the only ones that have these glucocorticoid-induced cytoskeletal changes. A more detailed structural analysis of these CLANs is possible using transmission electron microscopy of whole mount lamina cribrosa cells. The CLANs consist of microfilament bundles that are held together by electron-dense vertices (Fig. 5c). We are in the process of trying to understand and identify what actin binding protein(s) may be responsible for the cross-linked actin network formation. Glucocorticoids cause not only a change in the lamina cribrosa microfilament structure, but also cause changes in lamina cribrosa cell microtubules. Dexamethasone treatment leads to a much more tangled microtubule network in the lamina cribrosa cells (Fig. 5c).

There is an intimate association between the cytoskeleton and the extracellular matrix. Therefore, we asked the question whether the steroid-induced changes in the lamina cribrosa cytoskeleton are also associated with changes in the lamina cribrosa extracellular matrix. We have morphological evidence that glucocorticoids cause

c. 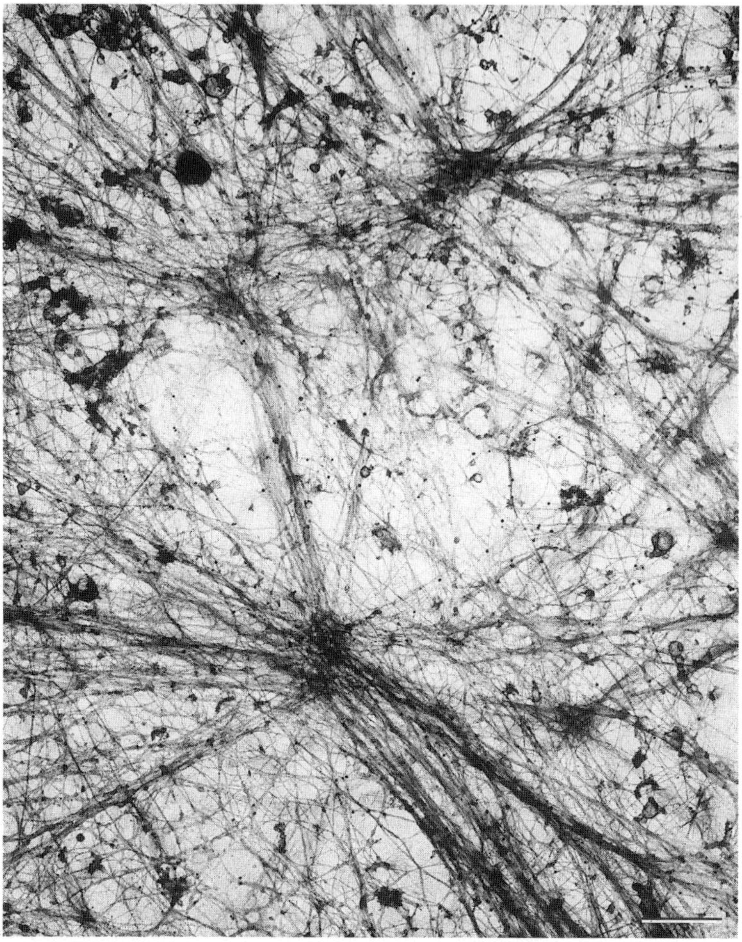

*Fig. 5.*

changes in the extracellular matrix of cultured lamina cribrosa cells. This indirect evidence for dexamethasone-induced effects comes from transmission electron microscopy studies. Cultured lamina cribrosa cells often have overlapping cell processes as can be seen in trabecular meshwork cross sections (Fig. 6a). Control, normal lamina cribrosa cells have typical mitochondria, nucleus, and endoplasmic reticulum with what appear to be secretory vesicles as well as cytoskeletal elements (Fig. 6a-c). Cells that are exposed to $10^{-7}$ M dexamethasone for 14 days have a marked proliferation of their endoplasmic reticulum and of their Golgi apparatus (Fig. 6d-e). Both the endoplasmic reticulum and the Golgi are responsible for the synthesis and post-translational modification of secreted proteins such as extracellular matrix proteins. There appears to be a deposition of extracellular material in the steroid-treated cells (Fig. 6f), and we are in the process of identifying this material using electron microscopy immunohistochemical techniques. Preliminary biochemical analysis suggests that at least a portion of this increased extracellular matrix material is fibronectin and laminin.

Although so far we have been talking mainly about glaucomatous changes to the

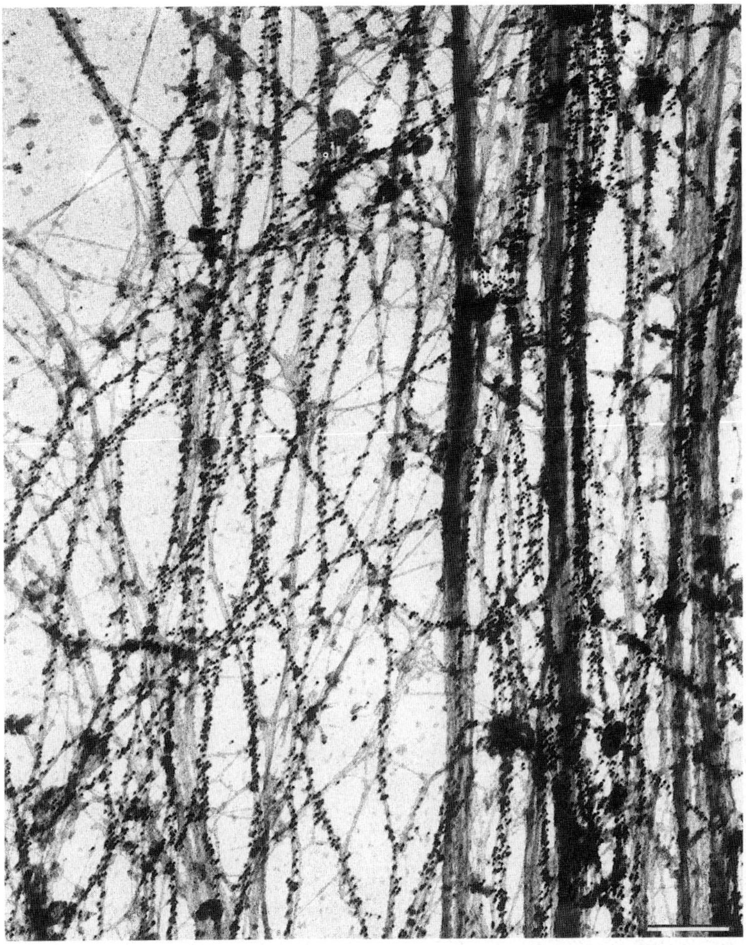

d.

Fig. 5.

optic nerve head, open-angle glaucoma actually affects two regions of the eye: the trabecular meshwork and the lamina cribrosa. We have previously shown that glucocorticoids can induce many changes in cultured human trabecular meshwork cells which are very similar to the steroid changes we see in dexamethasone-treated lamina cribrosa cells[24-25]. We would therefore like to hypothesize that the trabecular meshwork and lamina cribrosa are biochemically similar tissues and that the cells cultured from these two tissues may also be similar. We would further suggest that primary open-angle glaucoma may result from a common defect(s) in these two cell types. The idea of trabecular meshwork and lamina cribrosa similarity has been previously proposed[32-33]. We are now generating considerable evidence to support this hypothesis. Both the trabecular meshwork and lamina cribrosa form a reticulated network of extracellular matrix material of similar biochemical composition[3-5,27,31]. The biochemical and morphological characteristics of trabecular meshwork and lamina cribrosa cultured cells are also very similar. The cells produce an identical extracellular matrix consisting of collagens I, III, IV, V, and VI, fibronectin, laminin, and have a very similar proteoglycan profile. Both cultured trabecular

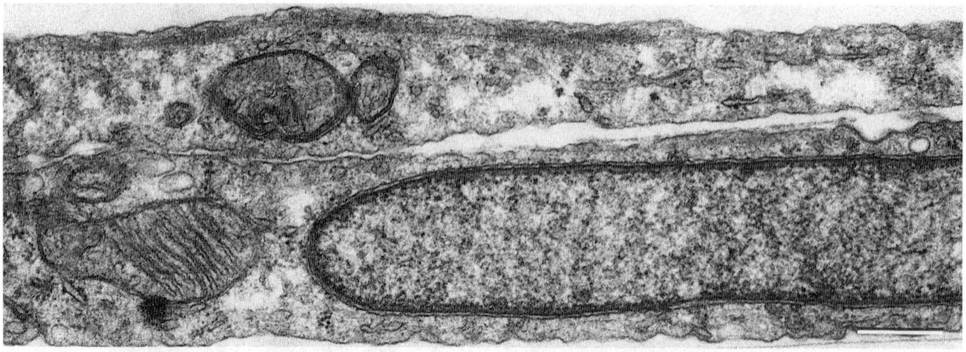

*a.*

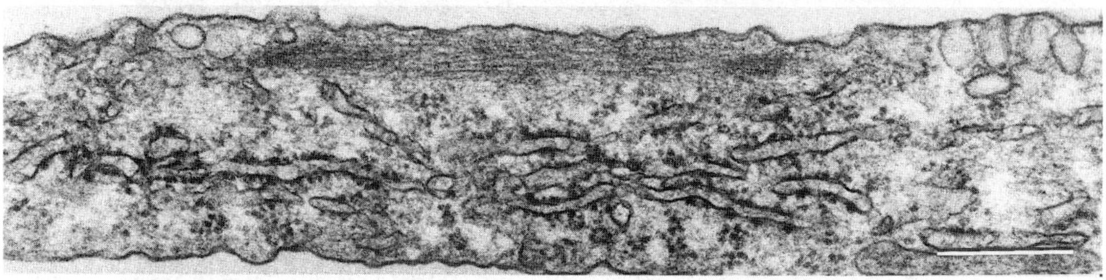

*b.*

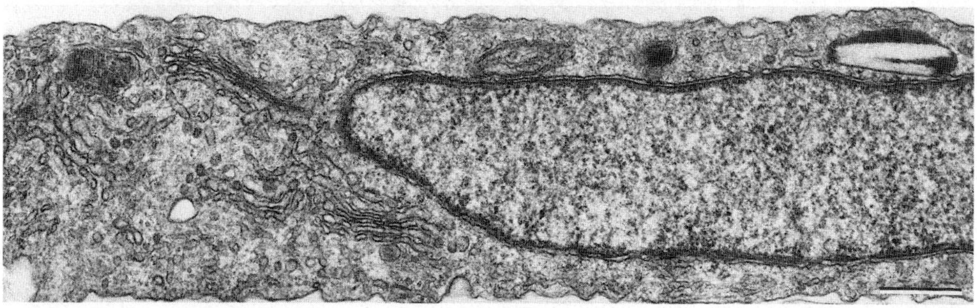

*c.*

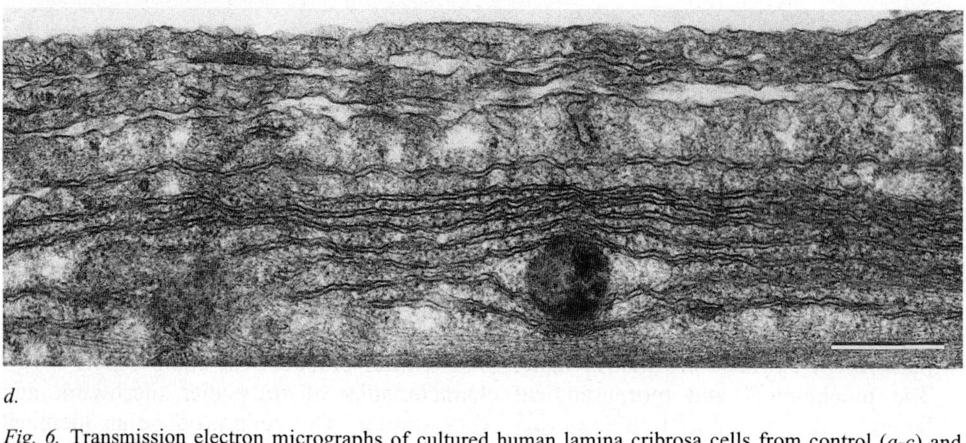

*d.*

*Fig. 6.* Transmission electron micrographs of cultured human lamina cribrosa cells from control (*a-c*) and DEX-treated (*d-f*) cultures. DEX treatment casued a proliferation of endoplasmic reticulum (*d*) and Golgi apparatus (*e*) as well as an increased deposition of extracellular matrix material between cells (*f*). Bar = 0.5 μm.

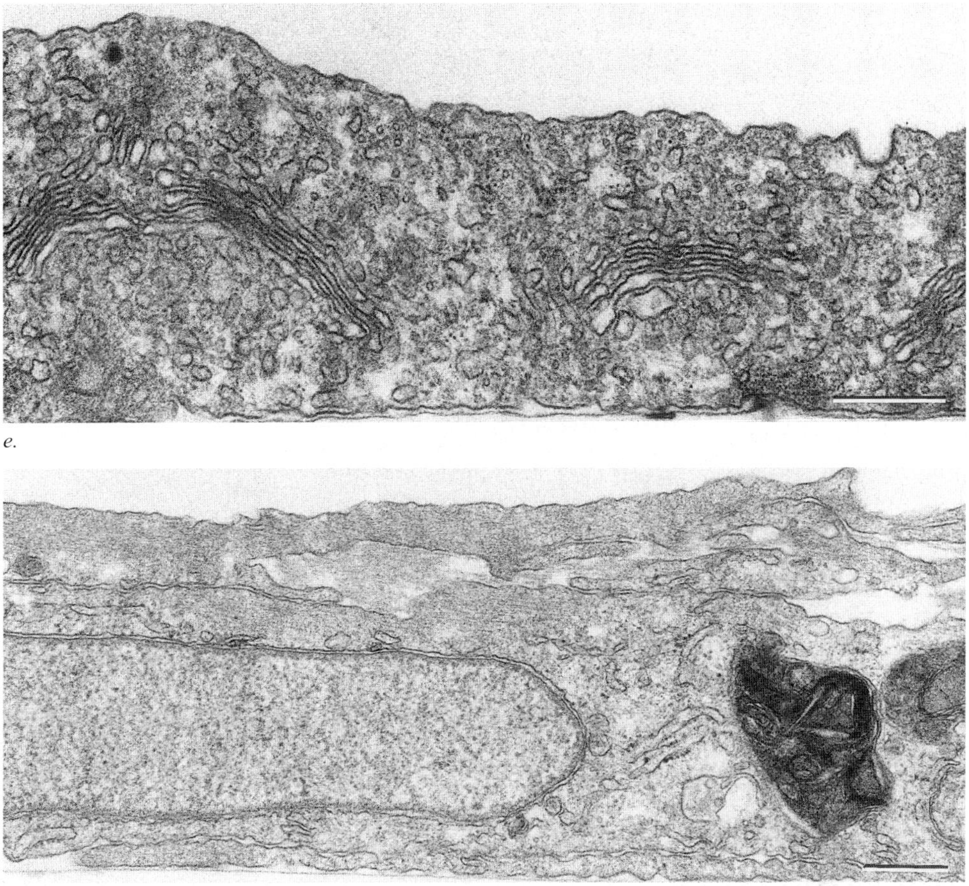

*e.*

*f.*

*Fig. 6.*

meshwork and lamina cribrosa cells undergo similar steroid-induced morphological, cytoskeletal, and extracellular matrix changes. The most convincing evidence for trabecular meshwork and lamina cribrosa similarity comes from studies comparing the patterns of protein expression between these two tissues as well as cultured cells. We have radiolabeled lamina cribrosa and trabecular meshwork proteins from dissected tissue or cultured cells by placing them in labeling media containing $^{35}S$-methionine or $^{3}H$-leucine for 24 hours. The cells/tissues were washed and the proteins were extracted in a buffer containing urea and NP40. The radiolabeled lamina cribrosa and trabecular meshwork proteins were then subjected to either one-dimensional SDS-polyacrylamide gel electrophoresis (1D-PAGE) or high resolution two-dimensional PAGE. The resulting gels were characterized by computerized image analysis of autofluorographs of the gels. Seven ocular tissues were radiolabeled and analyzed by SDS-PAGE: lens epithelium, lamina cribrosa, scleral fibroblasts, retinal pigment epithelium/choroid, trabecular meshwork, iris, and corneal endothelium (Fig. 7). SDS-PAGE separates proteins based on their size, with high molecular weight proteins at the top of the gel and lower molecular weight proteins at the bottom of the gel. There are certainly some similarities in the proteins that are ex-

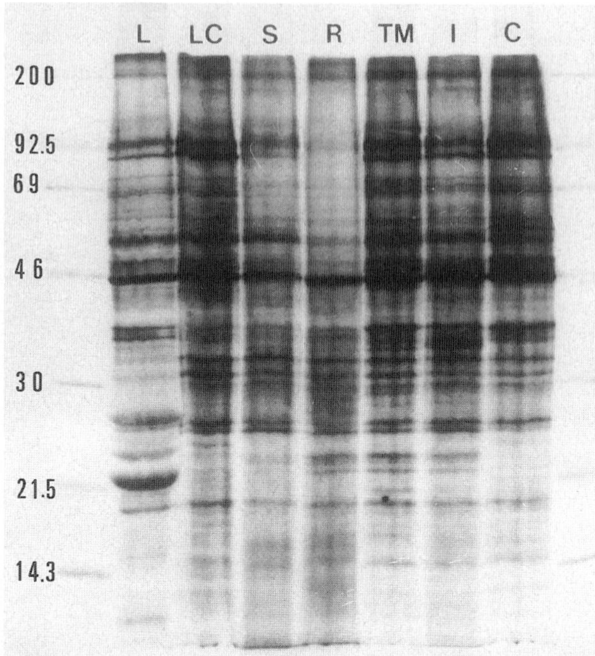


a.

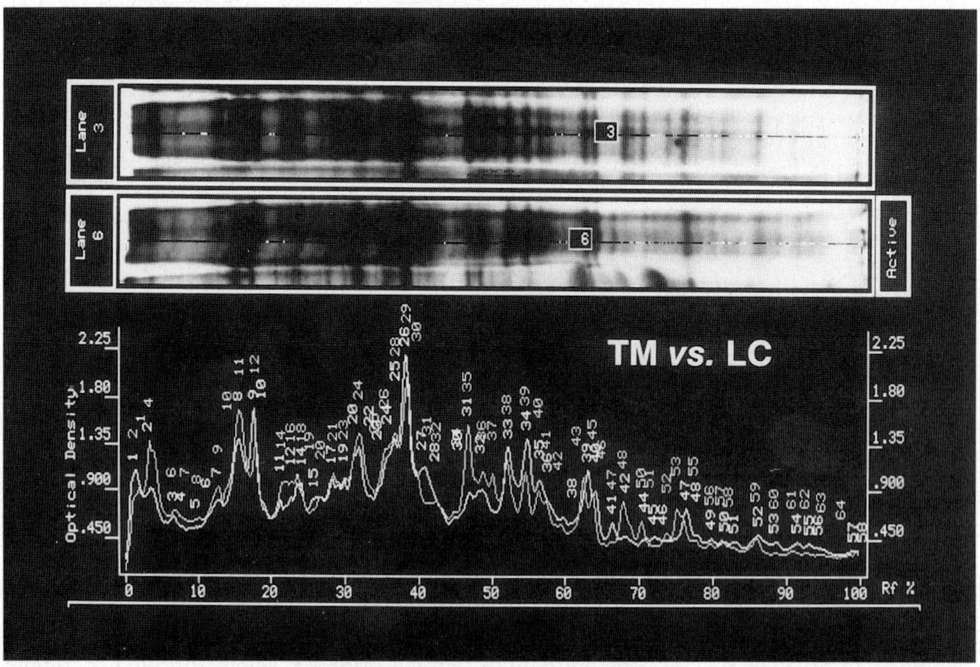


b.

*Fig. 7.* Polyacrylamide gel electrophoretic comparison of protein expression in various human ocular tissues. (*a*) Autofluorograph of radiolabeled proteins separated by SDS-PAGE from seven different ocular tissues. Lens (L), lamina cribrosa (LC), sclera (S), retinal pigment epithelium/choroid (R), trabecular meshwork (TM), iris (I), and corneal endothelium (C). Molecular weight standards (kiloDaltons $\times 10^3$) are

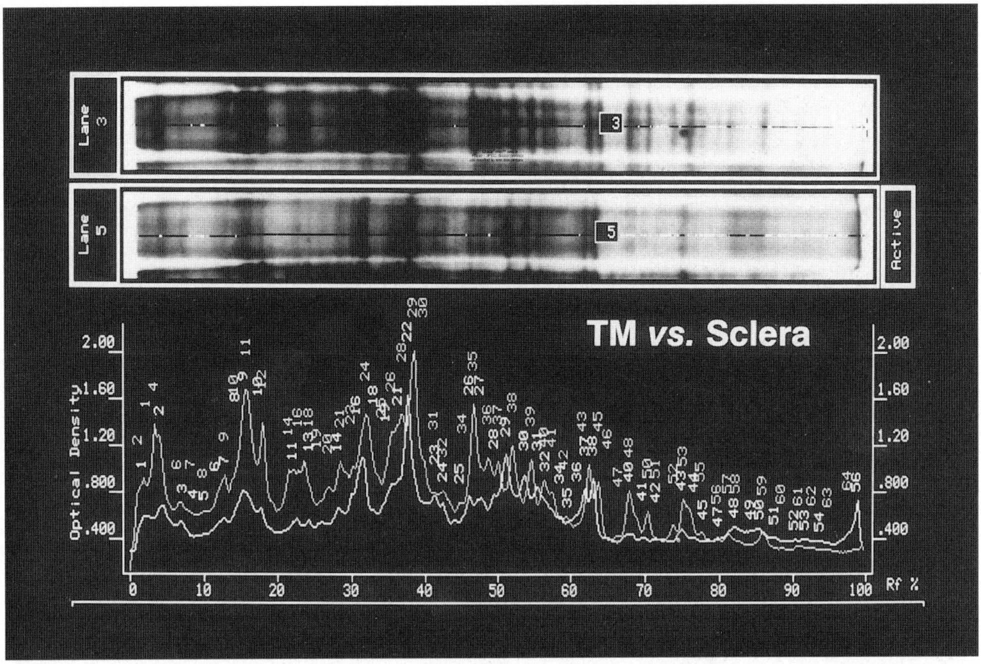


*c.*

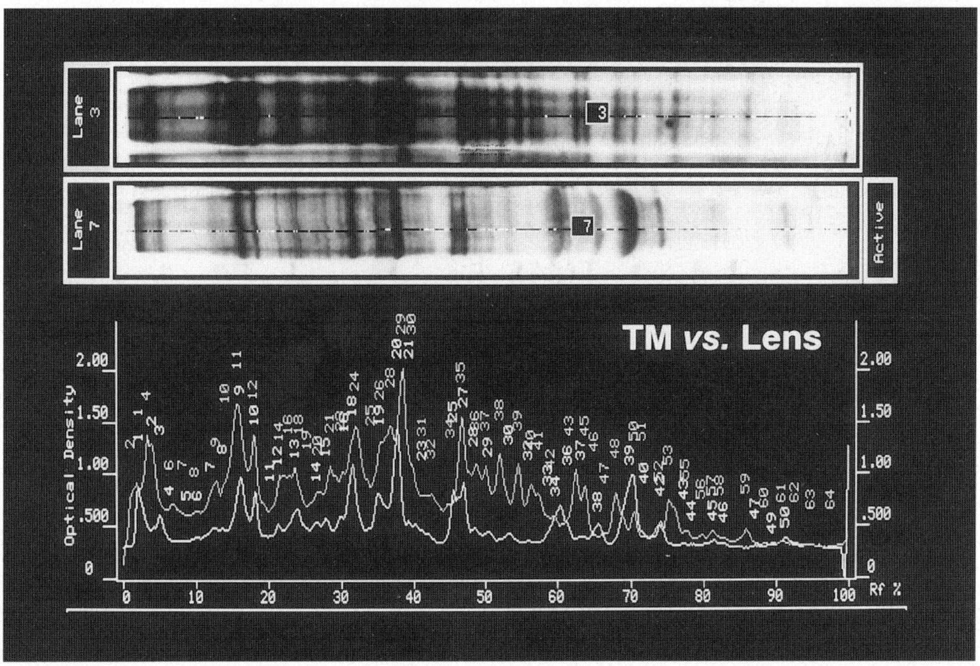


*d.*

←

shown in the left-hand lane. Computer image analysis comparing protein expression between: (*b*) TM and LC, (*c*) TM and sclera, and (*d*) TM and lens. Protein expression was most similar between the TM and the LC.

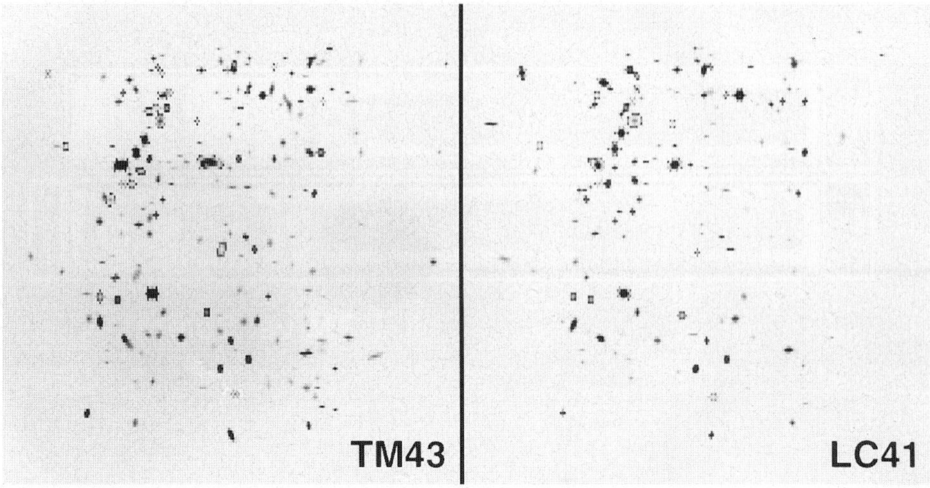


*a.*

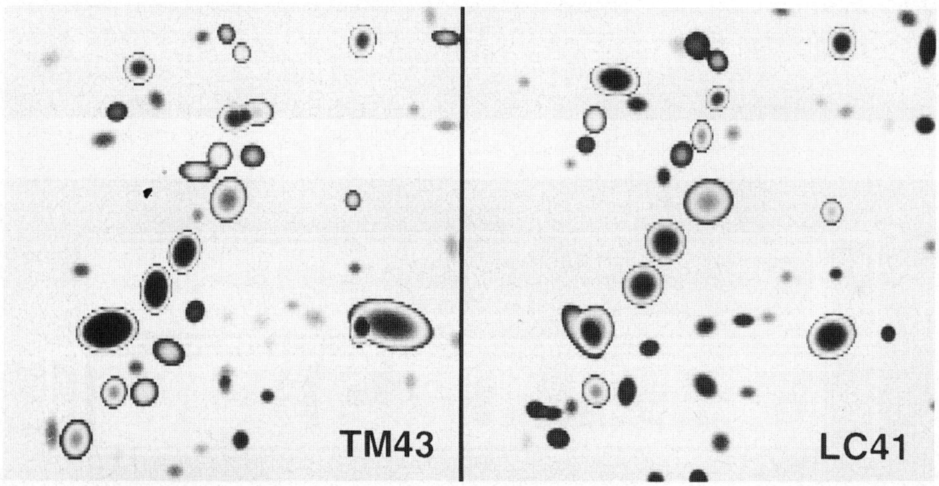


*b.*

*Fig. 8.* Two-dimensional polyacrylamide gel electrophoretic comparison of protein expression in cultured human lamina cribrosa and trabecular meshwork cells. Radiolabeled proteins were separated using high resolution 2D-PAGE and autofluorographs were analyzed by computer. The overall protein expression in the TM and LC was remarkably similar when analyzing the entire gel (*a*) or a randomly seleted region of the gel (*b*).

pressed in all seven of these ocular tissues. For example, some proteins such as actin are clearly expressed by all of these tissues. These are considered "housekeeping" proteins and are expressed in all cells to the body. However, it is also apparent that there are proteins which are differentially expressed in each tissue. For example, the major proteins expressed in the lens, the crystallins, are relatively unique for the lens and not evident in the other tissues. Computerized image analysis of protein expression allows a very careful comparison between each of these tissues. A comparison of the profiles of trabecular meshwork radiolabeled proteins versus lamina cribrosa radiolabeled proteins shows that the overall profile of protein expression is very similar between these two tissues although several minor differences in expression can be noted (Fig. 7b). In contrast to the similarity between the trabecular meshwork and lamina cribrosa, a comparison of the trabecular meshwork tissue to the adjacent scleral tissue shows many major differences in protein expression (Fig. 7c). Likewise, a comparison of trabecular meshwork versus lens epithelium shows many major differences in the protein profiles (Fig. 7d).

One-dimensional SDS-PAGE analysis provides an overall estimation of protein expression. A technique with higher resolution is two-dimensional polyacrylamide gel electrophoresis (2D-PAGE), in which proteins are separated in the first dimension based on their charge by isoelectric focusing, and in the second dimension based on their size using SDS-PAGE. The autofluorographs of radiolabeled proteins were analyzed by computer imaging. Using this technique we have analyzed the protein expression in seven different ocular cells[34]. The greatest similarity in protein expression is between trabecular meshwork and lamina cribrosa. A comparison of proteins expressed in cultured trabecular meshwork cells and lamina cribrosa cells, both derived from an individual donor, is shown in Figure 8. Overall, the spot patterns between these two cell lines is extraordinarily similar (Fig. 8a) even when we examine specific regions of the gel with high resolution (Fig. 8b). It should be noted that there appear to be a few differences where minor proteins are expressed in the lamina cribrosa that are not expressed in the trabecular meshwork, and vice versa. Sorting out specific differences in protein expression in the various tissues such as the trabecular meshwork, lamina cribrosa, as well as the other tissues of the eye is going to be a long, detailed process. But out of all the tissues that have been examined to date, the trabecular meshwork and lamina cribrosa are the most similar in their protein expression.

In summary, we have used the *in vitro* culture of lamina cribrosa cells to examine the cell biology and biochemistry of the human lamina cribrosa. The cultured cells are synthetically capable of making the extracellular matrix that is characteristic of lamina cribrosa tissue. Glucocorticoids cause a cytoskeletal reorganization of the cultured lamina cribrosa cells which involves both the microfilaments and microtubules and appears to alter extracellular matrix synthesis. In addition, we have suggested that the lamina cribrosa and trabecular meshwork may be biochemically similar which may have important implications in our understanding of the pathogenesis of glaucoma. There are a number of additional studies for which cultured human lamina cribrosa cells will be useful. For example, we have been able to culture lamina cribrosa cells from glaucomatous donors and will be comparing how these cells differ from age-matched control lamina cribrosa cells. In addition, there may be important differences in the type of extracellular matrix or function of the lamina cribrosa cells that are cultured from donors of various ages. We now have 20 lamina cribrosa cell lines from donors of different ages and are in the process of trying to look at potential differences. We are also examining the effects of hydrostatic pressure and "stretchability" of the lamina cribrosa cells, looking at changes in protein and gene expression as well as cellular morphology. Another important area of research will be to examine the effects of other hormones and growth factors on lamina cribrosa cells. Ultimately, it may be possible to set up a lamina cribrosa organ culture model analogous to what has been done with the trabecular meshwork[35].

I would like to acknowledge my collaborators in this study as well as Lynne

Chapman for providing the pictures of the retinal vascular pericytes and vascular endothelial cells. I would like to thank the various regional eye banks who have provided us with the tissue essential for these studies, and Drs Lou DeSantis, Prem Mahendroo, and Bill York, who have supported and encouraged this work.

**Discussion of presentation**

**Dr. Kaufman**: You mentioned that the trabecular meshwork and the lamina cribrosa were the only two tissues that you had looked at or that you knew about that corticosteroids reorganized the cytoskeleton. I was going to ask, are you talking about in the eye, or are you talking about anywhere?

**Dr. Clark**: We have looked at a variety of different cultured cells, both from the eye and from non-eye sources. For example, we have looked at the ciliary epithelium, ciliary smooth muscle cells, retinal pigment epithelium, corneal stromal fibroblasts, corneal endothelial cells, and lens epithelial cells. In addition, we have looked at vascular endothelial cells, and have not seen the steroid-induced cytoskeletal changes in any of those cultured cell types, other than the trabecular meshwork and lamina cribrosa. I am not suggesting, by the way, that the glucocorticoids necessarily play a role in the glaucomatous pathogenic process at the optic nerve head. I think that it is an intriguing possibility, but we are currently just using glucocorticoids as a tool to try to understand how the lamina cribrosa cytoskeleton and extracellular matrix may communicate with each other.

**Dr. Kaufman**: But that seems a little strange? I mean, this should be such a fundamental biological phenomenon of corticosteroids. If they induced cytoskeletal changes in these tissues, they should also do it, or something like it, elsewhere.

**Dr. Clark**: I do not believe this unique effect of glucocorticoids on the trabecular meshwork and lamina cribrosa is at all strange. There are glucocorticoid receptors in all tissues in all cell types, and yet you get tissue-specific responses to the glucocorticoids. One tissue may regulate a whole different set of genes than another tissue when exposed to the same glucocorticoid. And I think that is what we are seeing here, that the trabecular meshwork and lamina cribrosa share very similar glucocorticoid response elements while other ocular cells have a different spectrum of glucocorticoid response elements accessible to the activated glucocorticoid receptor.

**Dr. Ransom**: Abe, I was interested in the cell identification slide that you showed us. It is becoming clear that it is not as easy to identify an astrocyte as we had once hoped that it would be. Glial filament acidic protein, for example, can occasionally stain oligodendrocytes in fish optic nerve during an early stage of development. I wonder if you had tried anything else, like YAL-C, on the slight chance that these astrocytes might be expressing oligodendrocytic markers.

**Dr. Clark**: We have not tested that. I think that needs to be done to better characterize what we have cultured from the lamina cribrosa and are calling lamina cribrosa cells.

**Dr. Ransom**: I would like to return to the question of glucocorticoid effects on different cell types. Since astrocytes have been emphasized this morning to bear important relationships to both the axons as well as to the lamina cribrosa itself, it has been pointed out in the past and demonstrated in experimental studies that glucocorticoids can have profound effects on astrocytes. Have you looked at astrocytes?

**Dr. Clark**: I think that that is a great question. Unfortunately, we do not have a lot of astrocyte cell cultures derived from our lamina cribrosa studies. Most of the cells that we have been able to grow out of lamina cribrosa have been what we have just described and call lamina cribrosa cells. I think that we should definitely look at the intimate relationship between these cells and the astrocytes, and how they may differentially respond to a variety of different factors, glucocorticoids being just one of them.

**Dr. Drance**: Dr. Ransom's suggestion of the astrocytes was not from the optic nerve, they were from elsewhere, were they not?

**Dr. Ransom**: Yes, that is true.

**Dr. Drance**: I was not belittling the observation, but I think you were referring to central nervous system astrocytes, were not you?

**Dr. Ransom**: That is correct, but I certainly would claim that these are also central nervous system astrocytes. But your cautionary note is well taken.

**Dr. Drance**: No, I was not injecting a cautionary note. On the contrary, what I was trying to say is that the comparisons that have been referred to have primarily been in ocular tissues, and I think Dr. Kaufman meant that there must be probably other systems in the body, including the one that you have already mentioned, that would probably have very similar responses. It would be most unusual that the eye would just be favored with this destructive process, or maybe constructive process.

**Dr. Clark**: This is a good point, as we do not yet know whether the glucocorticoid effects on the lamina cribrosa are constructive or destructive.

**Dr. Quigley**: Do you know the primarily level of steroid at which you saw this effect? Is it something that the cells would ever see physiologically?

**Dr. Clark**: The effects of glucocorticoid on the trabecular meshwork appear to be a physiological response. We have actually shown these cytoskeletal changes with physiological levels of cortisol. The response takes longer than using the higher pharmacological doses of a synthetic glucocorticoid such as dexamethasone. We have not yet evaluated the effects of cortisol on the lamina cribrosa cells, and we agree that this is essential to do.

**Dr. Anderson**: There seems to me there is a replication of what you have presented here and that is that cells that move from place to place and find themselves in different environments may find themselves expressing different things. For instance, the same cell placed in the trabecular meshwork beam might do something, while if you put the same cell in the cornea it might do something else. If you put it in a tissue culture it does yet something else. One of the problems with studying things in culture, is that they express things that they might not have in their native position. But the fact that you showed this corticosteroid response as being unique to this cell type indicates that it is not because of its environment, but something that happened during development and differentiation, to make it into a different cell type from that which is found in sclera and so on. And that is very puzzling to me, because I would have thought some of the features that you showed that relate trabecular meshwork to lamina cribrosa relate to the fact that they found themselves in an environment where they were forming holes through which fluid in one case and axons in another case went, and so that they simply had these features because they were in a similar kind of morphologic situation. But the fact that they preserve those features when they go to cell culture indicates that it is a differentiation, rather than a different expression in a new location. And I am puzzled by it and trying to figure out what that means in terms of the pathogenic process that we are trying to understand.

**Dr. Clark**: It could well be that the reason that the cells are in the environment they find themselves in is because they are responsible for making that environment. You can actually experimentally test that by taking the cultured cells and placing them in a different environment. For example, you can change the extracellular matrix on which they sit and see if you get a similar effect. We have not yet done that. But I believe that the cells are genetically programmed during differentiation and are to certain extent responsible for making their own environment.

**Dr. Anderson**: That is an interesting comment. I had not thought about that, but that would mean, then, that in culture, if they are responsible for making their environment, that they might then be made to do something different. So that in the right circumstance they would have arranged themselves so that they make holes, whereas scleral fibroblasts would arrange themselves to do something different because that is innately part of what they have been differentiated to do.

**Dr. Clark**: And in fact scleral fibroblasts in culture will grow in multiple layers, whereas the lamina cribrosa cells grow in monolayers even though both of these cell types are cultured under identical conditions.

**Dr. Quigley**: Embryologically these cells do not make holes in the area of the lamina cribrosa. The axons are there before these cells, as far as we know, ever get there. And certainly there is no sign of an extracellular matrix, lamina cribrosa at the time embryologically when the axons are already through and out into the brain. The nerve bundles presumably form early and later afterwards the extracellular matrix gets laid down and gets as big as we see it here. Can I ask, in the trabecular meshwork, are you talking about cells that we call the trabecular endothelial cells?

**Dr. Clark**: I do not call them trabecular endothelial cells because they do not have all the usual characteristics of endothelial cells. But, yes, others have called them this.

**Dr. Quigley**: Are these the cells that are on the outside of the beams of the trabecular meshwork?

**Dr. Clark**: I personally think that there are at least three different cell types in the trabecular meshwork, and, in fact, some of the trabecular meshwork cell cultures appear to have several cell types in them. And not all cells will respond identically to a variety of things such as glucocorticoids. We usually see only a subpopulation of those cells respond.

**Dr. Quigley**: Well granted that they are both apparently cell types that make collagen in culture, but in the lamina cribrosa, the cells that we showed pictures of here, are inside the beam, are actually living in the beam, they are completely surrounded by connective tissue. The cells in the trabecular meshwork... ?

**Dr. Clark**: Are just the opposite.

**Dr. Quigley**: The cells in the trabecular meshwork that line the beam have an extracellular glycocalyx on one side and the extracellular matrix on the other side; they are polar. So I would be very surprised if these cells wind up behaving in similar fashions if only because of that quite striking difference in their polarity; but maybe they do.

**Dr. Drance**: I just wonder if I could ask another question for the clinicians around the table. If corticosteroids were to have some detrimental effect, for instance, on the optic nerve, then it should be our impression that people who are on high doses of systemic steroids, for instance, for asthma therapy, one should be able to show epidemiologically that in fact these people have glaucoma more frequently or more severely. I do not think that that has been suggested.

**Dr. Clark**: If you look at the ability of glucocorticoids to cause glaucoma, usually topical ocular administration has been shown to give the highest....

**Dr. Drance**: That is pressure.

**Dr. Clark**: That is pressure as well as visual field defects. I think, because topical ocular glucocorticoid administration gets higher concentrations to the meshwork than does systemic administration, you may see ocular hypertension expressed earlier by topical administration than you would during systemic administration. I do not know whether systemic glucocorticoid administration causes changes in the lamina cribrosa and whether these changes would be good or bad. The fact that you see steroid-induced changes to both cytoskeletal and extracellular matrix may be bad in the trabecular meshwork but may be good in the lamina cribrosa. We just do not yet know.

**Dr. Kapin**: Could I follow up on Dr. Quigley's question, as well as Dr. Drance's question? Do you envision endogenous glucocorticoids induced by stress being enough to produce such changes?

**Dr. Clark**: Interestingly, there have been several suggestions over the course of 40 or 50 years that stress may be associated with an increased incidence of glaucoma[36-38]. I am not sure exactly how to put those studies in perspective, perhaps some of the clinicians in the audience can. There have also been three independent studies that suggest that, on an average, patients with primary open-angle glaucoma have a slightly higher level of cortisol in their plasma[39-41]. So there is suggestive evidence out there, but I do not think it is as yet definitive evidence.

**Dr. Anderson**: We talk about these differences in the cortisol level, but we now have to make sure we make a distinction between cortisol causing pressure elevation and cortisol causing something to happen in the optic nerve and alter its susceptibility to damage. We should not lump them together as cortisol causing glaucoma, because those are two separate elements, and if they both occur, we would like to know them separately, not lumped.

**Dr. Epstein**: Two questions. One, do you know anything about the embryological origin of the lamina cribrosa, in that I think most people think trabecular cells are of neural crest origin. And the second question, because it is interesting is this question of cells versus extracellular matrix. There are a number of new markers and cell associated antigens, some of which have just been described by John Morrison. I would think that these would be very interesting to look at. Are there a normal number of cells of these different types in the lamina cribrosa of glaucomatous eyes? I guess the old answer was that there is certainly a normal number of glial cells, but I do not know if we know about these other types of cells. Could these have been missed in the earlier qualitative analyses? How confident are we that there are normal cell numbers in the lamina cribrosa in glaucoma?

**Dr. Clark**: I do not think that the embryological origin of the lamina cribrosa is known. Much of the work that has been done tracing embryological origin of tissues has been done in animals like the mouse or the chicken which unfortunately do not have what we would classically call a lamina cribrosa. So, I do not think people know what the embryological origin of the lamina cribrosa is. Does anyone else in the group know? Now to answer your second question. Since the lamina cribrosa is anatomically a very complex tissue, I think it would be very difficult to do quantitative cell number experiments. The experiments that have been done in the trabecular meshwork were studies involving painstakingly serial sections to actually count cell number per trabecular meshwork beam area. I think that the anatomy of the trabecular meshwork is probably a lot simpler than the anatomy of the optic nerve head. So I do not think the studies that you suggest have been done in conclusive manner.

**Dr. Quigley**: Talk about counting things, I guess everybody points at me, David, since I've spent my career counting little things. I would love to know how many of these resident lamina cribrosa cells there are inside the extracellular matrix of the average optic nerve head. I would guess there is fewer than a thousand. Now, that might be very important, those thousand cells, but it depends on what the turnover in the matrix is. Let us imagine this matrix is a pretty boring, quiet, low turnover kind of a tissue, and once that stuff gets made it just sits there and thumps with the normal pulsations of the eye, and normally nothing much happens. In that case how many cells you have might be trivial. I mean, ten of them might be enough to keep it all going, compared to the hundred that were there before. I am not even sure how to design an experiment to count the number of lamina cribrosacytes. John Morrison might have some ideas. I guess you could attempt to count those cells, but you would have to be sure you were not counting a pericyte, a vascular cell, an astrocyte ... Very tricky to do. I think the issue of the dynamic nature of this extracellular matrix, though, is at least as important as the cells, and in part because Dr. Clark's work is looking at how you can count that, is good. Reed, you have something to add, I hope.

**Dr. Pyeritz**: I would like to emphasize the burgeoning utility of transgenic animal models whereby one could take a mouse, for example, and knock out any particular gene that you thought might be important in the lamina cribrosa, and then breed the animals to homozygosity and look to see what is happening anatomically and, one would hope, be able to analyze this physiologically as well.

**Dr. Clark**: I think that is a terrific idea. The problem is we do not know what is uniquely expressed in the lamina cribrosa. And hopefully, with the approach of culturing lamina cribrosa cells, we can try to identify what is uniquely expressed in the lamina cribrosa versus the astroglial cells versus the scleral fibroblasts, and then do those exact studies that you are referring to.

**Dr. Pyeritz**: But I would be, not only open minded, inventive, in what you choose to examine. For example, who could have thought that individuals who are heterozygous for a deficiency of elastin, would have the Williams' syndrome?

**Dr. Quigley**: Which is what?

**Dr. Pyeritz**: The Williams' syndrome is a disorder of abnormal facies and mental retardation and supravalvular aortic stenosis and perinatal hypercalcemia.

**Dr. Quigley**: I certainly would not have thought of that.

**Dr. Pyeritz**: There you go. And yet, here is a human model of elastin deficiency, and I bet dollars to donuts that no one has ever looked at the lamina cribrosa in somebody with Williams' syndrome.

**Dr. Quigley**: The strength of the mouse is absolutely spectacular for various kinds of issues, until you find out that the mouse has absolutely no extracellular matrix to speak of in his optic nerve head. Now, John Morrison pointed out some subtle structures in the lamina cribrosa of the rat that you can call extracellular matrix, but the mouse is even tinier. We have been very excited about studying ganglion cell behavior in mouse, in transgenic models, and I think we may find that is more useful to us. The mouse sclera is so thin that you can see through it. And as John Morrison may find when he raises the pressure chronically in a rat, do they not get big eyes? As opposed to a monkey, where the effect on the eye is not to make the eye get dramatically larger, in the rodent it does. So we will have some minor troubles there, but point well taken about transgenic mice.

## References

1. Hernandez MR, Igoe F, Neufeld AH. Cell culture of the human lamina cribrosa. *Invest Ophthalmol Vis Sci.* 1988; 29:78-89.
2. Nayak RC, Berman AB, George KL, Eisenbarth GS, King GL. A monoclonal antibody (3G5)-defined ganglioside antigen is expressed on the surface of microvascular pericytes. *J Exp Med.* 1988; 167: 1003-1015.

3. Hernandez MR, Luo XX, Igoe F, Neufeld AH. Extracellular matrix of the human lamina cribrosa. *Am J Ophthalmol.* 1987; 104: 567-576.
4. Morrison JC, L'Hernault NL, Jerdan JA, Quigley HA. Ultrastructural location of extracellular matrix components in the optic nerve head. *Arch Ophthalmol.* 1989; 107:123-129.
5. Goldbaum MH, Jeng S, Logemann R, Weinreb RN. The extracellular matrix of the human optic nerve. *Arch Ophthalmol.* 1989; 107:1225-1231.
6. Shields MB. *Textbook of Glaucoma*, 3rd Edition. Williams & Wilkins: Baltimore. 1992; pp. 172-197.
7. Hernandez MR, Luo XX, Andrzewska W, Neufeld AH. Age-related changes in the extracellular matrix of the human optic nerve head. *Am J Ophthalmol.* 1989; 107:476-484.
8. Shin DH, Becker B, Kolker AE. Family history in primary open angle glaucoma. *Arch Ophthalmol.* 1977; 95:598-600.
9. Leske MC. The epidemiology of open-angle glaucoma: a review. *Am J Epidemiol.* 1983; 118:166-191.
10. Davies TG. Tonographic survey of the close relatives of patients with chronic simple glaucoma. *Brit J Ophthalmol.* 1968; 52:32-39.
11. Tielsch JM, Sommer A, Katz J, Royall RM, Quigley HA, Javitt J. Racial variations in the prevalence of primary open-angle glaucoma. *JAMA.* 1991; 266:369-374.
12. Andrzejewska W, Hernandez MR, Neufeld AH. Racial differences in the extracellular matrix of the lamina cribrosa. ARVO Abstract. *Invest Ophthalmol Vis Sci.* 1989; 30:428
13. Chi T, Ritch R, Stickler D, Pitman B, Tsai C, Hseih FY. Racial differences in optic nerve head parameters. *Arch Ophthalmol.* 1989; 107:836-839.
14. Pohjanpelto PEJ, Plava J. Ocular hypertension and glaucomatous optic nerve damage. Acta Ophthalmol. 1974; 52:194-200.
15. Sommer A, Tielsch JM, Katz J, *et al.* Relationship between intraocular pressure and primary open angle glaucoma among white and black Americans. *Arch Ophthalmol.* 1991; 109:1090-1095.
16. Gaasterland D, Tanishima T, Kuwabara T. Axoplasmic flow during chronic experimental glaucoma. I. Light and electron microscopic studies of the monkey optic nervehead during the development of glaucomatous cupping. *Invest Ophthalmol Vis Sci.* 1978; 17: 838-846.
17. Quigley HA, Addicks EM. Chronic experimental glaucoma in primates. II. Effect of extended intraocular pressure elevation on optic nerve head and axonal transport. *Invest Ophthalmol Vis Sci.* 1980; 19:137-152.
18. Morrison JC, Dorman-Pease ME, Dunkelberger GR, Quigley HA. Optic nerve head extracellular matrix in primary optic atrophy and experimental glaucoma. *Arch Ophthalmol.* 1990; 108:1020-1024.
19. Fukuchi T, Sawaguchi S, Hara H, Shirakashi M, Iwata K. Extracellular matrix changes in the optic nerve lamina cribrosa in monkey eyes with experimentally chronic glaucoma. *Graefe's Arch Ophthalmol.* 1992; 230:421-427.
20. Quigley HA, Brown A, Dorman-Pease ME. Alterations in elastin of the optic nerve head on human and experimental glaucoma. *Brit. J Ophthalmol.* 1991; 75:552-557.
21. Yang JL, Neufeld AH, Zorn MB, Hernandez MR. Collagen type I mRNA levels in cultured human lamina cribrosa cells: effects of elevated hydrostatic pressure. *Exp Eye Res.* 1993; 56:567-574.
22. Hernandez MR, Andrzejewska WM, Neufeld AH. Changes in the extracellular matrix of the human optic nerve head in primary open glaucoma. *Am J Ophthalmol.* 1990; 109:180-188.
23. Kass MA, Johnson T. Corticosteroid-induced glaucoma. In: Ritch R, Shields MB, Krupin T, eds. *The Glaucomas*. St. Louis: CV Mosby. 1989; pp. 1161-1168.
24. Wilson K, McCartney MD, Miggans ST, Clark AF. Dexamethasone induced ultrastructural changes in cultured human trabecular meshwork cells. *Current Eye Res.* 1993; 12:783-793.
25. Clark AF, Wilson K, McCartney MD, Miggans ST, Kunkle M, Howe W. Glucocorticoid-induced formation of cross-linked actin networks in cultured human trabecular meshwork cells. *Invest Ophthalmol Vis Sci.* 1994; 35:281-294
26. Steely HT, Browder SL, Julian MB, Miggans ST, Wilson KL, Clark AF. The effects of dexamethasone on fibronectin expression in cultured human trabecular meshwork cells. *Invest Ophthalmol Vis Sci.* 1992; 33:2242-2250.
27. Yun AJ, Murphy CG, Polansky JR, Newsome DA, Alvarado JA. Proteins secreted by human trabecular meshwork cells: glucocorticoid and other effects. *Invest Ophthalmol Vis Sci.* 1989; 30:2012-2022.
28. Tripathi BJ, Tripathi RC, Swift HH. Hydrocortisone-induced DNA endoreplication in human trabecular meshwork cells in vitro. *Exp Eye Res.* 1989; 49:259-270.
29. Polansky JR, Kurtz RM, Fauss DJ, Kim RY, Bloom E. In vitro correlates of glucocorticoid effects on intraocular pressure. In: Kriegelstein GK, ed. *Glaucoma Update IV.* Berlin: Springer-Verlag. 1991; pp. 20-29.
30. Samples JR, Alexander JP, Acott TS. Regulation of the levels of human trabecular meshwork matrix metalloproteinases and inhibitor by interleukin-1 and dexamethasone. *Invest Ophthalmol Vis Sci.* 1993; 34:3386-3395.
31. Hernandez MR, Weinstein BI, Schwartz J, Ritch R, Gordon GG, Southren AL. Human trabecular

meshwork cells in culture: morphology and extracellular matrix components. *Invest Ophthalmol Vis Sci.* 1987; 28:1655-1660.

32. Rehnberg M, Ammitzboll, Tengroth B. Collagen distribution in the lamina cribrosa and the trabecular meshwork of the human eye. *Brit J Ophthalmol.* 1987; 71: 886-892.
33. Tengroth B, Ammitzboll T. Changes in the content and composition of collagen in the glaucomatous eye – basis for a new hypothesis for the genesis of chronic open angle glaucoma. *Acta Ophthalmol.* 1984; 62:999-1008.
34. Steely HT, Wilson K, Clark A, Knepper PA. Biochemical similarities of human trabecular meshwork and lamina cribrosa. ARVO Abstract. *Invest Ophthalmol Vis Sci.* 1990; 31:2233
35. Johnson DH, Tschumper RC. Human trabecular meshwork organ culture. *Invest Ophthalmol Vis Sci.* 1987; 28:945-953.
36. Van Alphen GW, Stokvis B. Psychosomatic aspects of intraocular pressure. *Nederl Tijdschr Geneesk.* 1951; 95:2246-2256.
37. Weinstein P. Nervism in ophthalmology. *Ophthalmologica* 1954; 127:164-178.
38. Tassman IS. The role of stress in ocular disease. *Trans Am Acad Ophthalmol Otolaryngol.* 1957; 61:179-193
39. Ray S, Mehra KS, Misra S, Singh R. Plasma cortisol in glaucoma. *Ann Ophthalmol.* 1977; 9:1151-1154.
40. Rozsival P, Hampl R, Obenberger J, Starka L, Rehak S. Aqueous humor and plasma cortisol levels in glaucoma and cataract patients. *Current Eye Res.* 1981; 1:391-396.
41. Schwartz B, McCarty G, Rosner B. Increased plasma free cortisol in ocular hypertension and open angle glaucoma. *Arch Ophthalmol.* 1987; 105:1060-1065.

# 6. BIOMECHANICAL PROPERTIES OF THE OPTIC NERVE HEAD

RAN ZEIMER, Ph.D.

**Dr. Quigley**: Our next speaker is Ran Zeimer, who was at the University of Illinois, Chicago, and is now at Johns Hopkins University. Ran is going to try to synthesize for us, at least his charge was to try to synthesize for us, a lot of the fibrils and strands we saw this morning into behavior of the tissue. And he is a biomedical engineer.

**Dr. Zeimer**: I would like to use an approach based on my training as a physicist and propose a model for susceptibility to glaucoma damage. I will base myself on the little amount of facts available to us on the biomechanical properties of the optic nerve head and mostly on theoretical considerations. A model is a simple-minded way to organize thoughts and facts into one framework which can then be used to direct scientific inquiries. I hope that you will examine it critically.

But before I present my model I would like to comply with Harry's request and give a quick overview of viscoelasticity.

The relationship between the strain (the elongation) and the stress (the tension) can be complex in biological tissues. I will touch only on a few basic phenomena such as relaxation, creep, and preconditioning, all of which have been observed in connective tissues such as the skin.

The first noticeable property of viscoelastic tissues is the non-linear nature of the stress (tension) –strain (elongation) relationship. As shown in Figure 1 viscoelastic tissues respond with a decreasing amount of elongation as the tension increases. This is in contrast to elastic material that have a linear relation.

The next property exhibited by viscoelastic tissues is 'creep', illustrated in Figure 2. A tissue exposed to a constant force continues to elongate over time. Conversely, as shown in Figure 3, if one subjects a tissue to a constant elongation, the tissue rearranges itself leading to a reduction in stress. This phenomenon, which is also time dependent, is termed relaxation.

Finally, a tissue subjected to a first cycle of stress increase and decrease does not revert to its original elongation. As shown in Figure 4, after a few cycles, the tissue settles in a repetitive pattern different from the original one. This change in behavior induced by initial cycles is termed conditioning. This phenomenon must be kept in mind when performing measurements since the first few will not represent the behavior of the subsequent ones. In other words, the tissue exhibits memory and behaves differently if it was previously stretched. This phenomenon is observed in athletes and dancers, such as the one shown by Dr. Pyeritz, who can exhibit remarkable and reversible flexibility after having conditioned their connective tissues.

**Dr. Drance**: I would like to ask a question. When you say that there is this conditioning and you are referring to the phenomenon of the young lady who showed remarkable flexibility, is there a variation, or is there a physical law, which applies to the tissues. Is there a variation, is this biological phenomenon?

**Dr. Zeimer**: This a very good question which I was going to address next. The

*Optic Nerve in Glaucoma, pp. 107–121*
*edited by S.M. Drance*

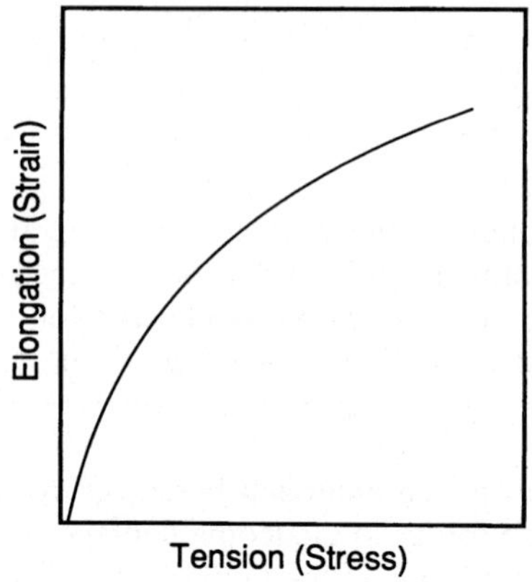


*Fig. 1.*

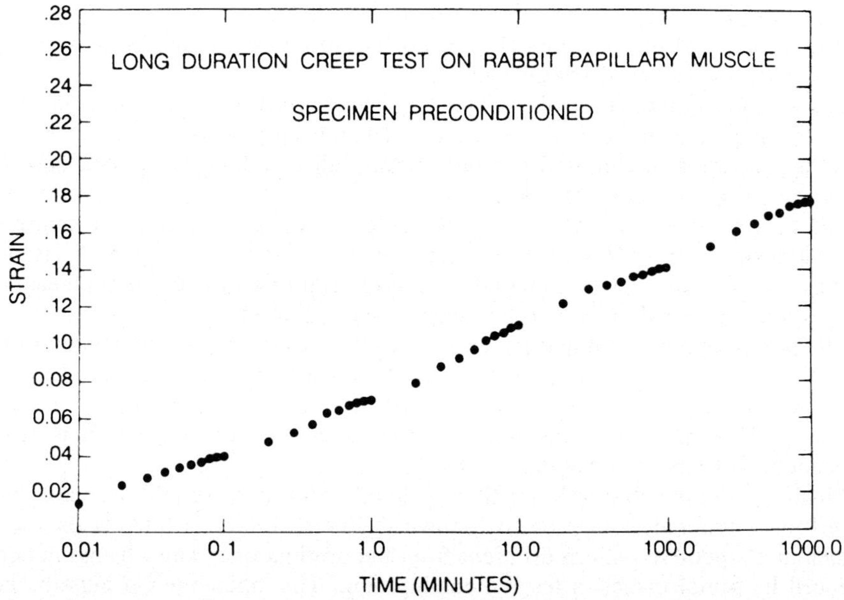


*Fig. 2.*

strength of connective tissues is basically due to collagen and elastin fibers. Tissues behave differently according to the composition and arrangement of these fibers. Elastin behaves like an elastic material. It elongates reversibly within the physiological range and shows little creep. On the other hand, collagen behaves more like a viscoelastic material. It is prone to creep, relaxation and conditioning. The combination of these two components into one tissue like the skin yields a complex behavior that a number of investigators have begun to model and elucidate. One such model, shown in Figure 5, assumes that the tissue is a combination of elastin fibers that run straight and collagen fibers that are wavy. When one applies some stress, the straight elastic fibers first carry the load and an elastic response is ob-

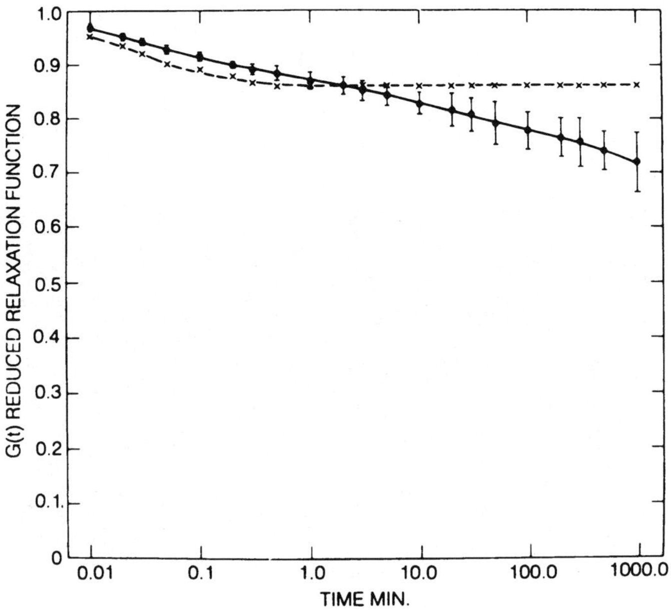


*Fig. 3.*

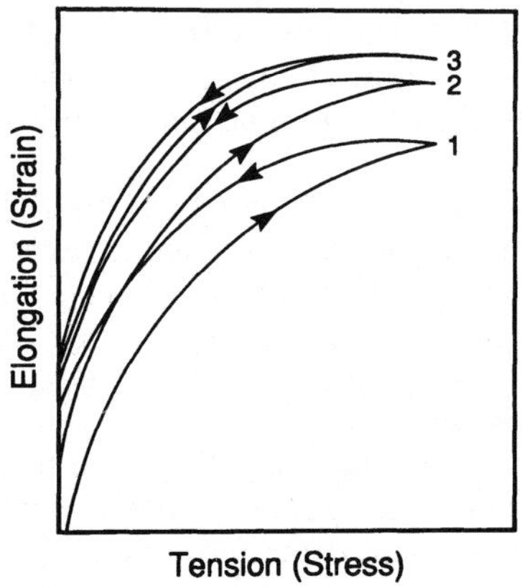


*Fig. 4.*

served. As the stress increases the collagen fibers straighten, carry more of the load and exhibit a viscoelastic behavior. Thus, the behavior of a given tissue depends on the range of stress applied to it and on the composition of elastic and collagenous fibers.

**Dr. Anderson**: Can I get you to clarify here. You are talking about elastic and viscoelastic, and I think also about biologic modification of the tissue in response to something as a third phenomenon perhaps. Is the increased flexibility due to "conditioning" in the sense of athletic training, or is there a biologic remodeling by the tis-

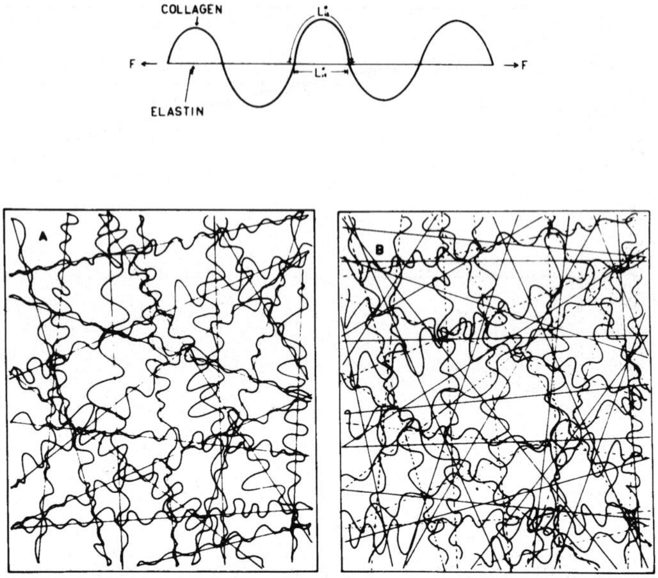


*Fig. 5.*

sue as a repair process after repetitive stretch? In this particular model that you are now describing, if the elastin has already been stretched to its elastic limit before you get a viscoelastic stretch of the collagen, the elastin must be stretched beyond its elastic limit so that it no longer would function when you relax it again.

**Dr. Zeimer**: You basically took one of my punch lines. That is right, one can anticipate that if the elastic range of the elastin fibers is exceeded because the stress is not taken over sufficiently by the wavy collagen fibers, then some irreversible change should occur in the elastin fibers. There seems to be little information on the skin, probably due to the limited clinical concern, but we will see that this concept can be applied to the lamina cribrosa.

Now, I would like to focus the talk specifically on the optic nerve head. As I mentioned before, my intention is to propose a model that incorporates the properties discussed above and experimental data, into a possible explanation for the susceptibility of some individuals to damage related to pressure.

I propose that glaucoma patients do not have an abnormal lamina cribrosa or an abnormal sclera, but rather suffer from a mismatch between the properties of their lamina cribrosa and their scleral canal.

To explain the model we can refer to Figure 6. I have simplified the terms and relate to elongation and pressure rather than to stress and strain. To illustrate my point I have plotted the effect of pressure on the deformation of the scleral canal as if there was no lamina cribrosa attached to it and, similarly, of the lamina cribrosa as if it was on its own. As the pressure increases, there is first a linear elastic behavior due to the elastin fibers, and at higher pressures, as the collagen fibers sustain more of the load, the behavior becomes viscoelastic. The scleral canal behaves in a similar fashion. It must be stressed that the scleral canal is dramatically different from the bulk of the sclera. Dr. Quigley has told us how the scleral canal at the level of the

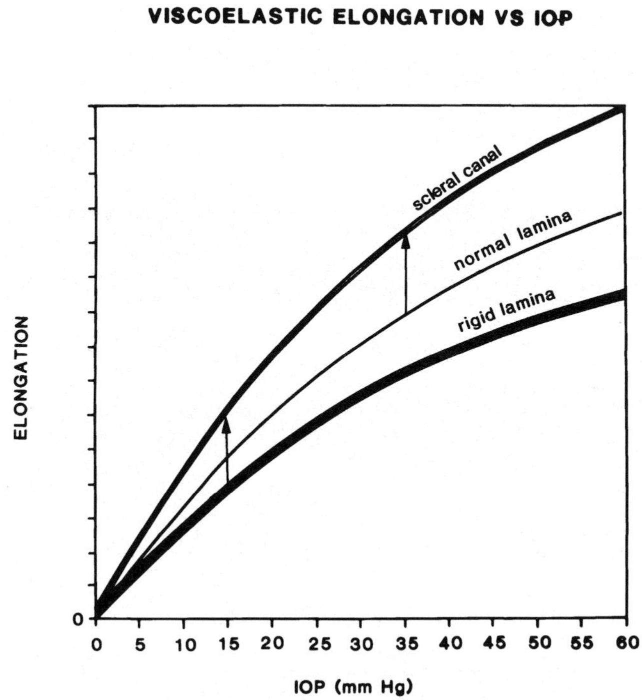


Fig. 6.

lamina cribrosa is reinforced by dense elastin fibers that run along the circumference.

The figure illustrates a case in which the scleral canal is less rigid than the lamina cribrosa. Since the two tissues need to be connected, an equilibrium must be reached. In our case, the lamina cribrosa needs to be stretched to reach the equilibrium and the scleral canal must be constricted. The lamina cribrosa can extend to some degree without reaching the stage described in Dr. Anderson's question, namely without being accompanied by damage to the elastin fibers. If this range is equal to the vertical bar shown in the figure, the intraocular pressure (IOP) can be increased to 40 mm Hg and yet the lamina cribrosa can reach the diameter at equilibrium without damage. However, in the case of a normal but more rigid lamina cribrosa, illustrated in the figure, the diameter mismatch is larger and only an IOP of 15 mm Hg can be sustained without damage.

A model based on a mismatch between the properties of the two tissue thus implies that individual differences in the relative properties of the scleral canal and the lamina cribrosa determine the range of pressure that an individual can sustain without reaching the point at which the elastin fibers have reached their elastic limits.

What will happen when the above limit is reached? Since, as Dr. Quigley told us, the elastin fibers are very resilient, it is likely that they will not rupture but rather snap from their point of insertion. The tension will now be partially transferred to the viscoelastic collagen fibers and phenomena such as creep, relaxation and conditioning will take place. Under the sustained tension, the lamina cribrosa will creep and its diameter will enlarge. Moreover, the tissue will tend to exhibit relaxation. These mechanisms may have two consequences: transfer of the tension back to the

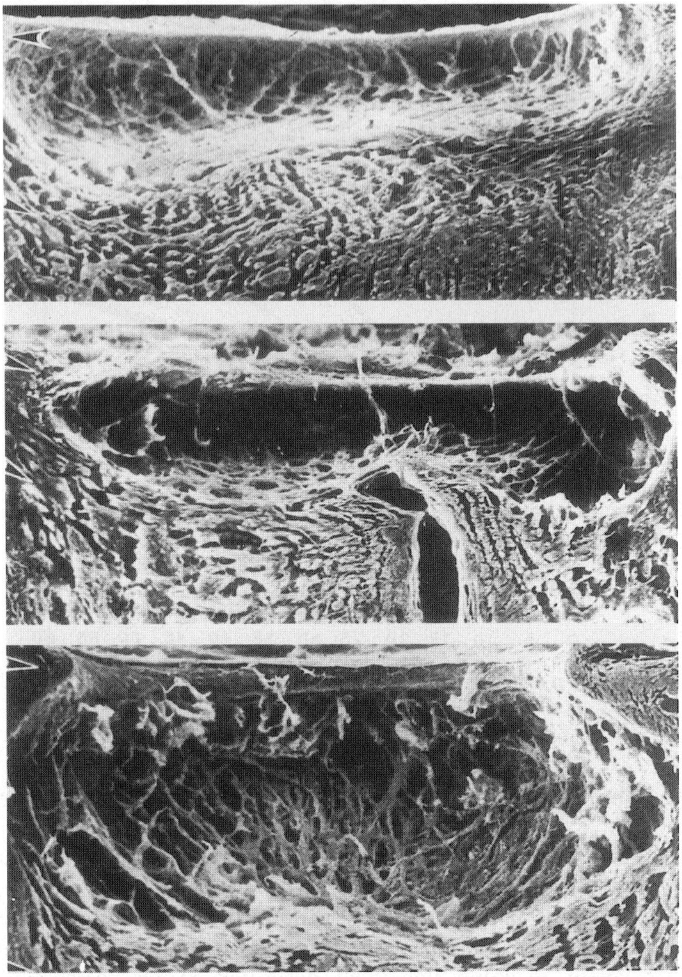

*Fig. 7.*

remaining elastin fibers and reduction of the inward pull on the scleral canal. The loading of the elastic fibers that are already at the end of their elasticity range will make the tissue appear stiffer and will increase the likelihood of further snapping. The release of the inward pull on the scleral canal will cause it to enlarge.

The enlargement of the scleral canal is compatible with observation in glaucoma specimen. Dr. Quigley has shown cross-sections of human optic nerve head at different stages of glaucoma damage as shown in Figure 7. It is readily apparent from the sections that the scleral canal at the level of the lamina cribrosa is larger in more advanced cases. It is important to stress that the enlargement occurs at the level of the lamina cribrosa and not at the level of Bruch's membrane. This explains the unchanged diameter of the disc as viewed clinically and the excavation of the disc. The remaining neural tissue now has to configure to the enlarged scleral canal once and therefore, it appears excavated as it passes beyond the opening in Bruch's membrane.

We have performed a study of our own in which we obtained post mortem glau-

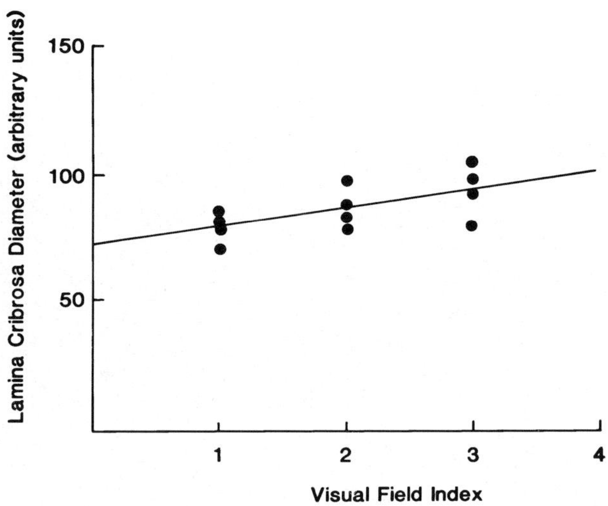


*Fig. 8.*

coma eyes and examined them histologically. Also, some rough clinical data were obtained from the clinicians who saw the patients prior to their death. As shown in Figure 8, the scleral canal was larger in patients who had worse visual field losses. On the other hand, there was no enlargement at the level of Bruch's membrane.

**Dr. Quigley**: Can you tell us how you measure the diameter of the scleral canal? It was histological measurements, I take it, in human eyes that had a history of glaucoma during their lifetime. How did you measure the scleral canal diameter?

**Dr. Zeimer**: As mentioned above, it was measured from the histologic section at the level of the insertion of the lamina cribrosa. This is illustrated in Figure 9.

**Dr. Quigley**: You had an anterior limit and a posterior limit. Was the diameter measured at the anterior limit, at the posterior, or the average of the two, what was it?

**Dr. Zeimer**: We measured the diameter at the anterior and posterior location and found no noticeable difference.

We also measured the thickness of the lamina cribrosa in these patients. As shown in Figure 10, the thickness decreases as the diameter increases. This also agrees with the findings of Dr. Quigley who observed a thinner lamina cribrosa in more advanced cases.

In addition to the study of the anatomy at different degree of glaucoma damage, we investigated the mechanical properties of the optic nerve head. We hoped that if we could measure the mechanical properties of the optic nerve head we could predict if an individual is susceptible to glaucomatous damage. In a nutshell, we developed a system to measure noninvasively the displacement of the optic nerve head under an induced short rise in IOP. The motion was measured by laser Doppler velocimetry by sending a laser into the optic nerve head and combining the outgoing light with a reference beam. The motion was induced by inflating the eye for a very short time with a suction contact lens. As shown in Figure 11, we obtained a curve

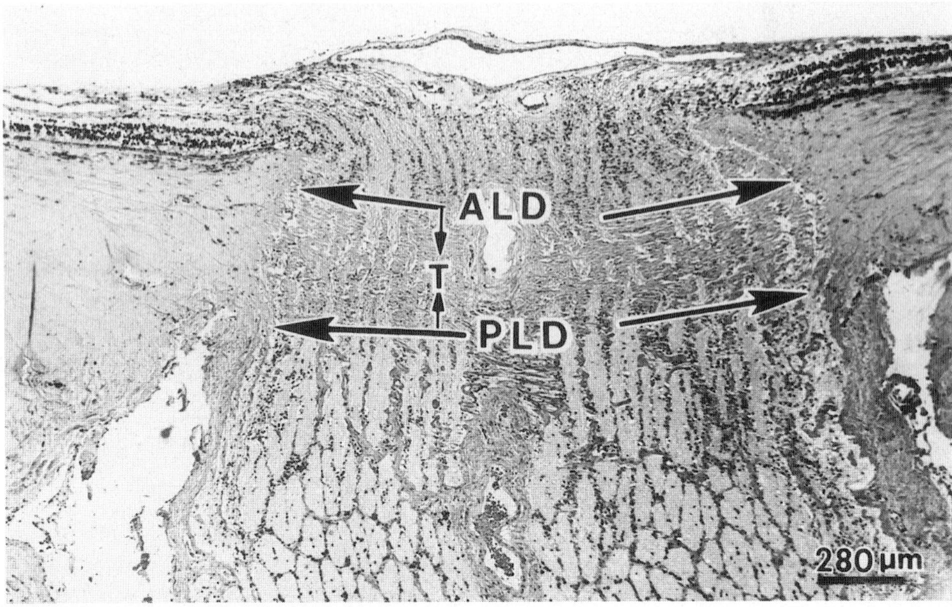


*Fig. 9.*

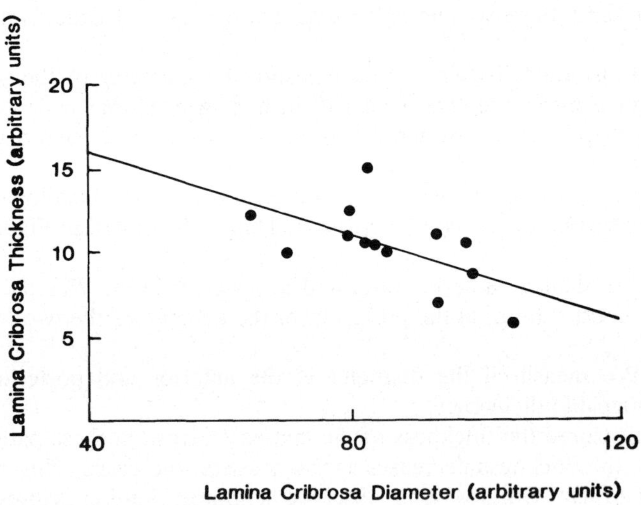


*Fig. 10.*

of the velocity of recession of the optic nerve head as a function of time. The area under the curve yielded the amount of displacement for a given induced pressure. We were able to measure deformations in humans with a reproducibility of 16 microns by averaging up to four measurements. The results in humans indicated that the backward deformation was very low (20 microns) in normals. A very preliminary study in glaucoma patients indicated that the displacement was equal or lower. Thus, in glaucoma, the values fell below the detection limit implying that they could

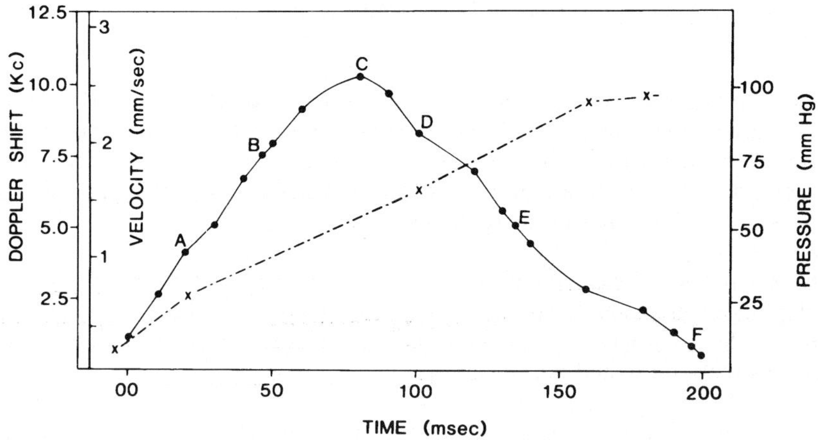


*Fig. 11.*

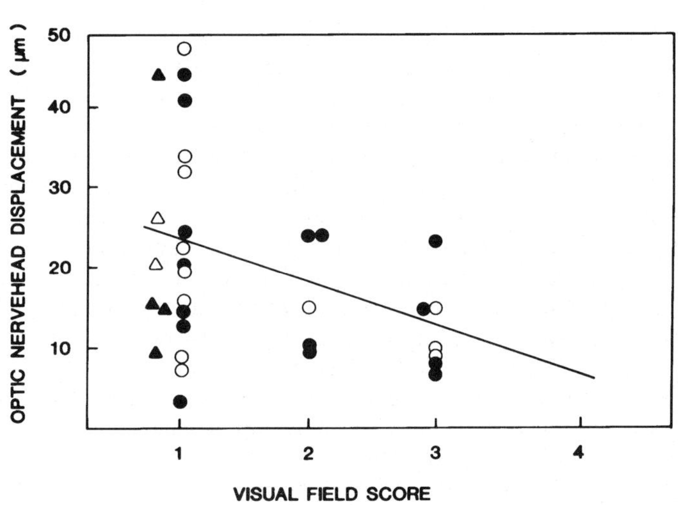


*Fig. 12.*

not be differentiated from those of normals. To verify the observation we initiated a study in post mortem human eyes using the same technique.

The major finding is shown in Figure 12 in which the results of measurements in glaucoma patients are marked with dots and those of normals with triangles. The empty symbols indicate the contralateral eyes, so the filled symbols represent results of one eye per patient. The results indicate that the optic nerve head displacement decreases with the progression of visual loss. In other words, the optic nerve head support becomes stiffer as the damage is more pronounced. This was confirmed by the following observation: in eyes with equal degree of visual field loss the average difference in displacement was 4.5 ± 3 microns; while in eyes with asymmetry the difference was 20 ± 6 microns, the eye with less damage being always the one with more motion.

**Dr. Alm**: On what part of the optic nerve head displacement were the measurements made?

**Dr. Zeimer**: In living eyes we wanted to avoid large blood vessels because the dynamics of a large blood vessel filled with blood under pressure may not reflect the behavior of the lamina cribrosa. Therefore, we measured on a central area devoid of large vessels. In the postmortem eyes we did not have problems with blood vessels and measured at the center of the optic nerve head.

**Dr. Alm**: But if you consider the pictures that you showed and Harry Quigley showed with sloping edges of the lamina cribrosa, is not that where the movement would be of interest, that is where the remaining axons are, and you could easily have large movements that you would not detect.

**Dr. Zeimer**: Local measurements may indeed be more interesting but they were not pursued once we doubted that the method could be applied clinically.

**Dr. Quigley**: We have just tried to do some measurements, following up on what Ran is doing, presenting to you here, using the image analysis systems that a number of the people here are familiar with, that is, you are optically bouncing light off the surface of the optic nerve head and changing the eye pressure on a minutes to hour length basis. In monkey eyes, where you put a needle in the eye, you raise a reservoir of fluid, raise the eye pressure for periods of time, image the optic nerve head surface, or at least what you think is the surface, or at least what light reflects from. And Albert, in this case you can do some regional measurements. Let me just briefly tell you what you find. The first thing you find is that the optic nerve head surface does move away from you as you raise the eye pressure to 45 mm Hg. It comes back at you when you lower the pressure to 10 again, 10 being where we started. The movement over a 45-minute period of instantaneously raising the pressure to 45 in a normal monkey eye, you get an immediate backward movement which is rapid, and then a slower, continued movement to an asymptote that looks like it would finish its creep in about an hour. If you then lower the eye pressure you get an immediate movement backward toward the original position and again, the slowly declining slope of movement, returning almost elastically to the original position. Regionally the movement is greater above and below than it is through the middle of the nerve head. That is in the normal, and we have produced the pressure damage in the monkey eyes, and that data is being analyzed right now. So I can not tell you yet whether it actually is going to be stiffer, as Ran's original measurements were, but our initial experiments indicate that it is, in fact, stiffer. That the glaucoma nerve head is not behaving in the same viscoelastic way as the normal.

**Dr. Alm**: Well, my concern is mainly, you started by showing that you could almost point your finger at the excavation of the disk in glaucoma. That would be hidden to your measurements, what is in the periphery, and now you are talking about movement backwards and forwards, but did you also have some radial movement that you may stretch the peripheral part of the lamina cribrosa, which in fact may do even more damage to the axons?

**Dr. Zeimer**: Exactly. The backward motion is apparently not a good indicator of the deformations that lead to damage of the axons.

**Dr. Quigley**: Does everybody understand Albert's point? If we are talking about the scleral canal goes this way, and if he is saying the scleral canal enlarges in that orientation, but we are measuring movements with a beam that is coming in this way, that can only see things going in this direction, it could go this way indefinitely and we would never know any movement happened unless the movement in this direction had a component of posterior stretching associated with it

**Dr. Kaufman**: The only question I have, and I realize that with your visual field score, you know, you are trying to get into all the three categories, but the slope is really dependent on two points, maybe even one point in your category #1. Otherwise it would be a straight line with no relationship with severity. So I think one needs to be a little cautious. I know that is not the main part of your argument, but I think, based on those data, to imply that there is a severity relationship somehow with the disease and the displacement based on those data is reaching perhaps a little bit more than maybe what you ought to.

**Dr. Zeimer**: Paul, the reason I do not show you only the average, is indeed to let you assess the reliability of the data. There is no doubt that the numbers are small and for that very reason they can be affected either way by few data points. If one deletes points we could obtain any result, we could actually increase the slope if we deleted points in the other categories. The tentative conclusion proposed here is supported by Harry's data in monkeys which point to the same trend.

**Dr. Caprioli**: Ran, did you try to correlate your optic nerve head displacement with either refractive error or some estimate of scleral rigidity? I am thinking that the myopes may have a less rigid sclera and the hyperopes may have a more rigid sclera, and maybe this had something to do with your displacement. I mean, there is an old theory that myopes are more susceptible to glaucoma damage, than others...

**Dr. Zeimer**: We did not measure scleral rigidity and have no information on the refractive error. However, I would like to remind you that we measure the displacement of the optic nerve head relative to the sclera and thus, one cannot anticipate an influence of the scleral rigidity on the measurements themselves. On the other hand, as explained in my model, a more flexible sclera, as suspected in myopes, could indeed increase the mismatch and increase the risk to glaucoma damage.

The increase in rigidity, if present in advanced glaucoma, could be due to a number of pathologic changes. As mentioned above, it is partially due to the fact that the elastin fibers are at the limit of their elastic range, but cellular mechanisms may also play a role. The cells responsible for renewal of collagen tissue are likely to be affected by the deformation of the supporting beams or alteration in blood supply and they may produce abnormal connective material which increases the rigidity.

I would now like to finish the presentation of the model by mentioning a few more observations that the model could incorporate.

The increased rigidity accompanied with the damage may initiate a close loop mechanism. As the lamina cribrosa stiffens the mismatch increases and thus, as explained above, smaller IOP increases are sufficient to cause it to reach its limit. This may explain why glaucoma patients are more susceptible to damage in the more advanced phases.

The model could also explain the behavior after intraocular pressure reduction. When an elevated IOP is reduced while the lamina cribrosa is still in its elastic mode, the appearance could be reversed as the elastin fibers are intact. This may be the case in younger individuals or those who have suffered intraocular pressure injury for a shorter period. However, if the IOP is reduced after the lamina cribrosa has crept, the scleral canal will constrict and the lamina cribrosa will not. This will cause the lamina cribrosa to bow backward as observed in advanced glaucoma.

**Dr. Pyeritz**: Ran, I think that medical geneticists are often accused of focusing too much on the outliers, but if you look at your two outliers there and remove them from the data pool, I suspect your regression slope would be close to zero.

Let us focus on the two that really are outliers. And I think my point is that the message may be in those two eyes rather than in the mass of the other data, and that they may be telling you something important about how to interpret this.

**Dr. Zeimer**: As I mentioned in my response to Dr. Kaufman, it is not quite justified to isolate cases when the numbers are limited as points may seem to be outliers due the scatter of the data.

**Dr. Caprioli**: Ran, what you have offered here is a hypothesis about the conformation of the connective tissue, skeleton if you would, of the optic nerve head. But what I would like to hear is your hypothesis about how the nerves are killed.

**Dr. Zeimer**: I suppose that once the lamina cribrosa is deformed, a number of mechanisms could take place to cause damage to the neuronal tissue. The blood supply could be impaired because the laminar beams carrying the vessels creep. The deformation of the beams and the increased rigidity could also cause direct strangulation and kinking of the axons.

**Dr. Morrison**: Maybe I could rephrase Joe's question a little bit. You mentioned the rigidity of the tissue; do you think a rigid lamina cribrosa is bad for the optic nerve, or is it good for the optic nerve fibers?

**Dr. Zeimer**: Going back to the original thought, the lamina cribrosa should not be judged by itself. The issue is, does a given lamina cribrosa match a given scleral canal? Thus, a rigid lamina cribrosa could coexist with a rigid sclera without inducing a susceptibility to IOP damage. This would not be the case if the scleral canal is pliable.

**Dr. Quigley**: John, I did not use to think that I knew the answer to your question. But we began studying the nerve head and we found that it has this tremendous complement of elastin. The elastin is only present in the scleral ring around the lamina and through the lamina, and as you go 2, 3, 4 millimeters off into the sclera in any direction there is no elastin to speak of at all. So this tissue is endowed naturally with a material that is designed to provide tremendous elastic behavior. Now, if you have seen the mires on an application tonometer, you know what the eye wall is doing every time your heart beats. And I think I know why all that elastin is there. So, I now think that the nerve head had better be elastic or something nasty is going to happen, because it is naturally built that way. So I now think that we do not want to have a rigid lamina as opposed to an elastic one. And if the glaucomatous nerve head, by either its effect of the first damage or as the original cause becomes rigid, I strongly suspect it is bad for either axons or their blood supply. I want to add one more little thing, and, to Joe's list or the list that Ran made of ways nerve fibers could die because of this process' starting, another is one that really comes out of things that Doug has suggested, namely, the capillaries are within the beams. A capillary breaks open and you lose the blood–brain barrier at that point, as the endothelial cell gives up, just as you would with a disc hemorrhage happening more anteriorly where you can see it. So that materials that are within the serum normally are suddenly in much higher concentration in the extracellular space around the nerve fiber than they used to be before. That is not to say there is a lack of oxygen, or a lack of glucose being delivered, it is to say there is a nastiness being delivered to a neural tissue that should not see those things.

**Dr. Van Buskirk**: I am still a little confused by your mechanical hypothesis. Are you differentiating stretchability from flexibility? In other words, end-to-end stretch from side-to-side stretch?

**Dr. Zeimer**: What I am looking at is elongation, what you call stretchability.

**Dr. Van Buskirk**: That stretchability is that something separate from its flexibility, its ability to bend, so to speak?

**Dr. Zeimer**: Much like the skin there is no force involved in bending. We are only dealing with the ability to elongate under tension.

**Dr. Van Buskirk**: I guess I am trying to understand why, it is basically the same tissue, the scleral canal and the lamina.

Also, I guess I just do not understand why the scleral canal is enlarging. It seems to me no matter how weak or strong the laminar fibers are, that the scleral canal would not enlarge.

**Dr. Zeimer**: The scleral canal is a hole and it is reinforced, as Harry showed, by a ring of elastin fibers. The lamina cribrosa is completely different. It is a mesh with large openings with elastin and collagen fibers that run across it.

**Dr. Quigley**: Let me speak to the issue. Are the areas of the lamina, the immediate sclera next to the lamina, and the sclera somewhere away from there, are they similar tissues? This is cross-sections of the collagen in the lamina beams. So this is within the lamina itself, the picture on the left. The next picture is the cross-sections of the collagen just alongside it in the insertion region. That is the typical distribution of collagen right next to the disc but not within the lamina. And the next is the cross-sections of collagen in the sclera, some distance away in the equator. Now, I have no idea what collagen type these are. We tried to do immunogold staining in the cross-sections, and cross-sections of collagen will not stain with the antibody, they only stain in longitudinal sections and you can not look at diameter. So I do not know if these are different collagen types, but I know they are very different in the diameter distribution.

**Dr. Zeimer**: Harry, could you comment more on the elastin? You have slides showing the elastin distribution within the laminar beam and in the scleral connection, which I think are very relevant.

**Dr. Quigley**: This is elastin staining. As you go into the lamina cribrosa, this is a beam of neural tissue, that is a laminar strut, that is the connective tissue going in, you can see all the stained elastin within it, this is this insertion ring going around it, you can see the beam comes straight off the insertion ring there, and if you head off into the sclera going this direction down to the bottom, you will see less and less and less elastin as you go, so there is a different orientation of elastin and collagen, by the way, in this zone, compared to where you just entered the lamina. That is an anatomic fact. I do not know how it fits with his theory or not.

**Dr. Van Buskirk**: .... whether you have mismatch or not, you have a ring of scleral canal, and you have laminar fibers going from one side of the ring to the other. So I do not understand why the scleral ring is enlarging at the same time that these fibers are under stress and becoming more rigid. It seems to me that the ring would get smaller. Unless they are breaking their insertion into the side of the ring.

**Dr. Zeimer**: You are absolutely right. If the elastin snaps the collagen fibers will creep and relax and thus allow the scleral canal to enlarge toward the size that it would assume if it was by itself. As the lamina cribrosa assumes a new elongation it also undergoes structural and composition changes which make it more rigid. As I mentioned, the stretch of the remaining elastin fibers to their elastic limit will make the tissue appear stiff. The composition changes may be similar to scaring and likely to also increase the stiffness. Thus, the process of enlargement of the scleral canal and of the lamina cribrosa are not necessarily contradictory to the presence of increased rigidity.

I would like to conclude by continuing to enumerate potential causes for a mismatch. There could be a mismatch due to maturation: as the lamina cribrosa and the scleral canal are created at a different stage of maturation, the diameter and their properties may not be set in a matching manner. Another reason is the scleral canal can be too pliable for its diameter due to a lack of elastin at the insertion. A large opening requires more reinforcement to hold the same amount of pressure. But during development or as a consequence of aging the elastin reinforcement may be insufficient for that particular diameter. Alternatively, the scleral canal could be weakened by insufficient collagen resulting in a thin sclera. The tension in the sclera is related to other factors by the following equation:

$$\text{tension} = \frac{\text{IOP} \times \text{radius of globe}}{\text{scleral thickness}}$$

Dr. Drance co-authored a paper (*Graefes Arch Clin Exp Ophthalmol* 227:17-20, 1989) in which a significant difference in the estimated scleral tension was reported between glaucoma suspect and eyes that developed glaucoma. A thin sclera would imply that the scleral canal is pliable. This may be the case in myopia which is also aggravated by the increase in radius and the consequent larger tension.

On the other hand, the lamina cribrosa could be relatively too rigid due to inherent or acquired properties of the connective tissue. Cross-linking of fiber could be one such acquired change that stiffens the lamina cribrosa. We heard today that with age there is more cross-linking between the elastin and the collagen.

# 7. AXONAL DAMAGE

PAUL N. HOFFMAN, M.D., Ph.D.

I am going to compare the response to axonal injury in peripheral neurons, which support axon regeneration, and retinal ganglion cell neurons, which are normally incapable of effective regeneration. This discussion will focus on how these two systems differ with respect to the synthesis and axonal transport of tubulin. Recent evidence indicates that microtubules, polymers composed primarily of tubulin, play an essential role in axon elongation by stabilizing cytoplasmic processes arising from growth cones at the tips of elongating axons[1]. The disassembly of these microtubules by colchicine or other pharmacological agents results in the retraction of elongating axons[2].

Axonal growth occurs in two phases, elongation followed by growth in diameter (radial growth). Radial growth does not begin until after elongating axons have reached their targets (Fig. 1). Neurofilaments, the major intermediate filaments in mature neurons, are intrinsic determinants of axonal diameter which are intimately involved in the radial growth of large-caliber myelinated nerve fibers[3]. Microtubules and neurofilaments are the principal cytoskeletal polymers in myelinated nerve fibers[4].

Axon elongation occurs in mature neurons during peripheral nerve regeneration. When an peripheral axon is cut or crushed, the portion disconnected from the cell body undergoes Wallerian degeneration. Regenerating sprouts arising from the distal end of the proximal stump elongate towards their targets at rates of 3-6 mm/day depending on the metabolic state of the neuron. Prior axonal injury (*i.e.*, a conditioning lesion [CL]) increases the rate of regeneration in response to a test lesion several weeks later[5] (Fig. 2). The rate of axon regeneration also declines with age[6,7].

The absence of ribosomes in axons precludes cytoplasmic protein synthesis. Although the axon may have a volume several thousand times greater than that of the cell body, it depends on newly synthesized proteins produced in the cell body for its growth and maintenance. These proteins are translocated within axons via a process referred to as axonal transport[8]. Membrane-associated proteins (*i.e.*, vesicles and other membranous structures) are transported bidirectionally within axons at a rate of 400 mm/day via rapid axonal transport[9,10]. In contrast, actin, tubulin, and the neurofilament proteins, the principal cytoskeletal proteins in axons, are transported in the SCa and SCb components of slow axonal transport, which move at rates of 1-2 and 3-6 mm/day, respectively, in peripheral nerve fibers[11]. The neurofilament proteins are transported exclusively in SCa, while actin and tubulin are transported in both SCa and to a lesser extent SCb in peripheral nerve fibers (Fig. 3). SCb also contains clathrin, calmodulin, the enzymes of glycolysis, and a variety of other proteins[12]. It did not escape our attention that SCb contains two proteins known to be involved in the mechanism of regeneration (*i.e.*, actin and tubulin) and that the velocity of SCb is identical to the rate of regeneration[8]. (Fig. 4).

Tubulin is a dimer comprised of a single α- and β-subunit. α- and β-tubulin are encoded by multigene families[13]. At least 6 isotypes of β-tubulin can be distinguished on the basis of their amino acid sequences. Four of these isotypes are present in axons[14]. As we shall see, the level of expression of one of these isotypes, class II β-tubulin ($\beta_{II}$-tubulin), correlates closely with axon elongation during both development and regeneration[15,16]. Using hybridization with labeled cDNA probes, we have examined the expression of specific isotypes of β-tubulin in peripheral sensory neurons at various times

*Optic Nerve in Glaucoma, pp. 123–134*
*edited by S.M. Drance*

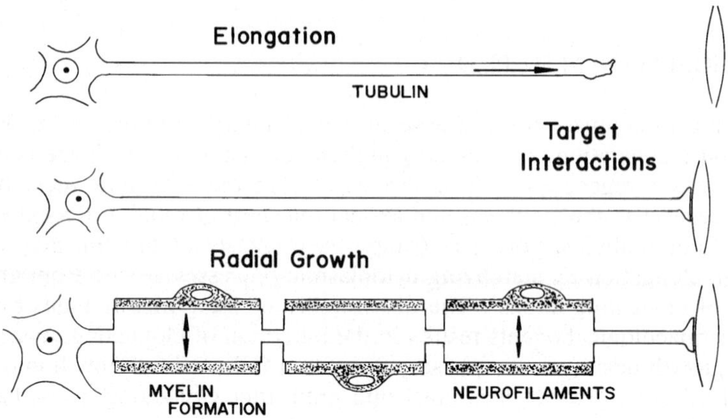


*Fig. 1.* The two phases of axonal growth.

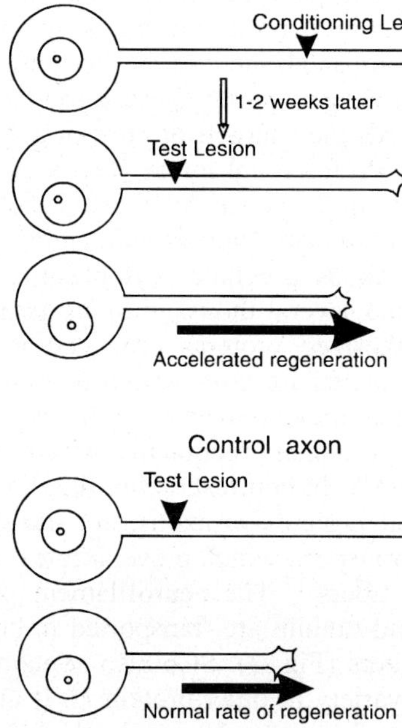


*Fig. 2.* Accelerated axon regeneration after a conditioning lesion.

after crushing the sciatic nerve (Fig. 5). In these studies, RNA purified from dorsal root ganglia (DRG), which contain the sensory neuron cell bodies, was analyzed on denaturing gels, transferred to nylon membranes, and hybridized with $^{32}$P-labeled cDNA probes (*i.e.*, Northern blot analyses)[17]. This analysis demonstrates that neurofilament expression declines, expression of $\beta_{II}$-tubulin increases, and the expression of $\beta_I$-tubulin and $\beta_{IV}$-tubulin changes relatively little (*i.e.*, <2-fold) after axotomy (Fig. 6). The expression of $\beta_{III}$-tubulin also changes relatively little after axotomy[18]. These ob-

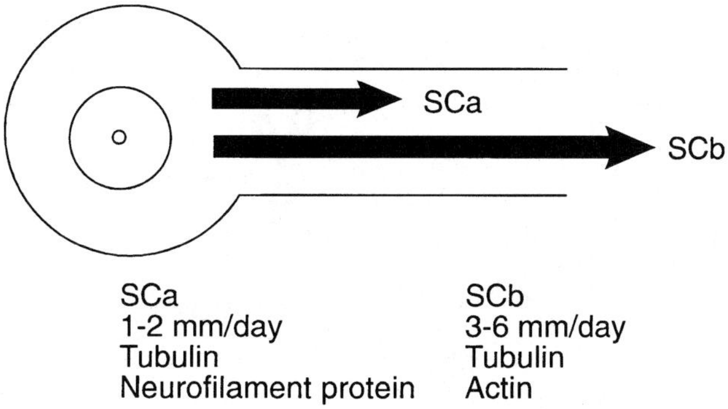


*Fig. 3.* The SCa and SCb components of slow axonal transport.

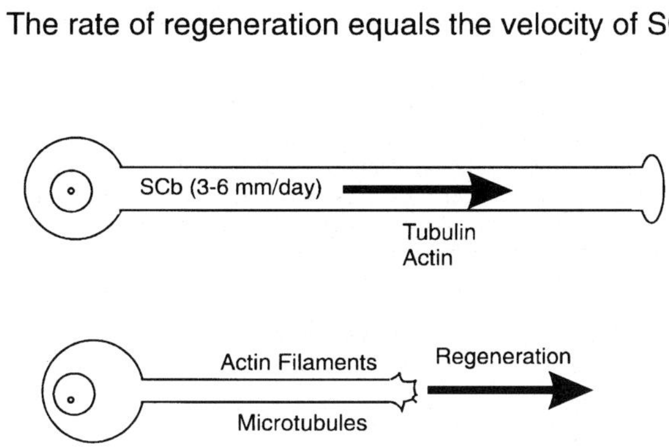


*Fig. 4.* The role of SCb in axon elongation.

servations indicate that accelerated regeneration after a conditioning lesion correlates with the increased expression of $\beta_{II}$-tubulin.

These changes in tubulin and neurofilament expression represent a recapitulation of the developmental pattern of gene expression (Fig. 7). $\beta_{II}$-tubulin is expressed at higher levels in developing than mature neurons, while the expression of $\beta_{I}$- and $\beta_{IV}$-tubulin change relatively little during development. In contrast, neurofilament expression is higher in mature than developing neurons[15,16].

The tubulin transported in sensory fibers can be pulse-labeled by injecting radioactive amino acids (*e.g.*, $^{35}$S-methionine) into the dorsal root ganglion. Nerves containing transported proteins can be harvested at various times after labeling and the distribution of radioactive tubulin along the nerve analyzed using immunoprecipitation and SDS-polyacrylamide gel electrophoresis (SDS-PAGE).

Using monoclonal antibodies (mAbs) which specifically recognize either $\beta_{II}$- or $\beta_{III}$-tubulin, we have been able to show that the increased $\beta_{II}$-tubulin expression is associated with a rise in the relative amount of tubulin transported in SCb in the proximal stumps of axotomized nerve fibers[19]. The distribution of labeled tubulin is compared

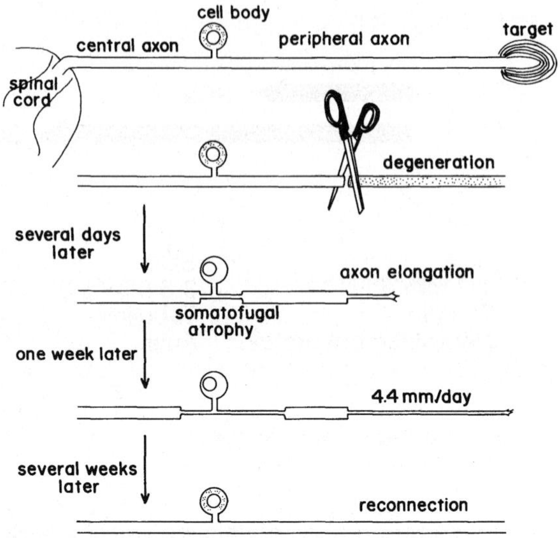


*Fig. 5.* Regeneration of peripheral sensory fibers. Peripheral sensory neurons give rise to a single axonal stem process which bifurcates into central and peripheral branches. Injury of the peripheral branch results in increased tubulin expression and reduced neurofilament expression in axotomized sensory neurons. Decreased neurofilament expression results in reductions in axonal neurofilament content and axonal caliber which start proximally near the cell body (soma) and spread somatofugally along the axonal branches at a rate equal to the velocity of neurofilament transport, which is two-fold greater in the peripheral than the central branch. This process is referred to as somatofugal axonal atrophy[3].

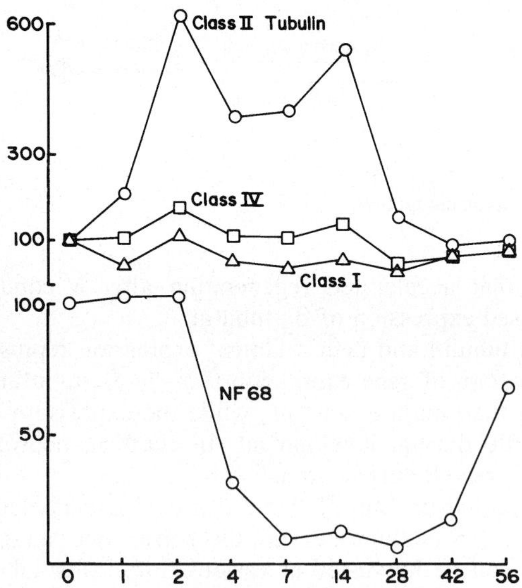


*Fig. 6.* Alterations in gene expression in axotomized sensory neurons. Hybridization with labeled cDNA probes was used to measure the abundance of mRNAs encoding $\beta_I$- (class I), $\beta_{II}$- (class II), and $\beta_{IV}$-tubulin (class IV) and neurofilament-L (neurofilament 68) in lumbar sensory neurons at various times after crushing the sciatic nerve. (From Hoffman and Cleveland[16].)

| NEONATAL | MATURE | AXOTOMY |
|---|---|---|
| High $\beta_{II}$-Tubulin | Low $\beta_{II}$-Tubulin | High $\beta_{II}$-Tubulin |
| Low NF | High NF | Low NF |

*Fig. 7.* Recapitulation of the developmental pattern of gene expression in axotomized peripheral sensory neurons.

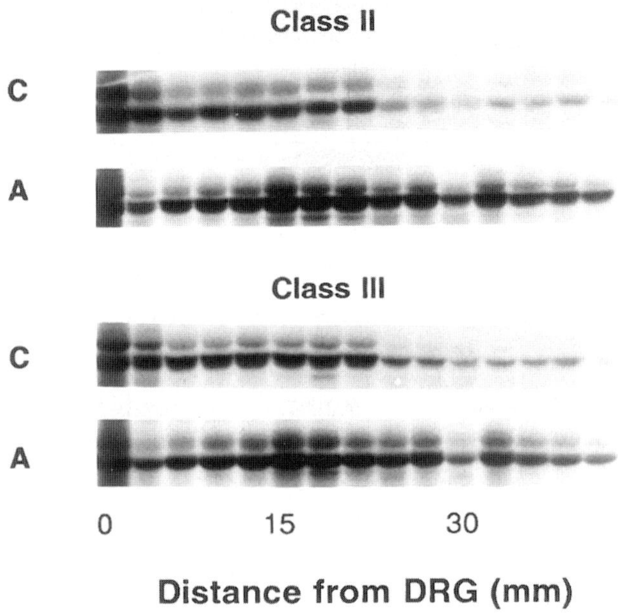


*Fig. 8.* Tubulin transport in intact and axotomized sensory fibers. In this gel fluorogram, the distributions of pulse-labeled $\beta_{II}$- (class II) and $\beta_{III}$-tubulin (class III) are compared in axotomized (A) and control (C) sensory fibers of the sciatic nerve seven days after labeling sensory neurons with $^{35}$S-methionine. Axotomized neurons were labeled seven days after crushing the sciatic nerve 50 mm from the dorsal root ganglion.

along intact and axotomized sensory fibers seven days after labeling sensory neurons with $^{35}$S-methionine in Figure 8. We found that the pulse-labeled neurofilament proteins, which are transported exclusively in SCa, extend 0-27 mm from the dorsal root ganglion seven days after labeling. Therefore, labeled tubulin located in this region of the nerve (0-27 mm) is associated with SCa, while tubulin located 27-45 mm from the dorsal root ganglion is associated exclusively with SCb. Comparison of the distributions of tubulin in intact and axotomized fibers demonstrates that increased amounts of both $\beta_{II}$- and $\beta_{III}$-tubulin are associated with SCb in axotomized fibers. Thus, the accelerated regeneration of sensory fibers after a conditioning lesion correlates with an increase in the relative amount of tubulin transported in SCb.

This suggests that the regenerative potential of axons is related to the amount of tubulin transported in SCb. According to this hypothesis, the relatively small amount of tubulin normally transported in SCb in peripheral nerve fibers is sufficient to support effective regeneration. Regeneration is enhanced when increased amounts of tubulin are transported in SCb (*i.e.*, after a conditioning lesion).

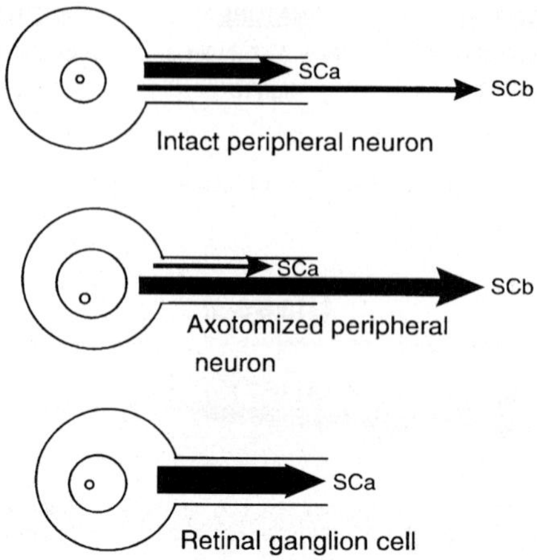


*Fig. 9.* Comparison of tubulin transport in peripheral nerve and optic nerve fibers.

| **NEONATAL** | **MATURE** | **AXOTOMY** |
|---|---|---|
| **High $\beta_{II}$-Tubulin** | **Low $\beta_{II}$-Tubulin** | **Low $\beta_{II}$-Tubulin** |
| **Low NF** | **High NF** | **Low NF** |

*Fig. 10.* Gene expression in retinal ganglion cell neurons.

How does this hypothesis account for the lack of effective regeneration of optic nerve fibers? Examination of tubulin transport in intact optic nerve fibers indicates that little, if any tubulin is normally transported in SCb in these axons[20] (Fig. 9). Surprisingly, all of the other proteins normally transported in SCb in peripheral nerve fibers, some of which may participate in axon elongation (*e.g.*, actin), are also transported in SCb in optic nerve fibers. Thus, there is a selective loss of tubulin from SCb in optic nerve fibers. This correlates with the inability of these axons to regenerate in the absence of a peripheral nerve graft.

A small proportion of optic nerve fibers are capable of regenerating into a segment of peripheral nerve attached to the cut optic nerve stump (*i.e.*, a peripheral nerve graft)[21]. In the absence of a peripheral nerve graft, no increase in tubulin expression is observed in axotomized retinal ganglion cell neurons[22,23] (Fig. 10). In fact, the rate of slow axonal transport declines 10-fold in the proximal stumps of axotomized optic nerve fibers, while the rate of rapid axonal transport is unchanged[24]. In contrast, an increase in tubulin expression is observed in retinal ganglion cell neurons which have regenerated axons into the peripheral nerve graft, but not in neurons which failed to regenerate their axons[25]. This increase in tubulin expression correlates with a 2-fold rise in the rate of tubulin transport in regenerating optic nerve fibers[26] which may reflect the transport of tubulin in SCb. These observations suggest that substances secreted by the peripheral nerve graft, which contains degenerating axons and replicating Schwann cells, may induce a rise in tubulin expression in axotomized retinal ganglion cell neurons. Replicating Schwann cells are known to synthesize and secrete a number of neurotrophic factors (*e.g.*, NGF, BDNF, and NT-3)[27]. These trophic factors may promote the regeneration of optic nerve fibers in peripheral nerve grafts by inducing the transport of tubulin in SCb in these axons.

It is important to remember that regeneration is a complex process which is also influenced by the local environment at the growing axon tip[28]. For example, Schwann cells, the myelin-forming cells in the peripheral nerves, promote regeneration, while proteins associated with central nervous system myelin, which is produced by oligodendrocytes, block axon elongation[29].

The evidence we have considered is consistent with a model in which the regenerative potential of axons is limited by the amount of tubulin transported in the SCb component of slow axonal transport. Increasing the relative amount of tubulin transported in SCb after axotomy is associated with accelerated regeneration, while the absence of tubulin in SCb in optic nerve fibers may preclude effective regeneration. We can speculate that the relative amount of tubulin transported in SCb may also correlate with an axon's ability to withstand chronic compression, as may occur in glaucoma. A goal of future studies is to develop strategies for promoting the transport of tubulin in SCb in intact optic nerve fibers, and determining whether this facilitates the survival of optic nerve fibers in experimental models of glaucoma.

**Dr. Costa**: Is there dexamethasone change in any of these rates? Because you have to go to the regulation of the gene of this. Could be, is this gene regulated by a steroid hormone?

**Dr. Hoffman**: I do not know. We have not yet identified the factors which regulate the level of tubulin expression

**Dr. Costa**: But giving methasone would be very simple to see whether this is regulated.

**Dr. Hoffman**: Absolutely. And we are open to all suggestions, and there are a number of trophic factors that may also influence the level of expression of tubulin or neurofilament protein in neurons.

**Dr. Bray:** Paul, to answer one of your questions, I think you would agree, and you could probably expand it further, Lisa McKerracher has data that the retinal ganglion cells that have grown into peripheral nerve grafts that I will be talking about, are expressing and do up-regulate their expression of the tubulin gene. It is true she has not looked at the subclasses. Do you want to expand on that?

**Dr. Hoffman**: Yes, I do. In the absence of a peripheral nerve graft, tubulin expression is not increased in axotomized retinal ganglion cell neurons. Only a small proportion of optic nerve fibers regenerate in peripheral nerve grafts. Lisa McKerracher has found that there is a selective increase in tubulin expression in neurons which have successfully regenerated axons into peripheral nerve grafts[25]. Increased tubulin expression is not observed in neurons which failed to regenerate axons into the graft. Lisa also found an increase in the rate of tubulin transport in regenerating optic nerve fibers (*i.e.*, in the graft) which may reflect the transport of tubulin in SCb[26].

As I mentioned, actin and tubulin are normally transported in SCb in peripheral nerve fibers. In contrast, actin, but not tubulin is transported in SCb in optic nerve fibers. These observations in regenerating optic nerve fibers support the hypothesis that the regenerative potential of axons is related to the amount of tubulin transported in SCb. According to this hypothesis, the absence of tubulin in SCb normally precludes the effective regeneration of optic nerve nerve fibers. In contrast, the effective regeneration of optic nerve fibers in peripheral nerve grafts reflects the transport of tubulin in SCb.

**Dr. Morrison**: The things you have described are in the myelinated portion of the optic nerve. The glaucoma damage occurs within the lamina, which is anterior to most of the myelin. Do you think that there is going to be any difference in this behavior based upon that difference?

**Dr. Hoffman**: I suspect that these neurons respond similarly to injury at the lamina and in the myelinated portion of the nerve. Since glaucoma may reflect the chronic compression of axons at the lamina, it would be of interest to know whether the transport of tubulin in SCb in intact optic nerve fibers makes these axons more resistant to compression. The up-regulation of tubulin expression in the presence of a peripheral nerve graft raises the possibility that substances released from the graft (*e.g.*, trophic factors secreted by denervated Schwann cells) are responsible for this induction. If so, it may be possible to promote the transport of tubulin in SCb in intact optic nerve fibers, and see if these axons were more resistant to damage in experimental models of glaucoma.

**Dr. Siesjö**: I wonder what is known about the expression of messenger RNA for, say, the immediate early genes for growth factors following injury to peripheral and central neurons.

**Dr. Hoffman**: Injury of peripheral axons is associated with increased expression of the immediate early genes. These genes are also up-regulated after ischemia and in models of seizure, suggesting that they represent a non-specific response to injury.

**Dr. Siesjö:** I wanted to try to explain what I meant with this about the immediate early genes. We know from some insults delivered to the brain that when you have adverse conditions, like pre-ischemic hypoglycemia, you can actually suppress the expression of say, C4's, and the question has arisen whether the inability of the cells to respond with gene expression and with synthesis of the proteins that are required for recovery following the insult might really play a role. And my question was whether your conditioning stimulus would lead to a change in the expression of genes.

**Dr. Hoffman**: Yes, Wolfram Tetzlaff has shown that the immediate early genes are expressed in axotomized facial neurons. I suppose that all synthesis is inhibited if an ischemic insult is sufficiently severe.

**Dr. Morrison**: Yes, but particularly if you can express the messenger RNAs but you have suppressed your protein synthetic machinery enough to suppress also the synthesis of proteins which are required for it.

**Dr. Hoffman**: There is no question that the effective regeneration of peripheral axons is associated with the increased expression and synthesis of some proteins (*e.g.*, tubulin) and the reduced expression and synthesis of other proteins (*e.g.*, the neurofilament proteins). This represents a recapitulation of the developmental pattern of expression of these proteins.

**Dr. Costa**: To elaborate a little bit more on the priming, second priming stimulus. Did you study changes in the messenger? Is there a further increase of the messenger RNA for the tubulins or not when you....

**Dr. Hoffman**: In other words, with the second lesion. We have not specifically looked at that, but that is a very good question. In other words, if you injure it a second time do you get a further induction?

**Dr. Bray**: Yes, my question was really a follow-up to Dr. Morrison's. Would you predict from what you know, Paul, about peripheral nerves, that in the unmyelinated portion of the retinal ganglion cell axons that their transport rates would be different than in the optic nerve, where they are myelinated?

**Dr. Hoffman**: The method we use to study axonal transport (*i.e.*, pulse-labeling with radioactive amino acids) lacks the resolution necessary to answer that question. I suspect that there may be differences in axonal transport in myelinated and unmyelinated portions of the same axon. Real-time imaging techniques have been used to examine the movement of fluorescent tubulin in cultured neurons. Perhaps these techniques could also be used to investigate transport in the intra-retinal portions of optic nerve axons.

**Dr. Ransom**: There has been a lot of complementary work that has been done on the fish nervous system. There is the capacity of the intact organism to regenerate an optic nerve that is perfectly functional and correctly connected afterwards. So it seems to me that there are a rich number of possibilities to study this further, say, for example, in the fish. Your theory predicts that there would be plenty of class $\beta_{II}$-tubulin normally transported in the fish nervous system. Moreover, Claudia Strummer, who has been doing a lot of this work, is showing that oligodendrocytes are absolutely critical to the capacity of fish as well as other nervous systems to regenerate. So there has to be a signal that is transported retrograde. I would be curious to have any of your comments on that point. There must be signals going in the other direction, and perhaps they can be studied by some of the same kinds of approaches that you have used to study transport in the other direction.

**Dr. Hoffman**: So your point is that there is something that is probably having an effect on the level of synthesis within the neuron cell body that is coming from either the target or from the ensheathing cells? There are two issues here. The first concerns the neuron's intrinsic capacity to support regeneration. The second is whether there are substances in the central nervous system, possibly associated with myelin, which actively block regeneration in much the same way that regeneration stops in the peripheral nerves when regenerating axons reach their targets. Sensory fibers are capable of effective regeneration in the dorsal root, where they are myelinated by Schwann cells. When these regenerating axons reach the root entry zone of the spinal cord (and encounter the central nervous system environment) regeneration stops. Thus, factors in the central nervous system environment can block the regeneration of axons which clearly have the capacity to regenerate in the peripheral nerves. The question is whether optic nerve fibers normally have the capacity to regenerate which is repressed in the central nervous system, or does the capacity of optic nerve fibers to regenerate in peripheral nerve graft reflect changes in retinal ganglion cell neurons (*e.g.*, up-regulation of tubulin expression) induced by the graft. Our hypothesis is consistent with the latter possibility.

**Dr. Anderson**: Whether an axon is incapable of growing or it has not been induced to grow and regenerate are separate. The optic nerve axons are thought incapable of regenerating, and yet when you put a peripheral nerve sheath there, they are induced to regenerate, at least some of the nerve fibers are, and I am a little puzzled as to what factor does that. I took the inference from what you said that Schwann cells produced some factors that induced some synthesis and made the nerve capable of growing. That is the same thing as saying it had induced its innate but dormant ability to regenerate. But what is different in the goldfish that allows them do this without a Schwann cell transplant sheath?

**Dr. Hoffman:** I think that there are fundamental differences between the goldfish and mammalian central nervous system. This may involve both the central nervous system environment and the intrinsic ability of these neurons to support regeneration.

**Dr. Anderson**: But, if they are different, it might be critical to know the nature of that difference, because it would tell you what it is that makes one able to grow and the other one not able to grow...

**Dr. Hoffman**: Our approach has been to compare the expression and transport of cytoskeletal proteins in peripheral neurons capable of effective regeneration (*i.e.*, peripheral sensory and motor fibers) and central nervous system neurons which lack effective regeneration (*i.e.*, retinal ganglion cell neurons) within the same species (rat). These comparisons have revealed major differences in tubulin transport in these two systems. This has led us to propose that the regenerative potential of axons is directly related to the amount of tubulin transported in SCb, which, in turn, reflects the level of $\beta_{II}$-tubulin expression. According to this hypothesis, $\beta_{II}$-tubulin is expressed at high enough levels in uninjured sensory neurons to assure the amount of tubulin transported in SCb is sufficient to support effective regeneration. In contrast, the normal level of tubulin expression in retinal ganglion cell neurons is too low to support the transport of significant amounts of tubulin in SCb in optic nerve fibers. Our hope is that factors released by peripheral nerve grafts are capable of increasing tubulin expression in intact retinal ganglion cell neurons, leading to the transport of tubulin in SCb.

**Dr. Anderson**: And so something that would induce it to regenerate. If we assume, as you say, that the ability to regenerate is simply an extreme example of the ability to make minor repairs of small injuries, then this becomes relevant to glaucoma, because glaucoma may be little injuries to the axon at critical points...

**Dr. Hoffman**: That is correct. There is some evidence that tubulin transport is retarded in experimental models of diabetes. Human diabetics appear to have increased susceptibility to compressive injury of peripheral nerve fibers. This raises the possibility that the increased vulnerability to compressive injury in these patients is a consequence of reduced tubulin transport in SCb. If so, increasing the amount of tubulin transported in SCb in intact optic nerve fibers may make these axons less vulnerable to compression, as may occur in glaucoma.

## References


1. Tanaka, E.M. and Kirschner, M.W., Microtubule behavior in the growth cones of living neurons during axon elongation, *J.Cell Biol.*, 115 (1991) 345-363.
2. Yamada, K.M., Spooner, B.S. and Wessels, N.K., Ultrastructure and function of growth cones and axons of cultured nerve cells, *J.Cell Biol.*, 49 (1971) 614-635.
3. Hoffman, P.N. and Griffin, J.W., The control of axonal caliber. In P.J. Dyck, P.K. Thomas, J.W. Griffin, P.A. Low and J.F. Poduslo (Eds.) *Peripheral Neuropathy*, W.B.Saunders, Philadelphia, 1993, pp. 389-402.
4. Friede, R.L. and Samorajski, T., Axonal caliber related to neurofilaments and microtubules in sciatic nerve fibers of rats and mice, *Anat.Rec.*, 167 (1970) 379-388.
5. McQuarrie, I.G., The effect of a conditioning lesion on the regeneration of motor axons, *Brain Res.*, 152 (1978) 597-602.
6. Black, M.M. and Lasek, R.J., Slowing of the rate of axonal regeneration during growth and maturation, *Exp. Neurol.*, 63 (1979) 108-119.
7. Komiya, Y., Slowing with age of the rate of slow axonal flow in bifurcating axons of rat dorsal root ganglion cells, *Brain Res.*, 183 (1980) 477-480.
8. Lasek, R.J. and Hoffman, P.N., The neuronal cytoskeleton, axonal transport and axonal growth, *Cold Spring Harbor Conf.Cell Proliferation*, 3 (1976) 1021-1049.
9. Ochs, S., Effects of maturation and aging on the rate of fast axoplasmic transport in mammalian nerve, *Prog. Brain Res.*, 40 (1973) 349-362.
10. Tsukita, S. and Ishikawa, H., The movement of membranous organelles in axons, *J.Cell Biol.*, 84 (1980) 513-530.
11. Hoffman, P.N. and Lasek, R.J., The slow component of axonal transport: Identification of the major structural polypeptides of the axon and their generality among mammalian neurons, *J.Cell Biol.*, 66 (1975) 351-366.
12. Lasek, R.J., Garner, J.A. and Brady, S.T., Axonal transport of the cytoplasmic matrix, *J.Cell Biol.*, 99 (Suppl.) (1984) 212s-221s.
13. Cleveland, D.W., The multitubulin hypothesis revisited: What have we learned?, *J.Cell Biol.*, 104 (1987) 381-383.
14. Joshi, H.C. and Cleveland, D.W., Differential utilization of β-tubulin isotypes in differentiating neurites, *J.Cell Biol.*, 109 (1989) 663-673.
15. Hoffman, P.N., Expression of GAP-43, a rapidly transported growth-associated protein, and class II β-tubulin, a slowly transported cytoskeletal protein, are coordinated in regenerating neurons, *J.Neurosci.*, 9 (1989) 893-897.
16. Hoffman, P.N. and Cleveland, D.W., Neurofilament and tubulin expression recapitulates the developmental program during axonal regeneration: Induction of a specific β-tubulin isotype, *Proc.Natl.Acad.Sci. USA*, 85 (1988) 4530-4533.
17. Hoffman, P.N., Cleveland, D.W., Griffin, J.W., Landes, P.W., Cowan, N.J. and Price, D.L., Neurofilament gene expression: A major determinant of axonal caliber, *Proc.Natl.Acad.Sci.USA*, 84 (1987) 3472-3476.
18. Moskowitz, P.F., Smith, R., Pickett, J., Frankfurter, A. and Oblinger, M.M., Expression of the class III β-tubulin gene during axonal regeneration of rat dorsal root ganglion neurons, *J.Neurosci.Res.*, 34 (1993) 129-134.
19. Hoffman, P.N., Lopata, M.A., Watson, D.F. and Luduena, R.F., Axonal transport of class II and class III β-tubulin: evidence that the slow component wave represents the movement of only a small fraction of the tubulin in mature motor axons, *J.Cell Biol.*, 119 (1992) 595-604.
20. McQuarrie, I.G., Brady, S.T. and Lasek, R.J., Diversity in the axonal transport of structural proteins: major differences between optic and spinal axons in rat, *J.Neurosci.*, 6 (1986) 1593-1605.
21. So, K.-F. and Aguayo, A.J., Lengthy regrowth of cut axons from ganglion cells after peripheral nerve transplantation into the retina of adult rats., *Brain Res.*, 328 (1985) 349-354.
22. Hoffman, P.N., Pollock, S.C. and Striph, G.G., Altered gene expression after optic nerve transection: reduced neurofilament expression as a general response to axonal injury, *Exp. Neurol.*, 119 (1993) 32-36.
23. McKerracher, L., Essagian, C. and Aguayo, A.J., In situ hybridization analysis of tubulin and neurofilament mRNAs after axonal injury to retinal ganglion cells in the adult rat, *J.Cell Biol.*, 115 (1991) (2299)-396a.
24. McKerracher, L., Vidal-Sanz, M., Essagian, C. and Aguayo, A.J., Selective impairment of slow axonal transport after optic nerve injury in adult rats, *J.Neurosci.*, 10 (1990) 2834-2841.

25. McKerracher, L., Essagian, C. and Aguayo, A.J., Marked increase in β-tubulin mRNA expression during regeneration of axotomized retinal ganglion cells in adult mammals, *J.Neurosci.*, 13 (1993) 5294-5300.
26. McKerracher, L., Vidal-Sanz, M. and Aguayo, A.J., Slow transport rates of cytoskeletal proteins change during regeneration of axotomized retinal neurons in adult rats, *J.Neurosci.*, 10 (1990) 641-648.
27. Meyer, M., Matsuoka, I., Wetmore, C., Olson, L. and Thoenen, H., Enhanced synthesis of brain-derived neurotrophic factor in the lesioned peripheral nerve: different mechanisms are responsible for the regulation of BDNF and NGF mRNA, *J.Cell Biol.*, 119 (1992) 45-54.
28. Liuzzi, F.J. and Lasek, R.J., Astrocytes block axonal regeneration in mammals by activating the physiological stop pathway., *Science*, 237 (1987) 642-645.
29. Caroni, P. and Schwab, M.E., Two membrane fractions from rat central myelin with inhibitory properties for neurite growth and fibroblast spreading, *J.Cell Biol.*, 106 (1988) 1281-1288.

# 8. OPTIC NERVE REGENERATION

GARTH M. BRAY, M.D.

**Dr. Caprioli**: For this session, we have gathered an outstanding group of researchers with international reputations, but in keeping with the flexibility established this morning and the desire to keep contiguous the last presentation with Dr. Bray's presentation about Retinal Ganglion Cell Regeneration, I would like to hold my few introductory comments and introduce Dr. Garth Bray who is at the Center for Neuroscience at McGill University in Montreal, Canada. He is going to tell us more about the extensive work on retinal ganglion cell regeneration.

**Dr. Bray**: My talk this afternoon can be divided into three parts. First, I will review published work concerning the attempts that have been made in Dr. Albert Aguayo's laboratory to reconstruct one part of the nervous system – the optic nerve, by using peripheral nerve grafts. Second, I will discuss our studies of retinal ganglion cell death and the attempts to rescue these injured neurons. Finally, I will describe some recent work on the correlations between retinal ganglion cell survival and axonal growth. This final part of my talk relates to what was said in the preceding talk and will certainly be relevant to some of the things that are going to be discussed in the talk that follows.

I should explain at the outset that we use a cut of the optic nerve in adult rats as our experimental model. The optic nerve is cut close to the eye as a caricature of various types of optic nerve injury. Attempts to entice retinal ganglion cell axons to regrow into segments of peripheral nerve are not new. For example, in 1914, Leoz and Arcaute, students of Ramon y Cajal, cut the optic nerve in rabbits and attached a segment of peripheral nerve. In one of ten animals, the peripheral nerve remained attached to the optic nerve[1]. Using Cajal's silver stains, Leoz and Arcaute found that some axons appeared to grow from the optic nerve stump into the peripheral nerve graft. Ramon y Cajal observed this phenomenon in other parts of the nervous system. After several years, however, these observations were challenged. In particular, Clark[2], the Oxford University anatomist, argued that most of the axons that grew into peripheral nerve grafts arose from peripheral nerves that had been interrupted at the time of grafting.

In the early 1980s, Albert Aguayo and colleagues[3-5] used retrogradely transported tracers to prove, in effect, that Ramon y Cajal and his students were correct. This was done by inserting segments of peripheral nerve into the brain or spinal cord and, after time to allow for axonal growth, applying a retrograde tracer to the end of the nerve graft and demonstrating that neuronal cell bodies in the CNS had extended their axons into the peripheral nerve grafts. Moreover, these axons extended for distances of 3–4 cm to the end of the graft[4,5]. In the visual system, it was subsequently demonstrated that retinal ganglion cells would also regrow their interrupted axons into peripheral nerve grafts[6,7]. As discussed earlier by Paul Hoffman, the results of these experiments established the principle that the non-neuronal environment of injured axons influences whether or not there is axonal regrowth: CNS axons regrow in the milieu of peripheral nerves but not in that of the central nervous system.

Let me describe the method of grafting peripheral nerve segments to the optic nerve in greater detail. Figure 1 illustrates the model for optic nerve reconstruction

*Optic Nerve in Glaucoma, pp. 135–149*
*edited by S.M. Drance*

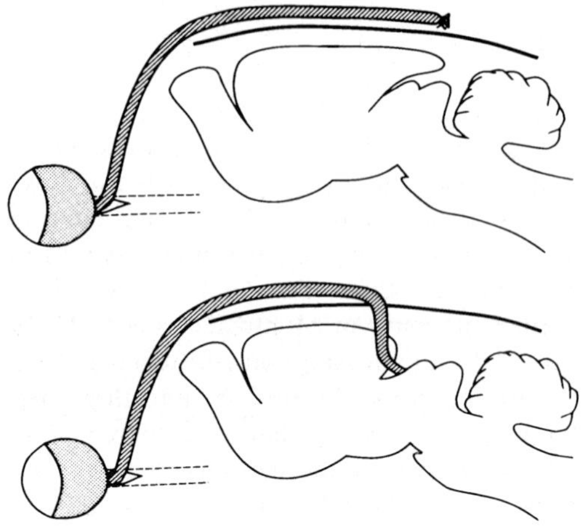

*Fig. 1.* Diagram of a peripheral nerve graft (hatched) connected to the ocular stump of an optic nerve transected close to the eye in adult rats or hamsters. *Top*: At the time of graft attachment, the distal end of the autologous graft is placed blind-ended between the scalp and the skull. *Bottom*: After eight to ten weeks to permit the growth of retinal ganglion cell axons, the end of the graft was inserted into the superior colliculus, the main target of these axons in rodents. Two to 18 months later, orthogradely transported tracers were injected into the vitreous to label regenerating retinal ganglion cell axons and their terminals. (Reproduced with permission from Aguayo *et al.*[12].)

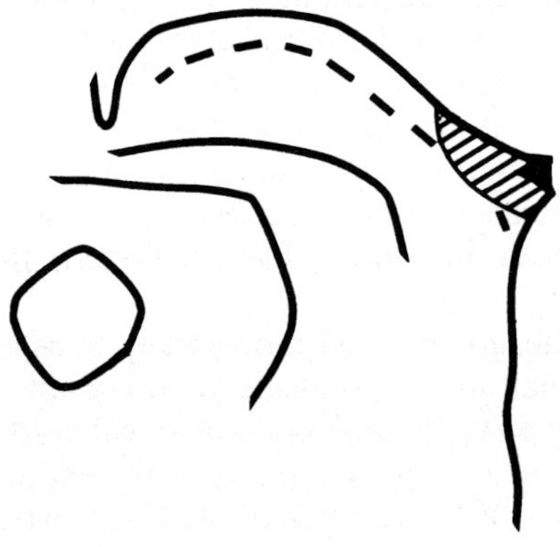

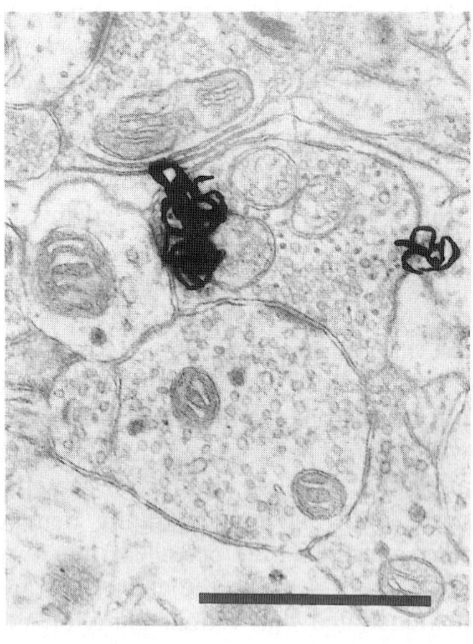

*Fig. 2.* Regeneration of retinal ganglion cell axons into the superior colliculus. *Left*: Camera lucida drawing of a transverse midbrain section illustrating the penetration of the superficial laminae (above the broken line) by regenerating axons and their terminals. The solid area represents the end of the nerve graft; the hatched area delineates the region in which there was labeling with HRP orthogradely transported from the eye. (Reproduced with permission from Carter *et al.*[8]). *Right*: Electron microscopic autoradiogram of a regenerated retinal ganglion cell axon terminal in the superior colliculus of a rat 16 months after the eye and the midbrain were connected by a peripheral nerve graft. The rat received [$^3$H]-labeled amino acids intraocularly two days before perfusion fixation. The regenerated terminal contains round vesicles and pale mitochondria, and contacts the vesicle-containing dendritic process of a collicular neuron. Bar = 1 μm. (Reproduced with permission from Vidal-Sanz *et al.*[13].)

that was developed by Manuel Vidal-Sanz. Taking advantage of the location of the ophthalmic artery in the infero-medial dura of the optic nerve, the whole optic nerve was cut as close to the eye as possible in adult rats. A segment of autologous sciatic nerve was attached to the short stump of the optic nerve. The remainder of the peripheral nerve graft was placed over the skull. After several weeks, HRP was applied to the end of the graft and two days later the retina was removed, flat-mounted on a glass slide, and stained for HRP activity. The presence of HRP-labeled ganglion cells in the retina indicated that their axons had grown to the end of the graft. By injecting anterogradely transported tracers (HRP, rhodamine isothiocyanate, or tritiated amino acids) into the vitreous chamber of the eye, we were also able to examine the growth of regenerating ganglion cell axons along the peripheral nerve grafts and into selected CNS targets[7-9].

Within the nerve grafts, the axonal growth cone was opposed to the Schwann cell basal lamina or to the Schwann cell cytoplasm itself. This finding may be explained by observations, mentioned by Paul Hoffman, that when retinal ganglion cells regrow their axons into nerve grafts, they change their expression of ß-tubulin[10]. When retinal ganglion cells regenerate their axons into peripheral nerve grafts, they also acquire the ability to express ß-integrin[11], a component of the receptor for components of the extracellular matrix of peripheral nerve.

To determine if these regenerating retinal ganglion cell axons would re-enter the central nervous system, the distal end of each peripheral nerve graft was inserted into the superior colliculus, which is the target of most retinal ganglion cell axons in rodents (Fig. 1, bottom). In adult rats or hamsters, the graft was left over the skull for several weeks and then inserted into the midbrain[7-9,13]. After intervals of several weeks to months, HRP was injected into the vitreous chamber and two days later, sections of the superior colliculi were processed to identify the axon terminals that had been labeled by anterograde transport of the tracer. Six to eight weeks after graft insertion into the superior colliculus, axon terminals were present up to 0.5 mm from the end of the graft[8]. At four to six months, this growth had extended up to 1 mm in hamsters[9]. These axon terminals were located in the superficial layers of the superior colliculus, which are retino-recipient (Fig. 2). Such terminals were capable of trans-synaptic activation of superior colliculi neurons in reponse to light flashed in the eye[14] and persisted for the life span of hamsters[9] and rats[13]. The properties of these regenerated retinal ganglion cell axon terminals in the superior colliculi are summarized in Table 1.

Early in the course of these studies, it became apparent that axotomy near the neuronal cell body was necessary if neurons were to extend their axons into peripheral nerve grafts[6,15]. But we also knew that the closer the lesion was to the cell body, the more likely was the axotomy to cause neuronal death. For this reason, we embarked upon a study to quantitate the effects of axotomy of retinal ganglion cell survival at various times after optic nerve lesion[16,17]. For these experiments, we used retrogradely transported tracers that, when applied to the superior colliculi and lateral geniculate nuclei, labeled all retinal ganglion cells. The number of retinal ganglion cells labeled with diI remains unchanged for up to 22 months while fluorogold-labeled neurons persist for at least 3 months.

Let me make five points about the fate of axotomized retinal ganglion cells (Table 2). First, retinal ganglion cell axotomy caused by cutting the optic nerve close to the eye causes a marked loss of RGCs. Approximately 90% of these neurons die by two weeks after the lesion. Second, the effect of axotomy on retinal ganglion

*Table 1.*

Regenerated Retinal Ganglion Cell Axons:
- growing along peripheral nerve grafts,
  - associate with Schwann cells,
  - can change retinal ganglion cell gene expression;
- re-enter the superior colliculus;
- form well-differentiated synapses that:
  - are functional,
  - persist,
  - show laminar specificity,
  - have appropriate post-synaptic domains,
  - increase in number,
  - mature in terms of their morphology.

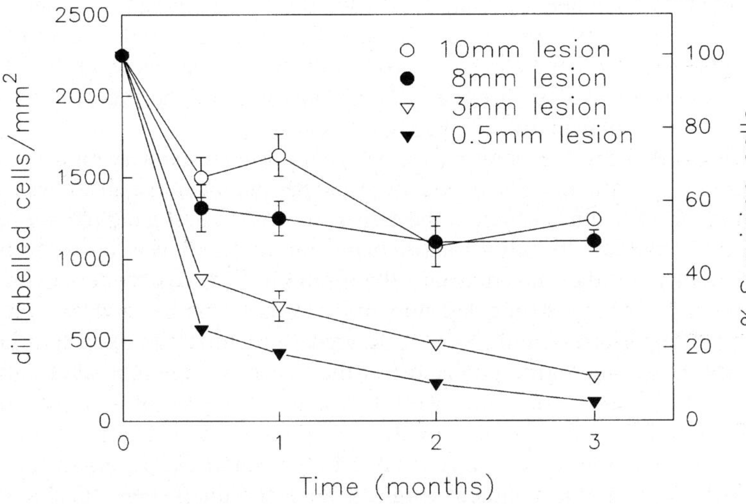


*Fig. 3.* Densities of retinal ganglion cells, expressed as numbers of diI-labeled cells/mm$^2$, in standard areas of adult rats two weeks to three months after optic nerve interruption. Data points represent the means of four to six retinas; standard errors of the mean are shown where greater than the size of the symbols. By two weeks after axotomy, there was an abrupt loss of retinal ganglion cells that was more severe when the optic nerve was cut close to the eye. This early retinal ganglion cell loss was followed by more gradual declines in retinal ganglion cell densities. (Reproduced with permission from Villegas-Pérez *et al.*[16].)

cell survival is related to the distance of the lesion from the eye (Fig. 3). We have quantitated this phenomenon[16] that was described in qualitative terms by earlier investigators[18-20].

**Dr. Quigley**: Could you explain more precisely where the optic nerve lesions were located?

**Speaker**: The distances in Figure 3 refer to the location of the optic nerve transection as measured from the back of the eye.

*Table 2.*

| Retinal Ganglion Cell Death after Axotomy is: |
|---|
| – severe, |
| – related to the site of lesion, |
| – characterized by early severe and later protracted phases, |
| – delayed in onset, |
| – apoptotic. |

**Dr. Quigley**: Your data show that 60% of the retinal ganglion cells were still surviving three months after optic nerve transection 10 mm from the eye in rats (Fig. 3). This result is different from that obtained in monkeys where nearly all RGCs would have died by this time[21].

**Speaker**: The third point about the retinal ganglion cell loss after axotomy is that there are two main phases that can be defined mathematically. There is an early acute phase, lasting approximately two weeks, followed by a more protracted phase of retinal ganglion cell loss (Fig. 3).

**Dr. Anderson**: May I interrupt? Just as Harry said, that does not happen in the monkey. When we transected the optic nerve, the axons survive the initial injury for six to eight weeks and then they all die[21]. There is not such a thing as lasting three months for any of them.

**Speaker**: Perhaps the difference between your data and ours reflects differences between rodents and monkeys.

**Dr. Quigley**: And the distal optic nerve that would undergo Wallerian degeneration was completely degenerate?

**Speaker**: Yes.

**Dr. Quigley**: Do you have any explanation for that? It would be almost unheard of for an axon that is cut to survive without hitting a target?

**Speaker**: There may be an answer to your question in the last part of my talk.

The fourth point concerning the effect of optic nerve transection is that the onset of retinal ganglion cell loss is delayed (Fig. 4). When the optic nerve is cut 0.5 mm from the eye, retinal ganglion cell densities remain normal for four days and then there is an abrupt loss of these neurons. On the other hand, if the optic nerve is cut intracranially (approximately 9 mm from the eye), the onset of RGC loss is delayed until Day 8. This delay is not just a matter of the retinal ganglion cells being dead but not disappearing; as Paul Hoffman mentioned in his talk, Lisa McKerracher has shown that retinal ganglion cell expression of mRNAs for tubulin as well as GAP-DH (an enzyme of the glycolytic cycle) remained at normal levels until approximately one week after an intracranial lesion[10].

The fifth point I wish to make concerning the death of axotomized RGCs concerns the type of death that affects these injured neurons. The onset of the abrupt decline in the number of retinal ganglion cells coincides with the development of retinal ganglion cells with the appearance of apoptosis[17]. Retinal ganglion cells are ob-

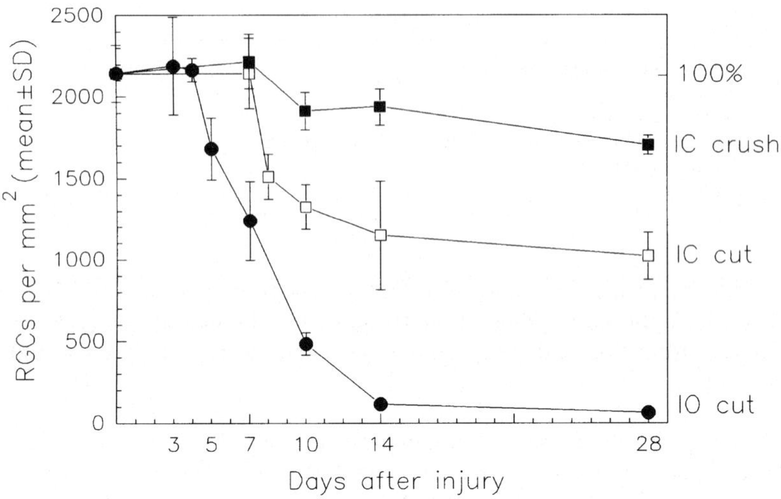


*Fig. 4.* Densities of fluorogold-labeled retinal ganglion cells in standard areas of flat-mounted retinas. Data points indicate mean ± SD for groups of three to six experimental rats and eight control (Day 0) rats. With intraorbital (IO) lesions, retinal ganglion cell loss was first noted on Day 5; with intracranial (IC) lesions, retinal ganglion cell loss began on Day 8. (Reproduced with permission from Berkelaar *et al.*[17].)

served that show fragmentation and shrinkage of their nuclear chromatin on Feulgen stains for DNA and, using the TUNEL reaction[22], show histochemical evidence for DNA fragmentation, a characteristic feature of apoptosis[23]. The appearance of apoptotic retinal ganglion cell implies that the death of these neurons is caused by an intrinsic cell process. In this experimental situation, this process has been initiated by the axotomy.

Apoptosis is a form of cell death that is seen in neurons as well as other cells during development, as well as neurons *in vitro* or *in vivo* that are deprived of their trophic factors. The finding of apoptotic retinal ganglion cells after optic nerve transection may indicate that the death of these neurons was precipitated by the loss of trophic support from the target and along the pathway of their axons in the optic nerve but other mechanisms may be involved as well.

**Dr. Choi**: Do you have evidence that the fragmentation is appropriate for apoptosis? Do you have any different size fragments on a gel or anything like that?

**Speaker**: We did not analyze these retinas for DNA "ladders", the biochemical criterion for DNA fragmentation. We were disuaded from doing such an analysis for two reasons: retinal ganglion cells represent only a small proportion of the cells in the retina and, because apoptotic cells disappear in a matter of hours (*e.g.* ref. 23), there are only a small number of apoptotic retinal ganglion cells in the retina at any one time. Thus, we used an *in situ* method[22] to demonstrate DNA fragmentation histochemically[17].

**Dr. Quigley**: We can corroborate that it is difficult to show the ladder pattern on a gel in an experimental glaucoma model looking for apoptosis, though the *in situ* method

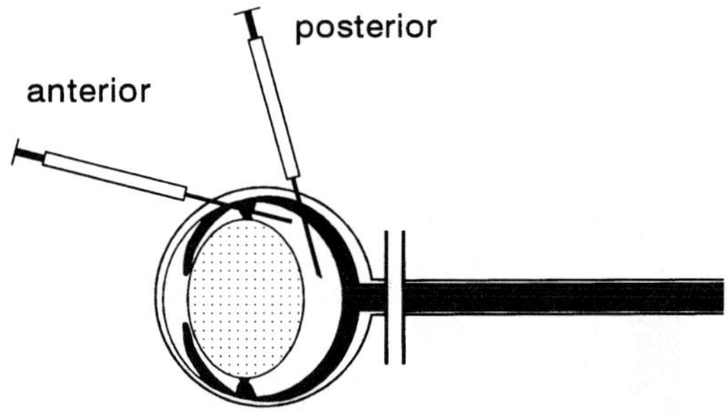


*Fig. 5.* Diagram illustrating the anterior and posterior routes of injection into the vitreous chamber. For anterior injections, the needle was inserted through the cornea-sclera junction and pierced the margin of the iris and the ciliary body to reach the vitreous chamber. For posterior injections, the needle was inserted through the sclera and retina at a distance of approximately three mm from the optic nerve. (Reproduced with permission from Clarke *et al.*[27].)

is another story. We hope to be able to figure out a way to do that even though there is only a selective amount of the DNA that is dying by that particular method.

**Speaker**: I want to move on now to a discussion of the possibility of rescuing these injured retinal ganglion cells. We turned to growth factors because there is *in vitro* evidence that brain-derived neurotrophic factor (BDNF) sustains these neurons in tissue culture[24,25]. We were also encouraged to study BDNF and related neurotrophins because retinal ganglion cells expressed *trk*B, the high affinity receptor for BDNF[26]. This was demonstrated immunocytochemically using an antibody to *trk*B and by *in situ* hybridization histochemistry using a probe for *trk*B mRNA.

Our methods for studying the effects of neurotrophins on retinal ganglion cell survival involved intraocular injections after optic nerve transection near the eye (Fig. 5). We label retinal ganglion cells by retrograde transport of a persistent fluorescent tracer and determine the densities of surviving retinal ganglion cells in standard retinal areas. The results of one series of such experiments are shown in Figure 6. In intact retinas, the density of retinal ganglion cells is 2200 to 2300/mm$^2$. With no injections, retinal ganglion cell densities decrease to approximately 50% by one week and to 10% or less by two weeks. A single injection of BDNF at the time of optic nerve transection leads to the survival of virtually all axotomized retinal ganglion cells at one week. Although retinal ganglion cells are progressively lost at 10 days and two weeks, significantly more of these axotomized neurons survive in the eyes that had received BDNF injections. Similar short-term "rescues" of axotomized retinal ganglion cells can be obtained with single intraocular injections of NT-4[27], a neurotrophin related to BDNF. In subsequent experiments, we have been able to expand the duration of this survival by continuous administration of the trophin with Alzet minipumps.

**Dr. Quigley**: I wonder if you could tell us whether or not any of the ganglion cells actually continued to survive beyond the control rate: in other words, beyond 14 days to 21 or 28 days. Where does the BDNF curve finally intersect the control curve?

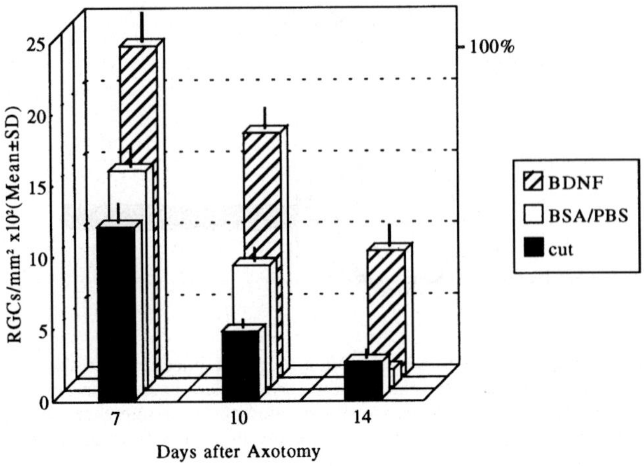


*Fig. 6.* Effects of BDNF injections (hatched bars), control injections (open bars), or no injections (solid bars) on retinal ganglion cell densities after optic nerve transection. One week after a single posterior injection of BDNF into the vitreous chamber, retinal ganglion cell densities were similar to those of intact retinas but were 77% and 57% respectively of the control-injected and uninjected retinas, respectively. At 10 and 14 days after axotomy, significantly more retinal ganglion cells survived with BDNF injections than with control or no injections. (Reproduced with permission from Mansour-Robaey *et al.*[28].)

**Speaker**: The answer to that question depends on the route of administration. If the BDNF was administered through the posterior retina, as is illustrated in Figure 6, there is no effect by 28 days. With the anterior route of administration, which I will discuss shortly, there is a more sustained effect that can last as long as 28 days: 15% of retinal ganglion cells survive with repeated anterior injections of BDNF but without any injection, only 3% of retinal ganglion cells survive for this time[28].

**Dr. Quigley**: It is terribly exciting to all of us who have always thought that ganglion cells could not make any kind of comeback after axotomy to see that growth factors can do this. I think one difficulty that has arisen in the literature is the use of the word “rescue”. That word has been used repeatedly in a number of laboratories to describe the prolonging of the cell survival, but it is not yet, unfortunately, rescuing these neurons. So that it is important, I think, when people look at these curves, not to think that the actual number that have survived has been prolonged yet, unfortunately.

**Speaker**: As mentioned earlier, our studies have also demonstrated that there is an intraocular source for sustaining the survival of retinal ganglion cells. In other words, some of the trophic effects of posterior administration of BDNF or NT-4 on retinal ganglion cells can be reproduced by anterior eye punctures or by anterior injections of PBS/BSA lacking neurotrophins[28]. These effects appear to be due to injury of structures in the anterior part of the eye, such as the iris and/or ciliary body (Fig. 5). We have some evidence the iris may be an important intraocular source of molecules that can support retinal ganglion cell survival. While it was previously demonstrated that the iris can release NGF[29], we have found that this structure also expresses BDNF and NT-4 mRNAs (Jelsma, Clarke, Bray and Aguayo, unpublished

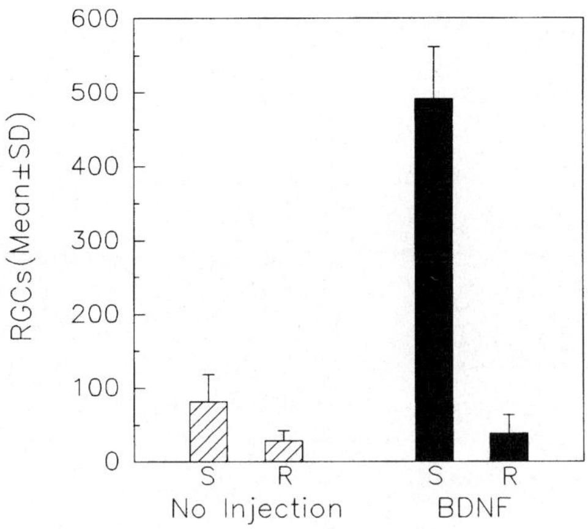


*Fig. 7.* Effects of intraocular injections of BDNF on retinal ganglion cell survival (S) and on the regeneration (R) of retinal ganglion cell axons into a peripheral nerve graft six weeks after optic nerve transection and graft attachment. In spite of the five-fold increase in the number of retinal ganglion cells that survived in the BDNF-treated group, the number of retinal ganglion cells that regenerated their axons into the peripheral nerve grafts was not significantly different in the two groups. (Data reproduced with permission from Mansour-Robaey *et al.*[28].)

observations). Thus, trophic factors produced by Schwann cells or muscle fibers in the iris may act intraocularly to influence neuronal survival and growth.

In addition to trophic factors for retinal ganglion cells within the eye, the mRNAs for BDNF and for NT-4 are also present within the optic nerve (Jelsma, Berkelaar, Bray and Aguayo, unpublished observations). We postulate that the presence of such trophic factors in the optic nerve explains the greater survival of retinal ganglion cells after optic nerve lesions far from the eye (Fig. 3). In other words, with lesions nearly 1 cm from the eye, there is a longer optic nerve to provide those retinal ganglion cells with this trophic factor.

Thus, we would propose that there are multiple sites of trophic support for retinal ganglion cells – in the eye, along the optic nerve, and from the target.

In the final part of my talk, I want to present the results of experiments designed to test the hypothesis that increasing the survival of retinal ganglion cells after axotomy would increase the number of retinal ganglion cell axons that grow into peripheral nerve grafts. For these experiments, we retrogradely labeled retinal ganglion cells by applying fluorogold to the superior colliculus, cut the optic nerve close to the eye, and attached a peripheral nerve graft with its distal end left under the scalp. At the time of optic nerve transection, and on Day 3 and 5, BDNF was injected into the vitreous. As illustrated in Figure 7, increasing the survival of axotomized retinal ganglion cells with BDNF did not result in the growth of a greater number of axons into the peripheral nerve graft.

Why could this be? The first clue came from experiments in which the intraretinal ganglion cell axons were immunostained with an antibody to neurofilaments (Fig. 8). These studies demonstrated that following BDNF injections, there was a proliferation of retinal ganglion cell axons around the optic disc when BDNF was given intraocularly. Thus, there was increased growth of intraretinal axons but these axons

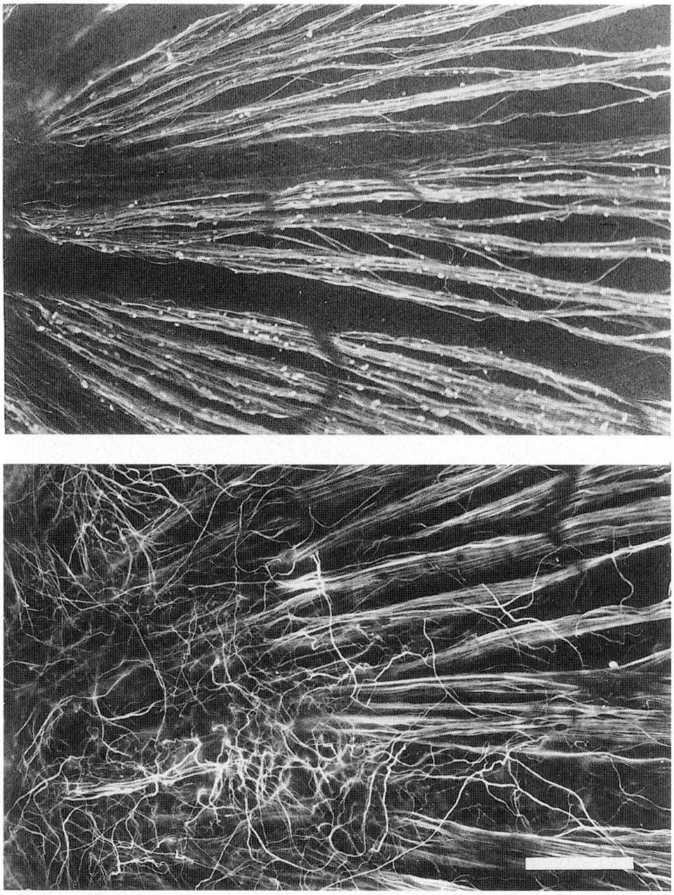

*Fig. 8.* Retinal flat-mounts showing retinal ganglion cell axons immunostained with an antibody (RT-97) that recognizes the phosphorylated 200-kDa neurofilament subunit. Retinal segments adjacent to the optic disc (on the left) two weeks after optic nerve transection. *Top*: Optic nerve transection without injections. The axon bundles are small and many degenerating fibers have a beaded appearance. There is no outgrowth of retinal ganglion cell axons at the origin of the optic nerve. *Bottom*: BDNF injections on Day 0, 3, 7, and 10 after optic nerve transection. There is a profusion of axonal processes near the optic disc. Bar = 100 μm. (Reproduced with permission from Mansour-Robaey *et al.*[28].)

did not make their way into the peripheral nerve grafts that had been attached to the short optic nerve stump.

To get a better understanding of what was happening to individual retinal ganglion cell axons in the retina, Dr. Hajime Sawai developed an *in vitro* method to label individual retinal ganglion cells and their axons. With this method of labeling, it is possible to trace the axons of individual retinal ganglion cells to the optic disc. We have studied retinal ganglion cells that were intact, axotomized, treated with BDNF or other neurotrophins, or had a peripheral nerve graft attached to the optic nerve stump.

If retinal ganglion cells are axotomized by transecting the optic nerve near the back of the eye, individual retinal ganglion cell axons retract from the optic disc within a few days. They subsequently make 180° turns and grow away from the retina. By increasing the number of retinal ganglion cells that survive for two weeks, administration of BDNF causes increases in the total number of axons that turn or branch at the optic nerve head.

Such results suggest that the environment of the optic disc is either inhibitory or non-permissive to axonal growth. Thus, you can appreciate my interest in this morning's discussion about the composition of the optic disc and the lamina cribrosa. During normal development, retinal ganglion cell axons grow directly through the optic disc and into the optic nerve. It has been assumed that the main reason that axons failed to grow into the optic nerve in adult animals was related to the presence of myelin-associated inhibitory molecules[30]. However, these results indicate that there is also a "block" to axonal growth at the level of the optic disc, where there is no myelin. We speculate that the growth-inhibiting cells at the optic disc are the astrocytes, which are present in great abundance at the disc as opposed to other parts of the retina.

**Dr. Quigley**: It seems to me that when you cut right at the back of the eye, it is possible that a certain portion of the axon, less than 1 mm, might die as a part of the crush injury. You then have an axon which, I was led to believe when I first looked at Dr. Sawai's beautiful tracings, had grown from the ganglion cell all the way across the retina but when it reached the disc, it turned around; that is, it almost made it. Rather, I think, is it not the case that the axon dies back just a little bit up into the eye and the growth cone starts near the disc? It is a question of whether the axon dies into the disc and then goes out. Maybe some of them do not do that but make a turn from where they were starting their new growth cone.

**Speaker**: The retinal ganglion cell axons that turn away from the optic disc are apparent by two weeks. If one looks at these retinas 1 week after the optic nerve has been cut, you see a retraction or dying-back of the retinal ganglion cell axons for approximately 600 μm from the optic disc with the appearance of growth cones. So Dr. Quigley is correct in suggesting that most axons may only die back into the retina for short distances. As they attempt to regrow, their growth cones appear to be unable to penetrate the optic disc. When a peripheral nerve graft is attached, some of these axons are able to grow into this environment.

So we have to consider two barriers to axonal regrowth in the optic nerve (Table 3). The first is at the level of the optic disc and the lamina cribrosa, where the axons are not myelinated. The second barrier is the one within the myelinated portion of the optic nerve[30]. The attachment of a peripheral nerve graft close to the eye presumably changes the environment that is responsible for the second barrier but the barrier at the optic disc may remain intact.

In summary, we view these experimental attempts to reconstruct the interrupted retino-fugal pathway as facing two important challenges: *1.* the development of approaches that lead to more persistent survival of axotomized retinal ganglion cells; and, *2.* overcoming the different barriers to regrowth that are present at the optic disc and in the optic nerve.

**Dr. Drance**: When you talked about the anterior injection of trophins, you had to go through iris or other structures. I assume, however, that you were aiming to put the material in the posterior vitreous.

*Table 3.*

| Different Growth Environments for Regenerating Retinal Ganglion Cell Axons |
|---|
| – within the retina, |
| – at the optic disc, |
| – in the optic nerve. |

**Dr. Bray**: That is correct. The injecting needle is inserted through the periphery of the iris into the vitreous body (Fig. 5). We try to avoid the lens because such an injury causes it to opacify and adhere to the retina.

**Dr. Quigley**: In every animal you would have a natural experiment of distance from the injury by looking in the more peripheral retina compared to the more posterior pole. Can you give us an idea of death rates peripherally versus centrally, and is there a difference in cell size in terms of death?

**Dr. Bray**: Your first question, concerning the survival of retinal ganglion cells at different distances from the optic disc, was addressed in the experiments of Villegas-Pérez *et al.*[16]. As our measure of retinal ganglion cell densities, we counted diI-labeled neurons in standard areas 1, 2, and 3 mm from the optic disc. Compared to the numbers of retinal ganglion cells in intact retinas, which are greater in the areas closer to the disc, more retinal ganglion cells survived at 3 mm than at 1 mm from the disc.

The second question relates to the possibility that certain classes of retinal ganglion cells are selectivity vulnerable to injury or to the rescue effects of neurotrophins. We have the impression that the largest retinal ganglion cells are most succeptible to injury and to rescue. However, this is difficult to prove in the intracellular labeling studies because it is much easier to label the large neurons with this technique.

**Dr. Choi**: Is the death rate following transection fast enough that you can do pharmacological studies? Can you predict at least that there are few cells that are supposed to die in an epoch, so that you could try to see if, for example, transcription or translation inhibitors would stop the death?

**Dr. Bray**: The loss of retinal ganglion cells begins five days after intraorbital lesions and eight days after intracranial lesions (Fig. 4). Prior to the onset of retinal ganglion cell loss, the retinas are normal in appearance. Thus, the death rates are quite predictable. Such retinal ganglion cell densities also correlate with the expression of tubulin mRNA in the retina[10]. However, the possibility of influencing the death of these neurons with inhibitors of protein transcription or translation *in vivo* is complicated. Thanos *et al.*[31] have reported that retinal ganglion cell death can be curtailed by the administration of substances that inhibit microglia and macrophages. Thus, if inhibitors of macromolecular synthesis had an effect, it could be an indirect one on microglia.

**Dr. Kapin**: Dr. Bray, are you aware of any cell salvage studies that have been done with crush injury as opposed to transection of the optic nerve?

**Dr. Bray**: I am not aware that such studies have been done. It is an important issue because of the substantial differences of cut and crush injury on the survival of retinal ganglion cells[17] (Fig. 4).

**Dr. Anderson**: You promised earlier on that you would explain the difference between rodents and monkeys with regard to the number of cells that survive long-term. In the meantime, I thought of an explanation. We observed that, after cutting the optic nerve, the cells were perfectly healthy within the retina, as we observed them, until some time between six or eight weeks, and then all of a sudden all of the cells died[21]. A possible explanation for the discrepancy between what we thought we observed and what you are observing is that 95% of them die and 5% survive, and we did not recognize the 5% that were surviving. But I thought you were going to say something on that there was a species difference that accounted for this.

**Dr. Bray**: In addition to the different methods used to assay the survival of the axotomized retinal ganglin cells[16,21], I was going to suggest that the longer optic nerve in the monkey might have an effect. I do not have an alternate explanation for the difference between the species. However, I do believe that the demonstration of the survival and growth of retinal ganglion cell axons within the retina (Sawai *et al.*, unpublished observations) represents a partial answer to Dr. Quigley's earlier question concerning the apparent paradox of the survival of neurons when axons are disconnected from their target. These studies, as well as those involving anterior eye injury, indicate that the intraretinal milieu is conducive to neuronal survival and axonal growth.

**Dr. Quigley**: I was going to guess that, in a rat, to get eight to ten mm away from the eye, do not you have to do it intracranially?

**Dr. Bray**: That is correct.

**Dr. Quigley**: So you are giving those cells an opportunity to retarget some other central nervous system cell and to find a new target. So my guess was going to be that if you had done serial sections and autoradiography from an intravitreal injection, you might have found that they ultimately wound up targeting some cell.

**Dr. Bray**: Although we have not done the precise experiments you mention, all our lesions were made before the optic nerve has any branches or its axons have the opportunity to contact other neurons. Thus, we think it is more likely that retinal ganglion cells may receive trophic support via their axons in the optic nerve stump rather than by developing new contacts.

## References

1. Leoz Ortin, G. and L.R. Arcuate (1914) Procesos regenerativos del nervio óptico y retina con ocasión de injertos nerviosos. *Trab. Lab. Invest. Biol.* 11: 239-254.

2. Clark, W.E.Legros (1942) The problem of neuronal regeneration in the central nervous system. I.The influence of spinal ganglia and nerve fragments grafted in the brain. *J. Anat.* 77: 20-48.
3. Richardson, P.M., U. McGuinness, and A.J. Aguayo (1980) Axons from CNS neurons regenerate into PNS grafts. *Nature* 284: 264-265.
4. David, S. and A.J. Aguayo (1981) Axonal elongation into PNS "bridges" after CNS injury in adult rats. *Science* 214: 931-933.
5. Benfey, M. and A.J. Aguayo (1982) Extensive elongation of axons from rat brain into peripheral nerve grafts. *Nature* 296: 150-152.
6. So, K.-F. and A.J. Aguayo (1985) Lengthy regrowth of cut axons from ganglion cells after peripheral nerve transplantation into the retina of adult rats. *Brain Res.* 328: 349-354.
7. Vidal-Sanz, M., G.M. Bray, M.P. Villegas-Pérez, S. Thanos, and A.J. Aguayo (1987) Axonal regeneration and synapse formation in the superior colliculus by retinal ganglion cells in the adult rat. *J. Neurosci.* 7: 2894-2909.
8. Carter, D.A., G.M. Bray, and A.J. Aguayo (1989) Regenerated retinal ganglion cell axons can form well-differentiated retinal ganglion cell axons in the superior colliculus of adult hamsters. *J. Neurosci.* 9: 4042-4050.
9. Carter, D.A., G.M. Bray, and A.J. Aguayo (1994) Long-term growth and remodelling of regenerated retino-collicular connections in adult hamsters. *J. Neurosci.* 14: 590-598.
10. McKerracher, L., C. Essagian, and A.J. Aguayo (1993) Marked increase in ß-tubulin mRNA expression during regeneration of axotomized retinal ganglion cells in adult mammals. *J. Neurosci.* 13: 5294-5300.
11. Knoops, B., S. Carbonetto, and A.J. Aguayo (1993) Beta-1 Integrin subunit expression by central nervous system neurons is regulated following contact with the environment of the peripheral nervous system. *Soc. Neurosci. Abstr.* 19: 679.
12. Aguayo, A.J., M. Vidal-Sanz, M.P. Villegas-Pérez, and G.M. Bray (1987) Growth and connectivity of axotomized retinal neurons in adult rats with optic nerves substituted by PNS grafts linking the eye and the midbrain. *Ann. NY. Acad. Sci.* 495: 1-9.
13. Vidal-Sanz, M., G.M. Bray, and A.J. Aguayo (1991) Regenerated synapses persist in the superior colliculus after the regrowth of retinal ganglion cell axons. *J. Neurocytol.* 20: 940-952.
14. Keirstead, S.A., M. Rasminsky, Y. Fukuda, D.A. Carter, A.J. Aguayo, and M. Vidal-Sanz (1989) Electrophysiologic responses in hamster superior colliculus evoked by regenerating retinal axons. *Science* 246: 255-258.
15. Richardson, P.M., V.M.K. Issa, and A.J. Aguayo (1984) Regeneration of long spinal axons in the rat. *J. Neurocytol.* 13: 162-184.
16. Villegas-Pérez, M.P., M. Vidal-Sanz, M. Rasminsky, G.M. Bray, and A.J. Aguayo (1993) Rapid and protracted phases of retinal ganglion cell loss follow axotomy in the optic nerve of adult rats. *J. Neurobiol.* 24: 23-36.
17. Berkelaar, M., D.B. Clarke, Y.-C. Wang, G.M. Bray, and A.J. Aguayo (1994) Axotomy results in delayed death and apoptosis of retinal ganglion cells in adult rats. *J. Neurosci.* 14: 4368-4374.
18. Leinfelder, P.J. (1938) Retrograde degeneration in the optic nerves and retinal ganglion cells. *Trans. Am. Ophthalmol. Soc.* 36: 307-315.
19. Mantz, J. and M. Klein (1951) Modifications histologiques de al retine après interruption du nerf optique. *Compt. Rend. Soc. Biol.* 145: 922-924.
20. Radius, R.L. and D.R. Anderson (1978) Retinal ganglion cell degeneration in experimental optic atrophy. *Am. J. Ophthalmol.* 86: 673-679.
21. Quigley, H.A., E.B. Davis, and D.R. Anderson (1977) Descending optic nerve degeneration in primates. Invest. *Ophthalmol. Vis. Sci.* 16: 841-849.
22. Gavrieli, Y., Y. Sherman, and S.A. Ben-Sasson (1992) Identification of programmed cell death *in situ* via specific labeling of nuclear DNA fragmentation. *J. Cell Biol.* 119: 493-501.
23. Bursch, W., L. Kleine, and M. Tenniswood (1990) The biochemistry of cell death by apoptosis. *Biochem. Cell Biol.* 68: 1071-1074.
24. Johnson, J.E., Y.-A. Barde, M. Schwab, and H. Thoenen (1986) Brain-derived neurotrophic factor supports the survival of cultured retinal ganglion cells. *J. Neurosci.* 6: 3031-3038.
25. Thanos, S., M. Bähr, Y.-A. Barde, and J. Vanselow (1989) Survival and axonal elongation of adult rat retinal ganglion cells. In vitro effects of lesioned sciatic nerve and brain derived neurotrophic factor. *Eur. J. Neurosci.* 1: 19-26.
26. Jelsma, T.N., H.H. Friedman, M.J. Berkelaar, G.M. Bray, and A.J. Aguayo (1993) Different forms of the neurotrophin receptor trkB mRNA predominate in rat retina and optic nerve. *J. Neurobiol.* 24: 23-36.
27. Clarke, D.B., Y.-C. Wang, G.M. Bray, M. Rasminsky, and A.J. Aguayo (1993) Effect of Neurotrophin-4 on the survival of axotomized retinal ganglion cells in adult rats. *Soc. Neurosci. Abstr.* 19: 1104.
28. Mansour-Robaey, S., D.B. Clarke, Y.C. Wang, G.M. Bray, and A.J. Aguayo (1994) Effects of ocular injury

and administration of brain-derived neurotrophic factor on survival and regrowth of axotomized retinal ganglion cells. *Proc. Natl. Acad. Sci.* USA 91: 1632-1636.

29. Ebendal, T., L. Olson, Å. Seiger, and K.-O. Hedlund (1980) Nerve growth factors in the rat iris. *Nature* 286: 25-28.
30. Schwab, M.E., J.P. Kapfhammer, and C.E. Bandtlow (1993) Inhibitors of neurite growth. *Annu. Rev. Neurosci.* 16: 565-595.
31. Thanos, S., J. Mey, and M. Wild (1993) Treatment of the adult retina with microglia-suppressing factors retards axotomy-induced neuronal degradation and enhances axonal regeneration in vivo and in vitro. *J. Neurosci.* 13: 455-466.

# 9. PRESSURE AND GLAUCOMA

JOSEPH CAPRIOLI, M.D.

**Dr. Caprioli**: I would like to take a few minutes to redefine the clinical question at hand. I do so at the risk of boring the glaucomatologists present, but the others may find it of some interest.

In this morning's introduction, Harry talked a bit about intraocular pressure, and he told us how he hated the phrase "elevated intraocular pressure". I am going to use it here, but I do put it in quotes. The majority of individuals with so-called elevated intraocular pressure never develop glaucomatous optic nerve damage. A considerable proportion of patients with what we would consider a "normal" intraocular pressure do develop glaucomatous damage. The quoted proportion of ⅓ to ½ is a ballpark figure; it may be higher in Japan. Shiosi has suggested this, but there are arguments about retesting the pressure for many of those patients that have low pressures at one time and have high pressures at another time. Measurements of intraocular pressure are not a good way to identify patients with glaucoma. About 10 to 15 years ago there was a resurgence of interest in visual field measurements with the advent of automated methods to measure the visual field. This has not really lived up to its promise to make a diagnosis of early damage because of very high rates of fluctuation in the test, and that reproducible visual field abnormalities often develop relatively late in the course of the disease.

Our thinking about glaucoma has really changed over the course of the last decade or so, and we think about glaucoma, appropriately now, as an optic neuropathy which may be more or less dependent on intraocular pressure. Early detection is important but, more to the point of this symposium direct treatment of neurons to delay or prevent premature death should be investigated.

Let me show you the optic nerve of a patient with glaucoma, and let me draw your attention to the inferior portion of the disc rim, and I would like you to look at its width. A year later the disc rim has become significantly narrower, a blood vessel has dipped into an inferior notch, excavation is a word we sometimes use to describe this change. This is acquired damage from glaucoma (Fig. 1). As physicians we are drawn to the attention that this kind of change alerts us to. There are visible changes in the disc rim, there are visible changes in the lamina, the depth of the cup and perhaps this has contributed to our belief that all of the action is at the level of the lamina cribrosa. Dr. Quigley had a slide up this morning that said that the lamina cribrosa is the site of damage from glaucoma. I think that is an assumption that we are burdened with, and it is not necessarily true. Perhaps not all the damage in all patients with glaucoma occurs at the site of the lamina cribrosa. It is appealing to think of it that way because there are the changes that we can see, and therefore it "must" occur there, but we need to rethink that whole issue.

**Dr. Quigley**: Joe, I agree with your qualifying that statement; however, it is not the only evidence that we can clinically see something happening at the disc. There is a ton of experimental evidence that that is where it is, in experimental models and in humans with high pressures. But that does not mean that it could not be happening in cell bodies as well.

*Optic Nerve in Glaucoma, pp. 151–156*
*edited by S.M. Drance*

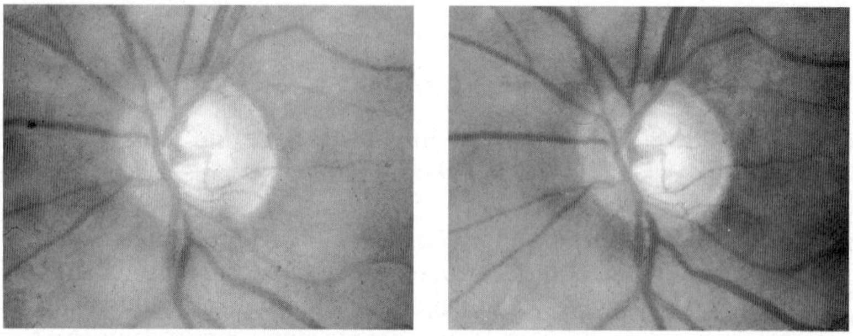

*Fig. 1.* The left optic nerve head of a patient with early primary open-angle glaucoma. The photographs are taken two years apart, the most recent one on the right. There is acquired damage to the inferior disc rim where an inferior notch has developed, and a blood vessel has dipped into the new area of excavation. Despite the structural change in the disc, the visual field, as tested by static threshold automated perimetry, remains normal.

**Dr. Caprioli**: The histopathological observations do not prove cause and effect; we have to be clear thinking about that. What I wanted to show you, in this same patient with this acquired change that I pointed out in the optic nerve, the visual field is normal. Even with the best methods that we have to measure visual fields, structural changes in the optic nerve often predate functional abnormalities. We talked a little bit about size of the optic canal, and I wanted to show you this example of two different patients; these are both photographed with the same camera, the same magnification, these patients had the same refractive error, and that this disc, you can see, is quite a bit larger than this one, in fact, the area is about four times as much (Fig. 2). However, if we measure the disc rim here, and compare it to this one, they are more nearly similar. There is, actually, more rim area in this larger disc, as Harry alluded to this morning, than there is in the smaller one, and there is a correlation between disc size and rim area and also number of ganglion cells. There is this great diversity in the size of a normal disc.

Here is a series of disc photographs of a patient showing progressive damage. These photographs are about one year apart, and a lot of the action is going on at the superior and inferior poles. Let me draw your attention to a couple of things. Here we have a disc hemorrhage and here is the disc rim which, if you follow it over the course of these five years, becomes more narrowed. It is not unusual for the disc rim to become more damaged subsequent to the appearance of a disc hemorrhage. Also, the disc rim in this location, inferior pole, has progressed. There is more damage, the disc rim has gotten thinner. This is a sick eye.

This is another patient with glaucoma, and you can see that there is a dense scotoma in the visual field here as a consequence of this. This is a patient we used to call a low-tension glaucoma patient although that is sort of a "dirty word" these days. This is a patient who has had pressures always below 15 mm Hg who has lost the disc rim completely inferiorly and you can see that this vessel is draped over a very sharp scleral edge, and that there is complete loss of ganglion cell axons in this area. What is amazing is that the superior rim, which is really quite thin, sustains a normal inferior visual field.

Disc hemorrhage has been the subject of clinical investigation and has been used by some to support a hypothesis that this may be an ischemic disease. That is, that disc hemorrhage may somehow reflect a primary abnormality in the circulation in

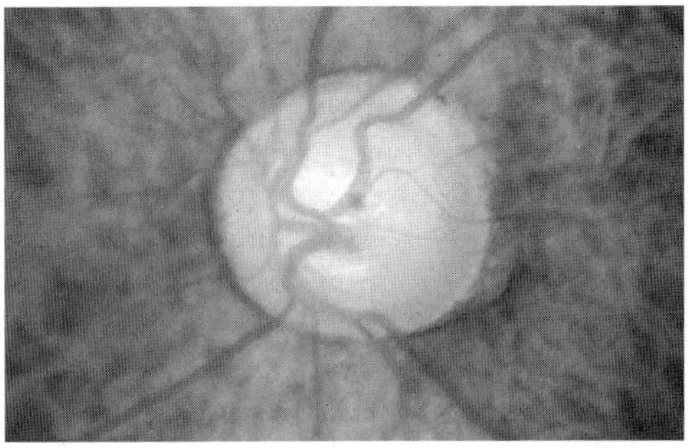

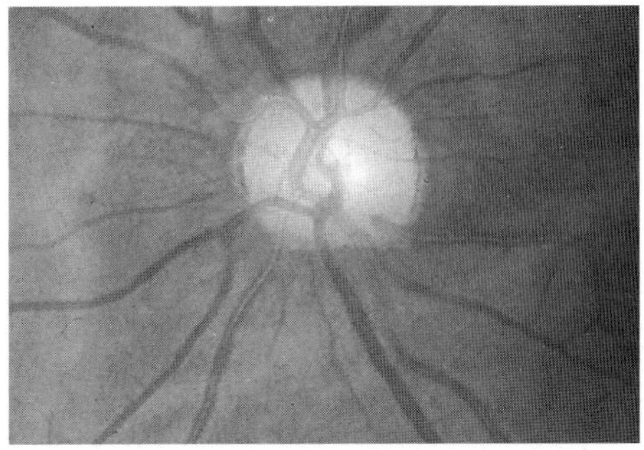

*Fig. 2.* The optic discs of two normal individuals. Both are emmetropic and have similar axial lengths; the photographs were taken with the same camera and at the same magnification. The eye with the larger disc has a larger cup. The measured disc-rim areas, however, are very similar.

that disc hemorrhages very often are followed by rather localized further damage in the disc. The appearance of these hemorrhages do not imply any mechanism in my view, but they are just associated with progressive damage, and which is cause and which is effect is not known.

There has been an attempt by clinicians to sort out what may be different mechanisms of damage through clinical observations of the optic nerve. This began when we were thinking more about low-tension glaucoma as a separate entity than the glaucoma caused by high pressure. Someone this morning used the word continuum, and it really does appear to be a continuum that we are dealing with. However, there have been some clues that there may be different patterns of damage, and if you believe that, it may be that there are different mechanisms as well. The next two eyes I am going to show you have the same amount of overall visual field loss, but they have quite different appearance of both the optic nerve and the visual field. The first is a patient who had sustained high pressures for some time, and has an evenly distributed disc rim. There is evidence that this cup was smaller in the patient years before. The visual field loss is widespread and rather shallow.

The second is a patient who has had low pressures and has extensive damage to one area of the disc rim associated with a rather focal scotoma. The history behind these observations becomes a bit controversial, but let me try to summarize a number of investigations that Dr. Drance and others have performed in that there appears to be different patterns of optic nerve damage and visual field loss. Certain patterns are associated with glaucomas that are progressive at low pressures, and some at high pressures. Perhaps in patients who have progressive damage at lower pressure there may be more of an ischemic mechanism than in patients with higher pressures. But in terms of pressure-independent and pressure-dependent damage, there is no reason to believe, for instance, that patients with high pressures do not also have some component of pressure-independent damage.

**Dr. Kaufman**: The term pressure-independent is sort of like waving a red flag in front of a bull.

**Dr. Caprioli**: That was the intent.

**Dr. Kaufman**: I figured it was. The fact that people do not have high pressure ever in their lives, and maybe the pressure is 8 mm Hg and they have horrible glaucoma and you have monitored the pressure with some device which has not been yet invented, 24 hours a day for 10 years, does not mean that the damage is independent of pressure, it simply means those people have suffered whatever it is they are suffering, at a pressure which 999 out of 1000 other people would tolerate. It does not mean that the damage is independent of pressure in that particular case, and so I do not know how one proves that the damage is independent of pressure. We have at least some evidence that says, from some of Stephen's studies and from one of Doug's studies, that even people who have so-called low-tension glaucoma and never had high pressures, still have some dependence of pressure in terms of the damage. This is the asymmetric, normal-tension glaucoma issue. I think to say that pressure-independent damage may be reaching a little bit, sort of the way you said Harry was reaching earlier in some of the issues. One needs to be careful when one chooses words at many levels. We all do this, we all fall into these kinds of things, I am as guilty as anybody in other areas. But I do not know that any case of glaucoma ever really is independent of the pressure.

**Dr. Caprioli**: Well, not anymore than we know for certain that any case of glaucoma has been dependent on pressure.

**Dr. Quigley**: Well, I disagree with that, because every statistical study that has ever been done, one risk factor which invariably comes up is the level of the intraocular pressure. Can we back up your slides one, because I want to show everybody the lamina cribrosa in the human. Everybody, if you looked at the scanning EM picture of this lamina cribrosa earlier today, you can see on this picture, right in here, and there, on the scanning electron microscopy where the pores are going through the lamina cribrosa. Notice in this picture of Joe's, in the inferior portion, the pores are long and strung out. Now, that was not what I showed you in the scanning microscopy of the normal human eye. So one of two things is true of this person. This person was born with a lamina cribrosa that looks quite unusual for the normal human pattern. Be it huge, long, oval pores, or, this person acquired that in the process of a disease. It is my hypothesis, and we can throw this up for Joe or others to discuss, that if there is a difference about these people who have lower eye pressure and develop this more localized damage, that there is something wrong with their connective tissues. And I think that lower pressure glaucoma patients are much more likely to be "mechanical" in that sense than those who have higher pressures who are probably more likely to be suffering from poor autoregulation against elevated eye pressure. I think the vascular theory of glaucoma is more likely to apply to those with higher pressures than to those with low pressures, and I am not denying that the vascular element is there at all, I am saying, let us look at the possibility, since it makes intuitive sense, that these folks have something wrong with their connective tissue.

**Dr. Kaufman**: But in neither case are you saying that they are independent of the intraocular pressure, are you?

**Dr. Quigley**: Pressure could still be a factor. It may not be a factor. I agree with Joe, there are probably patients in whom their eye pressure level will never turn out to have anything to do with their disease.

**Dr. Drance**: Paul, would you be happier with the expression that I used that there is a group of people who are less pressure-dependent?

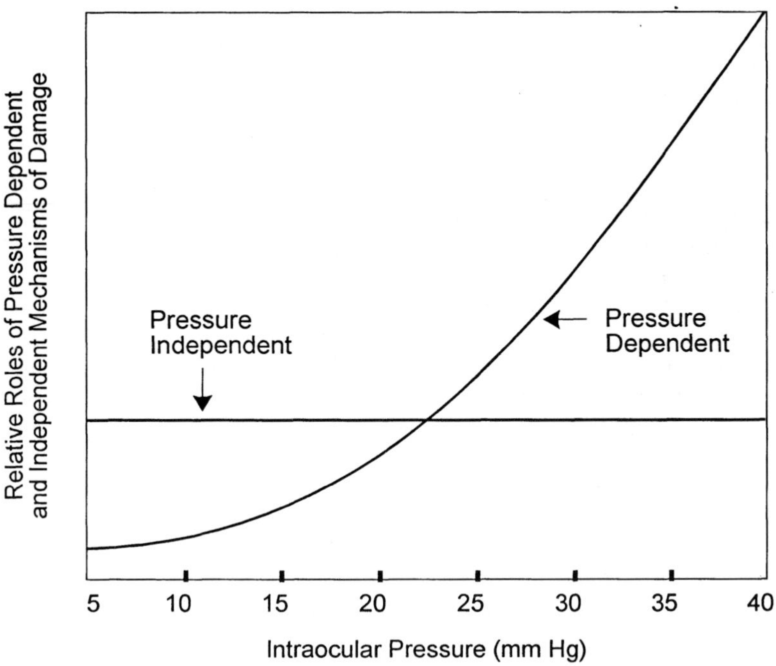


*Fig. 3.* A schematic diagram which proposes a hypothesis regarding the relative roles of pressure-dependent and -independent mechanisms of damage. Intraocular pressure is an important risk factor, and may be operative in patients even with low pressures. Pressure-independent components of damage may be operative across a whole range of intraocular pressures, in patients with high pressures and low pressures alike.

**Dr. Kaufman**: Yes, I am very happy with that.

**Dr. Caprioli**: I must make one comment, though, about these so-called normal- or low-tension patients. These patients often have evidence of vasospastic disorders. We can not show this in an epidemiologic sort of way, but I think the clinicians here have all seen cases of progressive nerve damage in patients who have Raynaud's disease, migraine headaches and so forth, in which you believe that pressure may not be such an important factor. But that is really anecdotal information.

This goes back to Paul's question about the role of pressure independence. I do not have direct evidence for that; it is a hypothesis that there are some pressure independent mechanisms that may be operative in some patients with glaucoma. Let me just show this one little sketch (Fig. 3).

What we have here, intraocular pressure, and this is some fuzzy thing we are calling mechanisms, and it is quite right that intraocular pressure certainly is an important risk factor for the development of glaucoma damage, even in patients with low pressures, as advanced by the two studies that Paul cited. But, it is likely to be more important, in patients with high pressure. So if there is a pressure-independent component of glaucomatous damage, it may be operative across the whole range of intraocular pressures, but in patients with higher pressures, of course, the pressure-dependent mechanism may be more important. So we are talking not about groups of patients with low-tension or high-tension glaucoma, but a spectrum of disease in which different mechanisms may be operating. That was one point I wanted to make. The other is, I do not think we need to be entirely wed to the concept that all of the damage takes place at the level of the lamina. I think we need to be open to the possibility that damage is occurring elsewhere to the retinal ganglion cells. Mike?

**Dr. Van Buskirk**: I just wanted to register my disagreement with what Paul said, and I thought I was agreeing with what you and Harry said, but what you just said here at the end was different from what Harry said. To disavow pressure independence is to suggest that pressure is the only factor, and I do not think we want to do that. So, if, you could call it pressure insensitive, or non-pressure factors, I think at least most of us would acknowledge that those exist. The question is whether or not pressure-independent factors are necessarily related to pressure, and I think Harry was saying something quite different than that. He was suggesting that if there is a vascular effect it may not be particularly related to low pressure. I do not know that pressure dependence is particularly related to the level of pressure. The only evidence we have heard about that was Abe's comment this morning about the association between the trabecular meshwork and the lamina cribrosa.

**Dr. Caprioli**: Well, certainly from an epidemiologic point of view the incidence of glaucoma rises dramatically with pressure. I am not equating pressure dependence with a correlation with elevated pressure.

# 10. PHARMACOPROTECTION OF NEURODEGENERATION

MICHAEL A. KAPIN, Ph.D.

The topic of this presentation is pharmacoprotection in neural tissue for the treatment of glaucomatous optic neuropathy. Pharmacoprotection implies the use of drugs to ameliorate cell injury or to prevent those processes that would lead to injury of the nerve cell. Much of what we understand about this subject has been derived from degenerative disease studies in the central nervous system. This is exemplified by the diversity of pharmacoprotective approaches that have been evaluated in disorders such as acute cerebral ischemia. In this disease, it has long been recognized that neurologic injury is vascular in origin, and the early clinical trials dealt with methods for enhancing perfusion. Strategies for modulating perfusion have included vasodilators, vasopressors, anticoagulants, spasmolytics and hemodilution. Modulation of metabolic demand through the use of barbiturates, benzodiazepines or the induction of hypothermia were neuroprotective approaches subsequently developed. Similarly, some success was achieved by reducing cellular or vasogenic edema with steroids or hyperosmolar agents. As our understanding of the pathophysiological consequences of neuronal injury expanded, novel ways of protecting the neurons were developed. Included in these protective strategies were manipulations of systems related to neurotransmitters, neuromodulators or signal transducers. Clearly, these are topics that will be covered by others in this session.

In keeping with the theme of this session, I would like to address pharmacoprotective strategies in the eye by means other than lowering intraocular pressure. To date, no cytoprotective strategies are indicated for the prevention of visual field deficits associated with glaucoma, although certain classes of drugs have been suggested for this purpose. This is illustrated by the use of calcium channel blockers for the amelioration of visual field deficits associated with some forms of glaucoma. Flammer and others were amongst the first to demonstrate the benefit of such agents to reduce visual field deficits in low-tension glaucoma (LTG) patients with peripheral vasospastic disorders[1-5]. The patients that showed a drug related improvement in peripheral vasospastic activity also showed an improvement in visual function. More recently, Netland and associates[6] asked whether the progression of glaucomatous injury in open-angle or low-tension glaucoma was altered in patients taking a calcium channel blocker for non-ophthalmic reasons. During a period of 3.4 years, only 11% of the treated low-tension glaucoma patients showed new visual field deficits as compared to 56% of the control subjects that showed similar changes. No change in the extent of optic nerve damage was reported in the treated low-tension glaucoma group; by comparison, 44% of the control patients showed progressive damage. The authors of these studies speculated that the improvement in visual function by the calcium channel blocker was related to a vascular mechanism. What is unclear is whether these agents provided some degree of protection by preventing calcium loading into the nerve cell. As will be discussed by Dr. Seisjö, excessive accumulation of calcium in the nerve cell is toxic.

With regard to neuroprotection and glaucoma, a number of questions arise. Firstly, can pharmacologic interventions aimed at the optic nerve head attenuate axonal degeneration? If injury to the non-myelinated axon traversing the lamina cribrosa is due to mechanical or pressure-induced distortion, then management of intraocular pres-

*Optic Nerve in Glaucoma, pp. 157–163*
*edited by S.M. Drance*

sure will continue to be an important avenue for the glaucoma patient. If injury to the neuron is related to ischemia of the optic nerve head, then understanding the effects of hypoxia on white matter or axonal injury is relevant to finding a cytoprotective drug. This topic will be addressed by Dr. Bruce Ransom. Another target for pharmacologic intervention is the retinal ganglion cell. It is common knowledge that the pathological changes of the optic nerve head are associated with the loss of retinal ganglion cells. The loss of these cells is thought by many to result from retrograde axonal degeneration that is initiated at the optic nerve head. Ultimately, the question can be asked as to whether the administration of an agent to the ganglion cell body can alter the progression of axonal degeneration. In studies where the optic nerve was transected, axonal degeneration was attenuated following intravitreal injection of growth factors, microglia protease inhibitors and anti-inflammatory agents[7-9]. Whether this situation has any relevance to the degenerative disease process in glaucoma is not clear; however, the pathological process leading to ganglion cell death in glaucoma may involve local changes at the cell soma or dendritic arbor. These local changes may be brought about by excitotoxicity (*i.e.* toxicity due to excessive glutamate stimulation) or microcirculatory disturbances. In the first case, elevations in glutamate concentrations in the vitreous have been measured in primary open-angle glaucoma (POAG) patients or in primates with pressure-induced optic neuropathy[10,11]. Excitotoxicity can occur by ischemia or other metabolic perturbations. Evidence linking circulatory disturbances in the retina to the initiation of glaucomatous changes is scarce for the following reasons. Firstly, circulatory disturbances in the inner retina may manifest only in some glaucoma patients or not exist at all. Secondly, it is possible that small blood flow changes may be overlooked because of resolution issues with blood flow technologies. Thirdly, circulatory disturbances may occur but not be observed in patients with episodic ocular hypertension or ocular hypertensive spikes. Finally, altered circulation may occur through impaired autoregulation. Autoregulatory capacity was tested by Grunwald in primary open-angle glaucoma and non-glaucoma controls[12]. In these studies, autoregulation was assessed using a suction cup to raise intraocular pressure (IOP) while blood flow was measured using the Blue Field Entoptic technique. Unlike the controls, blood flow decreased in POAG patients at lower pressures; typically above 25 mm Hg. It was also found that the majority of POAG patients were unable to demonstrate a hyperemic response as IOP was returned to baseline.

**Dr. Zeimer:** The autoregulatory failure or the fall in blood flow described in Grunwald's study was only at high pressures. How then at lower pressures of 15 mm Hg can one account for the loss of retinal ganglion cells by ischemia? If you want to make the point that the lack of autoregulation of blood flow could cause injury to the ganglion cells you have to work at a normal pressure to which the patient is subjected, and not stressing the system by raising the pressure.

**Dr. Kapin:** As aforementioned, it is not clear as to whether circulatory disturbances of the retina occur in any of the glaucomatous patients. However, it is possible that some glaucomatous patients that present with low intraocular pressures may exhibit episodic ocular hypertension or ocular hypertensive spikes. Under such circumstances, circulations to the optic nerve head and retina may become compromised.

**Dr. Alm:** I have another more serious problem with this theory. One of the reasons we are sitting here is that we have problems proving that intraocular pressure reduction really has an effect on the outcome of visual fields. If autoregulation was deficient, blood flow would be improved by reducing high pressure.

**Dr. Quigley:** One sentence, which is, as we looked at our mechanical factors earlier, Dr. Caprioli was kind to point out that the blood flow perturbation might have been an affect of the glaucoma, rather than the cause. Is this autoregulatory failure a cause or an effect?

**Dr. Kapin:** Good point. I don't know.

**Dr. Zeimer:** By analogy, it has been shown that in diabetes, there is a lack of autoregulation of blood flow; however, patients with diabetes do not have cupping and excavation as do glaucoma patients.

What I am addressing is the possibility that circulatory or excitotoxic disturbances of the inner retina may contribute to the degenerative loss of ganglion cells. Unfortunately, the mechanisms underlying ganglion cell death are not clearly understood and hence, it is not known whether neuroprotective strategies that target ischemic or excitotoxic injuries of the retina will benefit the glaucoma patient. It should be pointed out that in the brain and retina there have been many studies involving injury from hypoxia and excitotoxicity as well as the therapeutic approaches that have been taken to alleviate such injuries. Although models of retinal hypoxic injury are not glaucoma (*i.e.* they do not produce the clinical manifestations at the optic nerve head characteristic of glaucoma), they may produce pathologies in the ganglion cell layer similar to glaucoma. Drugs that are efficacious in ameliorating ganglion cell injury by ischemia or excitotoxicity may have application to glaucoma. For this reason, a review of retinal pathology following such insults will be presented.

It is known that oxygen debt of the region supplied by the retinal artery is associated with changes to the inner retina. Acute changes include swelling of the inner nuclear, inner plexiform, and ganglion cell layers. Typically, in a matter of days pyknotic nuclei are observed, which is followed by loss of ganglion cells and a thinning of the inner retina. Many of the histological changes observed in the inner retina following hypoxia were elucidated using the chick embryo retina preparation. David used this model to show that when subjected to anoxia, morphological changes occurred that were similar to the toxic effects of glutamate or potassium administration[13]. This is not surprising since it has been known for many years that high concentrations of glutamate are toxic to the inner retina. Interestingly, immunocytochemical and electrophysiological studies have unequivocally proven that glutamate is the major excitatory neurotransmitter in the retina as well as most other regions in the central nervous system[14,15]. Under normal conditions, neuronal release of glutamate is presynaptic and mediates an excitatory response on postsynaptic excitatory amino acid (EAA) receptors. Dissociation from these receptors as well as uptake into presynaptic neurons and/or glial cells is very rapid. Under certain conditions, glutamate release can be excessive and uptake mechanisms compromised. Excessive excitatory amino acid stimulation can result in neuronal injury and has been referred to as excitotoxicity[16]. In the central nervous system, it has been demonstrated that brief periods of ischemia can rapidly increase glutamate levels. Benveniste, using the *in vivo* dialysis technique, demonstrated increases in glutamate in the adult rat brain within minutes of global cerebral ischemia[17]. Excitotoxicity can occur in the absence of ischemia by other insults which include hypoglycemia or neuronal trauma[18]. As aforementioned, marked increases in glutamate concentrations have been measured in the vitreous of primary open-angle glaucoma patients or primates with pressure-induced optic neuropathy.

**Dr. Anderson:** This idea of ischemia-induced glutamate toxicity in the retina is relevant if we believe that ischemia in pressure-induced damage to the eye occurs in the inner retina. If we believe that ischemia occurs at the level of the lamina cribrosa, where these transmitters are not present because there are no synapses in that region, then of course, this does not apply. So, this concept or this direction of thought about the excitotoxicity mechanism applies only if we accept as a ground work that the ischemia is in the inner retina, not if the ischemia is in the optic nerve. Which is one of the things under consideration. I just want to point that this is relevant to one concept and theory, but not relevant to another.

**Dr. Kapin:** If ischemia mediates glutamate toxicity, we are likely talking about the inner retina. However, we should bear in mind that excitotoxicity can occur in the absence of ischemia, maybe by pressure-induced trauma.

**Dr. Siesjö:** I wonder if I could ask a question which I think would be nice for the discussion to follow. If you occlude the circulation to the brain and the head, there is a rank order of vulnerability among central neurons. And I wonder where in that rank order do we find the retinal ganglion cells, and which one of them would be knocked out first.

**Dr. Kapin:** I am going to address that.

**Dr. Siesjö:** The second question I have is related to a very old observation from people at high altitudes, and that is that one of the first functions in the brain which will be affected by a lowering of oxygen tension is visual acuity, and the question is, what is underlying this extreme sensitivity of vision up to moderate hypoxia, is it because of the vulnerability of the cells or is it because an inhibitory pathway or an inhibitory channel is turned on at moderate hypoxia? I think it would be nice to have answers to these questions.

**Dr. Kapin:** Unfortunately, I do not have an answer. I am not sure that the loss in visual function is related to perturbations of the inner retina or changes that occur centrally.

Glutamate toxicity to the inner retina has been extensively studied. Subcutaneous administration of glutamate to suckling mice resulted in ganglion cell loss, and in time, thinning of the inner retina[19-21]. Shortly after birth the integrity of the blood–brain barrier is achieved and toxicity is reduced. The retinal pathology following subcutaneous glutamate administration in suckling mice was similar to the pathologies observed following direct application of EAAs to the chick embryo retina[22-25] or following intravitreal injection of EAAs[26-28].

In the central nervous system, there are essentially two stages of EAA toxicity, swelling and subsequent cell loss[29]. This topic will be addressed by Dr. Choi. Typical of the brain, these same events are observed in the retina. In the rat, the first stage is characterized by marked edema of the inner retina which is observable for the first few hours and involves those cells in the ganglion cell, inner plexiform and inner nuclear layers. In the second stage, which corresponds to days after the excitotoxic event, there is a predominant degeneration of cells that may include ganglion, bipolar and amacrine cells. Overall, there is thinning of the inner nuclear and plexiform layers[27]. The extent of injury in the second stage appears to be dependent on the species, age, route of administration and dose of the EAA being evaluated.

EAA receptors are characterized as metabotropic or ionotropic. Activation of a metabotropic receptor affects cellular processes via G proteins. Ionotropic receptors affect the translocation of mono- and divalent cations across the cell membrane. There are at least three ionotropic receptors that have been named for the agonist that preferentially stimulates the receptor. These have been classified as N-methyl-D-aspartate (NMDA), kainate and AMPA (2-amino-3-[3-hydroxy-5-methylisoxazol-4-yl] propanoic acid). These EAA receptors are differentially localized to specific cells in the retina[14,15]. The localization of such receptors could account for the pathologies associated with glaucoma or inner retinal ischemia. For example cellular edema in the inner nuclear and ganglion cell layers may be related to stimulation of the AMPA or kainate receptor, whereas death of the retinal ganglion cell or some amacrine cells has to a large part been attributed primarily to excessive stimulation of the NMDA receptor[30]. The translocation of $Ca^{2+}$ through the activated NMDA receptor contributes greatly to the cytotoxicity on this cell.

The use of EAA antagonists to attenuate retinal pathology from ischemia or excitotoxicity has been extensively studied. Olney originally showed that the neurotoxic action of NMDA on the chick retina was blocked by competitive and non-competitive antagonists[22]. Using the same model, Price showed that the NMDA antagonist MK-801, and the AMPA receptor antagonist CNQX were only partially effective in blocking ischemic injury, but completely effective when administered together[24]. These findings supported the premise that both NMDA and non-NMDA receptors mediate injury in this model. Siliprandi and coworkers demonstrated that MK-801 attenuated ganglion cell loss in a dose-dependent fashion following intravitreal injection of NMDA[26]. The effects of excitotoxins on isolated rat ganglion cells in culture and the amelioration by selective antagonists has been studied by Caprioli. This topic will be addressed later in this session. It should be remembered that glutamate is the major EAA in the retina, and in this light it is not clear whether EAA antagonists will affect normal visual function. Finally, it should be noted that a number of models of retinal ischemia have been used to test a host of different therapeutics for preserving inner retinal morphology and function. Included were the use of metabotropic agonists such as 1S,3R-ACPD or non-competitive EAA antagonists such as MK-801 or dextromethorphan[31,32], antioxidants or free radical scavengers[33,34], PAF antagonists[34,35] and calcium channel blockers[36].

In summary, the mechanism by which ganglion cells and their axons degenerate in glaucoma is not clearly understood. There is evidence to suggest that degenerative changes may be related to excitotoxicity and perhaps, ischemia. What is not clear is whether the application of those agents that retard EAA toxicity can attenuate ganglion cell loss and prevent further deterioration of the visual field. While others have evaluated the acute effects of calcium channel blockers[6] or gangliosides[37] on visual function, longer and better controlled trials for preservation of visual field will be required. In this context, the EAA antagonists may be an appropriate therapeutic approach. Until we know the cause of the ganglion cell death, we will not know whether neuroprotective agents that target the ganglion cell will benefit the glaucoma patient.

## References


1. Flammer, J. Psychophysical mechanisms and treatment of vasospastic disorders in normal-tension glaucoma. *Bull. Soc. Belge Ophtalmol.* 244: 129-134, 1992.
2. Gasser, P. and J. Flammer. Short- and long-term effect of nifedipine on the visual field in patients with presumed vasospasm. *J. Int. Med. Res.* 18: 334-339, 1990.
3. Gasser, P., J. Flammer and F. Mahler. The use of calcium antagonists in the treatment of ocular circulation symptoms in the framework of a vasospastic syndrome. *Schweiz Med. Wochenschr* 118(6): 201-202, 1988.
4. Kitazawa, Y., H. Shirai and F.J. Go. The effect of $Ca^{2+}$-antagonist on visual field in low-tension glaucoma. *Graefe's Arch. Clin. Exp. Ophthalmol.* 227: 408-412, 1989.
5. Shirai, H., K. Asano, Y. Kitazawa and F.J. Go. The effects of calcium antagonist on visual field in low tension glaucoma . *Acta Soc. Ophthalmol. Jpn* 92(5): 792-797, 1988.
6. Netland, P.A., N. Chaturvedi and E.B. Dreyer. Calcium channel blockers in the management of low-tension and open-angle glaucoma. *Am. J. Ophthalmol.* 115: 608-613, 1993.
7. Carmignoto, G. and G. Check. Effect of NGF on the survival of rat retinal ganglion cells following optic nerve section. *J. Neurosci.* 9: 1263-1272, 1989.
8. Seniuk, N.A. Neurotrophic factors: role in peripheral neuronal survival and axonal repair. *J. Reconst. Microsurg.* 8: 399-404, 1992.
9. Thanos, S. and H.-J. Thiel. Mechanisms governing neuronal degeneration and axonal regeneration in the mature retinofugal system. *J. Cell Sci.* 15: 125-134, 1991.
10. Dreyer, E.B. and S.A. Lipton. A proposed role for excitatory amino acids in glaucoma visual loss. *Invest. Ophthalmol. Vis. Sci.* 34(4): 1504, 1993.
11. Schumer, R.A., S.M. Podos, S.A. Lipton and E.B. Dreyer. Increased glutamate in the vitreous of monkeys with induced glaucoma. *Invest. Ophthalmol. Vis. Sci.* 35(4): 1484, 1994.
12. Grunwald, J.E., C.E. Riva, R.A. Stone, E.U. Keakes and B.L. Petrig. Retinal autoregulation in open-angle glaucoma. *Ophthalmology* 91: 1690-1694, 1984.
13. David, P., M. Lusky and V. Teichberg. Involvement of excitatory neurotransmitters in the damage produced in chick embryo retinas by anoxia and extracellular high potassium. *Exp. Eye Res.* 46: 657-662, 1988.
14. Massey, S. Cell types using glutamate as a neurotransmitter in the vertebrate retina. In: *Progress in Retinal Research. Vol. 9* , edited by N.N. Osborne and G.J. Chader. Oxford: Pergamon Press, 1990, pp. 399-425.
15. Miller, R.F. and M.M. Slaughter. Excitatory amino acid receptors in the vertebrate retina. . In: *Retinal Transmitters and Modulators. Models For The Brain. Vol. II*, edited by W. W. Morgan. Boca Raton, FL: CRC Press, Inc., 1985, pp. 123-160.
16. Olney, J.W. Inciting excitotoxic cytocide among central neurons. *Adv. Exp. Med. Biol.* 203: 631-645, 1986.
17. Benveniste, H., J. Drejer, A. Schousboe and N.H. Diemer. Elevation of the extracellular concentrations of glutamate and aspartate in rat hippocampus during transient cerebral ischemia monitored by intracerebral microdialysis. *J. Neurochem.* 43(5): 1369-1374, 1984.
18. Beal, M. F. Mechanisms of excitotoxicity in neurologic diseases. *FASEB J.* 6: 3338-3344, 1992.
19. Hansson, H.-A. Ultrastructural studies on the long term effects of sodium glutamate on the rat retina. *Virchows Arch.* 6: 1-11, 1970.
20. Lucas, D.R. and J.P. Newhouse. The toxic effect of sodium L-glutamate on the inner layers of the retina. *Arch. Ophthalmol.* 58: 193-201, 1957.
21. Olney, J.W. Glutamate-induced retinal degeneration in neonatal mice. Electron microscopy of the acutely evolving lesion. *J. Neuropathol. Exp. Neurol.* 28: 455-474, 1969.
22. Olney, J.W., M.T. Price, T.A. Fuller, J. Labruyer, L. Samson, M. Carpenter and K. Mahan. The anti-excitotoxic effects of certain anesthetics analgesics and sedative-hypnotics. *Neurosci. Lett.* 68: 29-34, 1986.
23. Olney, J.W., M.T. Price, L. Samson and J. Labruyere. The role of specific ions in glutamate neurotoxicity. *Neurosci. Lett.* 65: 65-71, 1986.
24. Price, M.T., T. Honore, M.E. Mueller, J. Labruyere, E. Silverman and J.W. Olney. CNQX potently and selectively blocks kainate excitotoxicity in the chick embryo retina. *Soc. Neurosci. Abst.* 14: 418, 1988.
25. Reif-Lehrer, L., J. Bergenthal and L. Hanninen. Effects of monosodium glutamate on chick embryo retina in culture. *Invest. Ophthalmol. Vis. Sci.* 14(2): 114-124, 1975.
26. Siliprandi, R., R. Canella, G. Carmignoto, N. Schiavo, A. Zanellato, R. Zanoni and G. Vantini. N-methyl-D-aspartate-induced neurotoxicity in the adult rat retina. *Visual Neurosci.* 8: 567-573, 1992.
27. Sisk, D.R. and T. Kuwabara. Histological changes in the inner retina of albino rats following intravitreal injection of monosodium L-glutamate. *Graefe's Arch. Clin. Exp. Ophthalmol.* 223: 250-258, 1985.
28. Tung, N.N., I.G. Morgan and D. Ehrlich. A quantitative analysis of the effects of excitatory neurotoxines on retinal ganglion cells in the chick. *Visual Neurosci.* 4: 217-223, 1990.
29. Choi, D.W. Excitotoxic cell death. *J. Neurobiol.* 23: 1261-1276, 1992.

30. Sucher, N.J., E. Aizenman and S.A. Lipton. N-methyl-D-aspartate antagonists prevent kainate neurotoxicity in rat retinal ganglion cells in vitro. *J. Neurosci.* 11(4): 966-971, 1991.
31. Siliprandi, R., M. Lipartiti, E. Fadda, J. Sautter and H. Manev. Activation of the glutamate metabotropic receptor protects retina against N-methy-D-aspartate toxicity. *Eur. J. Pharmacol.* 219: 173-174, 1992.
32. Yoon, Y.H. and M.F. Marmor. Dextromethorphan protects retina against ischemic injury in vivo. *Arch. Ophthalmol.* 107: 409-411, 1989.
33. Nayak, M.S., M. Kita and M.F. Marmor. Protection of rabbit retina from ischemic injury by superoxide dismutase and catalase. *Invest. Ophthalmol. Vis. Sci.* 34(6): 2018-2022, 1993.
34. Szabo, M.E., M.T. Droy-Lefaix, M. Doly and P. Braquet. Modification of ischemia/reperfusion-induced ion shifts ($Na^+$, $K^+$, $Ca^{2+}$ and $Mg^{2+}$) by free radical scavengers in the rat retina. *Ophthalmic Res.* 25: 1-9, 1993.
35. Doly, M., M.T. Droy-Lefaix, M. Millerin and P. Braquet. Implication of platelet-activating factor (PAF) in retinal damage induced by ischemia-reperfusion. *Invest. Ophthalmol. Vis. Sci.* 32(Suppl.): 1031, 1991.
36. Takahashi, K., T.T. Lam, E.R. Buchi and D.P. Edward. Protective effects of flunarizine on pressure-induced ischemic injury in rat retina. *Invest. Ophthalmol. Vis. Sci.* 32(Suppl.): 864, 1991.
37. Brogliatti, B., T. Rolle, A. Cantatore and M. Bianco. Citicolina vs gangliosidi vs GM1 effetti sulla sensibilita centrale in pazienti glaucomatosi. *Boll. Ocul.* Anno 70 (Suppl. 1): 263-269, 1991.

# 11. NEURONAL INJURY

ERMINIO COSTA, M.D.

**Dr. Caprioli**: We would like to continue our discussion of the neurobiology of retinal ganglion cells, or at least the neurobiology of what might be pertinent to retinal ganglion cells. Dr. Erminio Costa, who is the director of the Georgetown Institute for the Neurosciences has kindly agreed to discuss his ideas about gangliosides and neuroprotection, among some other things. Dr. Costa.

**Dr. Costa**: I have so far been the beneficiary of an interesting learning experience. Since the days of my medical school studies I did not read much about glaucoma, therefore I badly needed an update on the progress that has occurred during the last four decades in our knowledge of glaucoma pathogenesis. Dr. Caprioli's visit to Georgetown University gave me an opportunity to share with him some of my views on the possibility of preventing neuronal death induced by a protracted stimulation by glutamate receptors without inhibiting the glutamate receptor function with competitive and uncompetitive antagonists. In fact, it is my intention to discuss with you that it is now possible to prevent neuronal death related to the pathological increase of glutamate content in extracellular fluids by targeting drugs to neuronal mechanisms operative in the homeostasis of free intraneuronal calcium $[Ca^{2+}]_i$, which is destabilized during glutamate excitotoxicity.

## 1. Glutamate: an important central nervous system neurotransmitter operative in excitotoxicity associated with central nervous system ischemia

Several lines of anatomical, physiological, biochemical and pharmacological evidence suggest that glutamate is a primary transmitter in the synaptic communication of retina neurons. Probably also in retina as it is the case in brain, virtually every neuron expresses glutamatergic receptors that are operative in mediating signal transduction in afferent glutamatergic synapses. These synapses include structurally different ionotropic receptors which regulate the increase of intraneuronal sodium or the simultaneous surge of sodium and calcium that follows the presynaptic release of glutamate. Several subtypes of glutamate ionotropic and metabotropic receptors regulate metabolic events in the postsynaptic neuron by increasing free intraneuronal calcium concentrations $[Ca^{2+}]_i$. This increase of $[Ca^{2+}]_i$ functions as an intracellular second messenger mediating the transduction of the extracellular signal (glutamate) into precise intraneuronal metabolic responses. This intermittent intracellular calcium signaling modulated by synaptic activity is promptly and intermittently quenched by a number of mechanisms located either intraneuronally or on the neuronal membrane. These include: *1.* $Ca^{2+}$ uptake into mitochondria via a $Na^+/Ca^{2+}$ exchanger; *2.* $Ca^{2+}$ uptake into specific endoplasmic storage sites via specific receptor mediated $Ca^{2+}$ channels or $Ca^{2+}$ ATPase; and *3.* $Ca^{2+}$ transport outside the neuron via $Ca^{2+}$ ATPase and the $Na^+/Ca^{2+}$ exchanger. If pathological events that increase glutamate content of brain interstitial fluids transform the physiological intermittent $Ca^{2+}$ signaling into a continuous long lasting stimulation of $Ca^{2+}$ permeable glutamate ionotropic receptors $[Ca^{2+}]_i$ leading to

*Optic Nerve in Glaucoma, pp. 165–180*
*edited by S.M. Drance*

a calcium homeostasis destabilization. When threshold values for the simultaneous stimulation of proteases, protein kinases and endonucleases are obtained, causing neuronal damage, delayed (hr) neuronal death may ensue if the $[Ca^{2+}]_i$ levels are consistently elevated for twenty minutes or longer. Hence in any neuron receiving glutamatergic synaptic inputs there is always the impending danger that in conjunction with a long-lasting increase of extracellular levels of glutamate coupled with an insufficient re-uptake of glutamate into neurons or glia cells, a $Ca^{2+}$ mediated neuronal degeneration may occur that might even lead to a $Ca^{2+}$ dependent neuronal death. This impending danger can become operative even in retina.

In connection with the emerging evidence that the destabilization of $[Ca^{2+}]_i$ homeostasis induced by paroxysmal stimulation of glutamate receptors may cause neuronal death it would seem of relevance to investigate whether an experimentally induced increase of the intraocular pressure coupled with a blockade of the glutamate re-uptake can cause damage to retina neurons greater than that elicited by only an identical increase of intraocular pressure in the absence of a pharmacological impairment of glutamate uptake. Support for the validity of this working hypothesis are reports that in several experimental models the pharmacological blockade of the glutamate re-uptake can increase neuronal damage[1] by prolonging the duration of $Ca^{2+}$ increase.

In this context one might mention that recently the proteins operative in glutamate re-uptake in glia and neurons were cloned[2]; the structure of these glutamate transporters substantially differs from that of the transporters for other neurotransmitters such as γ-aminobutyric acid, norepinephrine, dopamine or serotonin. This knowledge has paved the way for the discovery of specific and selective inhibitors of glutamate uptake[2].

## 2. Neuronal plasticity and glutamatergic synapses

A stimulation of glutamate receptors appears to be operative in the regulation of synaptic plasticity. This term designates a number of changes in synaptic function including the capability to change glutamatergic synaptic strength to adapt to environmental changes by increasing or decreasing for protracted time periods the maximal current intensity in a given glutamatergic synapse. Experimentally this phenomenon can be studied by applying a high frequency stimulation to glutamatergic afferents and measuring the duration of the long-term increase (long-term potentiation – LTP) or decrease (long-term depression – LTD) of synaptic currents. It is believed that during the physiological adaptation to environmental changes, LTP and LTD can occur in selected nodes of brain neuronal circuits and that these changes bring about neuronal circuitry modifications that can persist for hours or days. Present thinking tends to associate LTP and LTD with memory and learning.

In addition to LTP and LTD, synaptic plasticity can also be expressed by specific changes of synaptic morphology including the formation of dendritic synaptic spinulae. These changes may further prolong and strengthen neuronal circuitry modifications associated with the appearance of LTP or LTD. Probably in connection with these morphological synaptic changes triggered by environmental adaptation, modifications of the structural characteristics of the glutamate receptor maps expressed in postsynaptic membranes also may appear. Such a trend of thinking is supported by experimental evidence obtained in fish where persistent exposure of retina to dark or illumination causes the expression of synaptic spinulae linking horizontal cells to cone pedicles[3]. Thus one might suggest that changes in environmental conditions can bring about important modifications in synaptic structure occurring within short-lasting time constants and involving the participation of glutamate receptors. The term plasticity eminently applies to these dynamic changes of synaptic profile configuration. Moreover several lines of independent investigation give support to the view that this plasticity involving dendritic spinulae modifications is regulated by glutamatergic transmission because it can be prevented if an application of specific glutamate receptor antagonists is associated with illumination stimuli.

Figure 1(A) depicts an idealized glutamatergic synapse. We can distinguish presynaptic and postsynaptic sites separated by the synaptic gap. While it is possible to characterize histochemically catecholaminergic and serotonergic synapses by eliciting the formation of specific fluorescent derivatives of these transmitters, such a technology cannot be applied to the histochemical recognition of glutamatergic nerve terminals. The nerve endings of other transmitter systems can be recognized by the use of specific antibodies to specific enzymes operative in the transmitter synthesis. For instance in adrenergic endings one can detect immunohistochemically tyrosine hydroxylase, in acetylcholine terminals one can detect cholinoacetyltranspherase and finally in GABAergic terminals one can detect glutamic acid decarboxylase. However transmitter specific enzymes cannot be detected in glutamatergic terminals because the synthesis of glutamate occurs practically in every neuron as a part of energy metabolic processes that are unrelated to neurotransmission. A histochemical strategy that can be considered useful to recognizing and characterizing glutamatergic nerve terminals might be the use of specific antibodies against glutamate transporters operative in the neuronal uptake of glutamate. Alternatively one can recognize glutamatergic synapses with antibodies against specific postsynaptic glutamate receptors.

## 3. Structure and function of glutamate receptors

There is an astonishing diversity in the structure of receptors that transduce glutamate signaling into metabolic events regulating functional aspects of postsynaptic neurons. These transduction mechanisms can either lead to an increase of cationic influxes ($Na^+$ and $Ca^{2+}$) into neurons or to the activation of phospholipases or to the inhibition of adenylatecyclases. However the structural correlates to some of these transduction mechanism diversities sometimes consist of a single amino acid substitution which is virtually undetectable by immunohistochemical technologies. Nevertheless there are a number of other functionally significant differences in glutamate receptor structure that can be detected immunohistochemically. Several of these major differences in receptor structure are encoded by different genes. There are more than 16 different genes each encoding for either a family of glutamate receptor subunits or for structurally different monomeric glutamate receptors. There are two major classes of glutamate receptors: metabotropic[4] and ionotropic[5]. The metabotropic receptors are monomeric integral membrane proteins including seven hydrophobic domains that span the neuronal membrane. These monomeric receptors include three functional domains: extraneuronal, transmembrane and intraneuronal. The transmitter binds to the extraneuronal domain of metabotropic receptors which function by coupling the transmitter binding to the specific recognition site with the activation of a G protein bound to the receptor intraneuronal domain. These G proteins are oligotrimeric ($\alpha$, $\beta$, $\gamma$ subunits) structures that bind GTP and can metabolize it to GDP. Following the transmitter binding to a specific recognition site in the extraneuronal domain of the metabotropic glutamate receptors, the G protein coupled to the intraneuronal domain of this receptor dissoci-

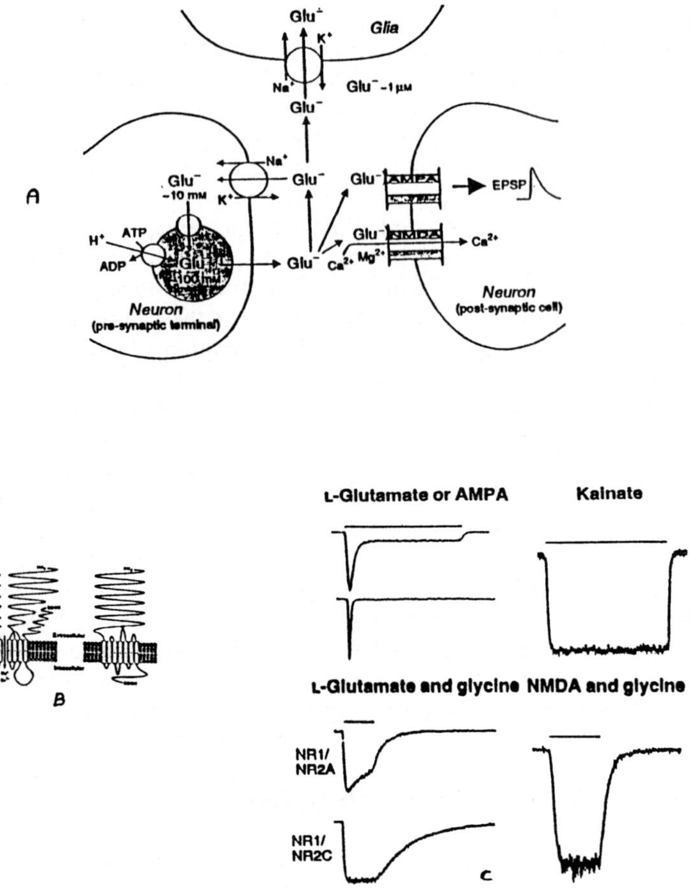


*Fig. 1.* A: dynamic processes operative in a glutamatergic synapse. Note high affinity neuronal and glia uptake mechanisms, low affinity glutamate uptake in synaptic vesicles. (Modified from Nanay *et al.*[2].) B: metabotropic (left) and ionotropic receptor structure. (Modified from Tanabe *et al.*[4].) C: Synaptic currents on recombinant AMPA (top left), kainate (top right) and NMDA receptors (two bottom traces). The time constant of the current recordings is identical. Please note the greatest responses obtained with NMDA which is not taken up or metabolized. (Modified from Szekely *et al.*[5].)

ates its α or ß subunit. By this dissociation a mechanism is triggered that links this receptor to either adenylate cyclase, and as a result the formation rate of cyclic AMP is reduced, or to a phospholipase C and as a result the formation rate of inositol triphosphate ($IP_3$) is increased. $IP_3$ regulates the uptake of $[Ca^{2+}]_i$ into specific endoplasmic reticulum stores by binding to specific intraneuronal $IP_3$ receptors.

Figure 1(B) depicts an idealized general structure for metabotropic glutamate receptors and contrasts its structural features with those of subunits of glutamate ionotropic receptors. There are three classes of ionotropic glutamate receptors which were classified several years ago on the basis of the chemical structure of three synthetic agonists each specific for one class of receptors[5]. The three classes are: kainate, AMPA and NMDA receptors. Also the ionotropic receptor subunits are integral membrane proteins that aggregate in heteropentameric complexes, each subunit including four hydrophobic transmembrane domains. There are at least 16 genes encoding for the different subunits of these three classes of receptors. The NMDA (N-methyl-D-aspartate) receptor subunits are encoded by two genes NMDA-R1 and NMDA-R2, four or five structurally different subunit isoforms originate from each gene. It is believed that there are several subtypes of native NMDA receptors, which are characterized by different assemblies of subunit isoforms, each assembly includes in their pentameric complex at least a subunit isoform of each of the two families.

Figure 1(C) shows that AMPA receptors autodesensitize promptly following agonist stimulation. The time constant of this desensitization is so fast that the $Na^+$ current is extinct before the glutamate has disappeared from the synaptic cleft. In contrast as shown in Fig. 1(C) the current generated from NMDA receptors lasts much longer. AMPA responses last about 3 milliseconds while those to NMDA last 80 to 90 milliseconds. Just to amplify some information given earlier about LTP at glutamatergic synapses, LTP induction is triggered by NMDA receptor stimulation, while the synaptic response that is strengthened by this stimulus is expressed by AMPA receptors. NMDA receptor stimulation causes a $[Ca^{2+}]_i$ increase larger than that mediated by AMPA receptor stimulation. Moreover it is important to reiterate a concept formulated yesterday by Dr. Siesjö: the activation of the NMDA receptors can convey a message to the nucleus. This message is probably encoded via a translocation to the nucleus of a protein kinase activated by the increase in $[Ca^{2+}]_i$, which very likely triggers the expression of early inducible genes. The induction of this class of genes is almost synchronous with the application of an appropriate stimulus to the NMDA receptor. The mRNA produced by these genes encodes transcription factors which immediately after their ribosomal synthesis in cytosol promptly revert to the nucleus where they promote the transcription of a number of genes, simultaneously[6]. These important transcription factors belong to the fos and jun families[6,7] and following their heterodimerization bind to specific promoter consensi to orchestrate the induction of a cascade of genes, which probably encode for proteins participating in the different aspects of synaptic plasticity, which as mentioned earlier is triggered by the glutamate activation of NMDA receptors.

Table 1 summarizes the major structural characteristics of metabotropic and ionotropic glutamate receptors. Obviously this summary only schematizes the present understanding of the structural correlates of the various subtypes of glutamate receptors that are presently known to participate in glutamatergic transmission.

The NMDA receptors are continuously blocked by $Mg^{2+}$ bound to specific amino acids located in the channel lining; this binding and the associated blockage are resolved by depolarizing stimuli. Probably in the postsynaptic membrane there is a mosaic of receptors including various molecular forms of NMDA, AMPA or kainate receptors. Obviously this association facilitates the resolution of the permanent inhibition of NMDA receptors by $Mg^{2+}$. Another characteristic feature of NMDA receptors is the presence of a recognition site for glycine. This amino acid plays the role of either an endogenous positive allosteric modulator of glutamate action at NMDA receptors or acts as an obligatory cotransmitter that allows the action of glutamate on NMDA receptors. This site can be also occupied by endogenous kynurenic acid which may act as competitive inhibitor of the positive alloseric action of glycine. In recombinant receptors this permissive action of glycine is maximized in NMDA receptors including isoforms of NMDA-R1 and of NMDA-R2 subunits.

*Table 1.* Structure and function information on ionotropic (A) and metabotropic receptors (B)

| A | | B | | | | | |
|---|---|---|---|---|---|---|---|
| *Subunit gene* | *Amino acids* | *% Homology GLU R1* | *Agonists* | *Permeability $Ca^{2+}$* | *Receptor gene* | *Amino acids* | *Effects* |
| GLU R1 | | | | Yes | MGLU $R_{10}$ | 1199 | $IP_3Ca^{2+}$ |
| | 1000 | 68-73 | AMPA | | | | |
| GLU R2 | | | | No | MGLU $R_{1ß}$ | 906 | $IP_3Ca^{2+}$ |
| GLU R3 | | | | Yes | MGLU $R_5$ | 1171 | $IP_3Ca^{2+}$ |
| GLU R4 | | | | Yes | | | |
| GLU R5 | | | | Yes | MGLU $R_2$ | 872 | cAMP |
| | 1000 | 38-40 | Kainate | | | | |
| GLU R6 | | | | Yes | MGLU $R_3$ | 879 | cAMP |
| GLU R7 | | | | – | MGLU $R_4$ | 912 | cAMP |
| $KA_1$ | | | | | MGLU $R_5$ | 871 | cAMP |
| | 1000 | 35 | Kainate | – | | | |
| $KA_2$ | | | | | | | |
| NMDA-R1 | 1600 | 22 | | Yes | | | |
| | | | NMDA | | | | |
| NMDA-R2A | | 1600 | 12-18 | None | | | |
| NMDA-R2B | | 1600 | 12-18 | None | | | |
| NMDA-R2C | | 1330 | 12-18 | None | | | |
| NMDA-R2D | | 1400 | 12-18 | None | | | |

## 4. NMDA receptors: NO formation and oxidative stress

The important increase of $[Ca^{2+}]_i$ following the glutamate binding to postsynaptic NMDA receptors can determine the activation of NO synthase, an enzyme which generates the gas NO (nitric oxide) by catalyzing the metabolism of arginine into citrulline. As shown in Figure 2 NO is a reactive molecule that can interact with superoxide forming free OH radicals which cause neuronal damage. In NMDA receptors the formation of NO is physiologically coupled with the activation of guanylate cyclase which in presence of NO promptly leads to the accumulation of cyclic GMP which like cyclic AMP acts as an affector of a specific protein kinase and thereby mediates some of the physiological responses regulated by glutamate. In the retina cyclic GMP in conjunction with a specific phosphodiasterase mediates the transduction of photons into $Na^+$ currents. NO can be also released from endothelial cells and mediates vasodilation, thus it might be a candidate to be studied in the vascular changes associated with modification of intraocular pressure. But as mentioned above in the presence of

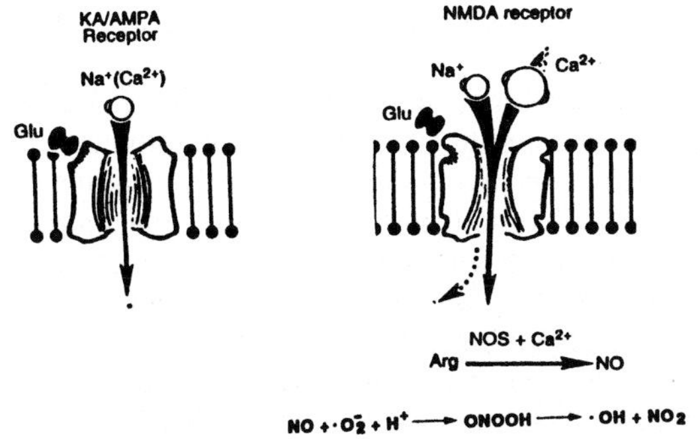


*Fig. 2.* Ionic events in AMPA/kainate and NMDA receptors. Please note the $Ca^{2+}$ dependency of NO synthesis and the chemistry of the interaction of NO with superoxide.

oxygen radicals it might trigger neurotoxicity. This additional neurotoxic component triggered by NMDA receptor activation adds to the neurotoxic actions of the persistent increases of $[Ca^{2+}]_i$ mediated by a pathological increase of glutamate in interstitial fluids. Thus among the consequences of the increase in intraocular pressure, oxygen radicals, NO and $[Ca^{2+}]_i$ increase may concur to determine degeneration and death of retina neurons.

When these processes are coupled, they can contribute to a progressive, slowly occurring neuronal damage via the action of OH radicals on mitochondria. As mentioned above, mitochondria participate in the regulation of $[Ca^{2+}]_i$ homeostasis. They can take up $Ca^{2+}$ via the $Na^+/Ca^{2+}$ exchanger located in the outer mitochondrial membrane. The continuous production of $H^+$ by the mitochondria which is associated with the synthesis of ATP creates the electrochemical condition that facilitates the influx of $[Ca^{2+}]_i$ into mitochondria which, as mentioned earlier, plays an important role in $[Ca^{2+}]_i$ homeostasis. Thus a precondition for this homeostatic function is that the oxidative phosphorylation of mitochondria proceeds at a brisk pace. However during a persistent pathological activation of glutamate receptors this buffering mechanism is impaired by the simultaneous influx of $Na^+$ which limits the efficiency of mitochondrial $Na^+/Ca^{2+}$ exchanger operative in mitochondrial $[Ca^{2+}]_i$ homeostasis. Moreover during oxidative stress, the free radicals can damage the mitochondrial DNA and because of a characteristic inability of mitochondria to repair this DNA damage, the synthesis of mitochondrial enzymes involved in oxidative phosphorylation which is mediated by mitochondrial DNA results impaired lowering the steady state level of enzymes attending the oxidative phosphorylation. The consequent decrease of mitochondrial oxidative phosphorylation generates an insufficient rate of mitochondria ATP biosynthesis and $H^+$ export. Such a reduction lowers the efficiency of mitochondrial $[Ca^{2+}]_i$ import and consequently decreases mitochondrial buffering capacity of $[Ca^{2+}]_i$. Hence a persistent oxidative stress promotes conditions that synergize the other causes of excitotoxicity elicited by glutamate and with time increases the impending excitotoxicity caused by persistent stimulation of glutamate receptors that are $Ca^{2+}$ permeable. In this situation even the smaller $Ca^{2+}$ influx mediated by persistent stimulation of AMPA receptors can become with time, a cause for chronic neurodegeneration. Thus the neurodegeneration deriving from chronic oxidative stress, and from glutamate induced $Ca^{2+}$ influx summate and might become of possible relevance in the pathogenesis of glaucoma during the persistent increase of intraocular pressure.

## 5. Neuronal $[Ca^{2+}]_i$ homeostasis destabilization: a target for neuroprotective drugs

These considerations obviously suggest that a blockade of glutamate receptors might be considered an appropriate strategy for a symptomatic therapy of the neuronal damage in glaucoma. However the visual pathway from retina to occipital cortex eminently functions via the utilization of glutamatergic transmission. Hence a protracted blockade of glutamate receptors with specific antagonists of various glutamate receptor subtypes is not encouraged by two orders of considerations. On the one hand, any visual deficit tends to be physiologically compensated by mechanisms that involve the activation of glutamatergic synapses, which are the main excitatory transmitter mechanism operative in neuronal pathways attending to visual function; of course one does not like to hamper physiological compensatory mechanisms in the presence of a progressive chronic damage to this function. On the other hand, the structural diversity of glutamate receptors imposes the use of a polypharmacy in order to assure that the variety of structurally different glutamate receptors operative in retina function are pharmacologically controlled. This polypharmacy for sure not only would limit the efficacy of synaptic plasticity attending to visual compensatory mechanism but also may cause a complex array of collateral side effects due to the involvement of glutamatergic synapses in the regulation of CNS cognitive and sensory motor functions. Ideally one would like to limit the excessive function of glutamate receptor only in the neurons that are the target for pathologically persistent glutamate receptor stimulation while leaving unharmed the physiological glutamatergic transmission that is operative in several brain structures. Of course ideal situations are hard to achieve, nevertheless one should attempt to work toward this strategic goal. The following part of this presentation is an attempt to work along this ideal approach.

## 6. Glycosphingolipids (GM1 and lyso GM1 synthetic derivatives) in the protection of $Ca^{2+}$ homeostasis destabilization

In a historical perspective the reasons that fostered the use of gangliosides and semisynthetic lysogangliosides in the treatment of neuronal damage deriving from a destabilization of $[Ca^{2+}]_i$ homeostasis, began about seven years ago. At that time Connor *et al.*[8], working with isolated pyramidal cells of adult guinea pig hippocampus kept in primary culture, demonstrated that a single glutamate application from a micropipette placed in the proximity of the neuronal membrane increases neuronal $[Ca^{2+}]_i$. This increase rapidly spreads from the neuronal areas close to the transmitter application and reaches the soma and dendrites of that neuron. The $[Ca^{2+}]_i$ increase and its diffusion was visualized using Flura 2 (a $Ca^{2+}$ sensitive fluorescent probe). They also showed that repeating the application of glutamate within appropriate short time intervals the $[Ca^{2+}]_i$ increase persists progressively longer after each successive glutamate application. As a tentative extrapolation from these results these authors[8] suggested that the rate of $Ca^{2+}$ influx elicited by repetitive glutamate applications was gradually overwhelming the neuronal homeostatic capacity to buffer $[Ca^{2+}]_i$ increases. The authors repeated similar experiments using NMDA, the specific agonists of the glutamate NMDA receptor which as mentioned earlier is highly permeable to $Ca^{2+}$ and could show that the successive applications of NMDA could duplicate the overwhelming of neuronal $[Ca^{2+}]_i$ homeostasis elicited by glutamate. Then they pretreated the neurons with sphyngosine and observed that these neurons were virtually resistant to the destabilization of $[Ca^{2+}]_i$ homeostasis induced by NMDA applications repeated at

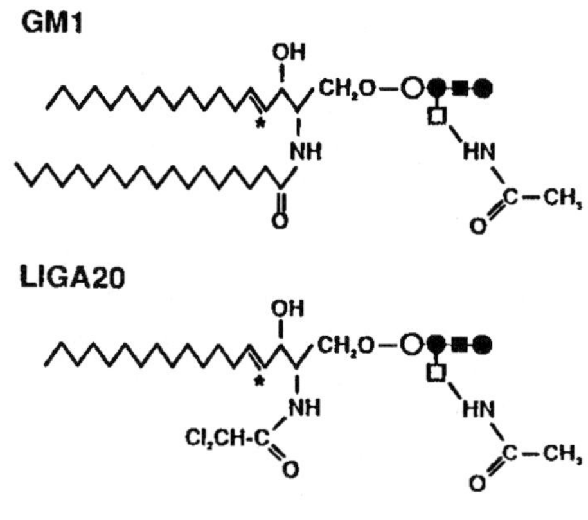


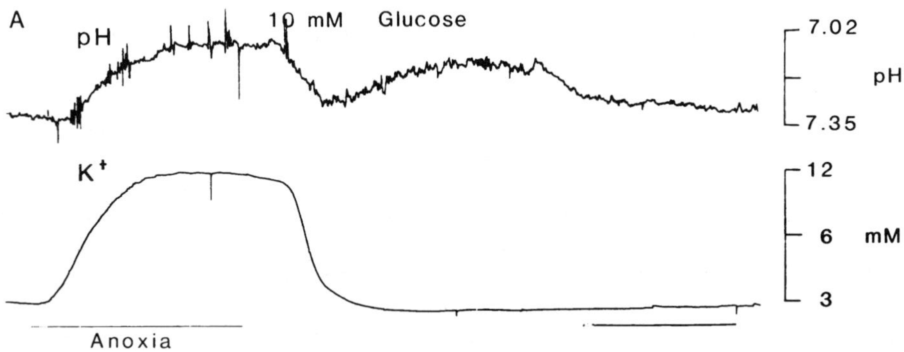


*Fig. 3.* Structure of GM1 and LIGA 20: the asterisk represents the position of tritium labeling in the compounds used for metabolic studies; □ = sialic acid; ○ = glucose; ● = galactose; ■ = N-acetylgalactosamine.

the same time intervals which in untreated neurons could overwhelm the homeostatic mechanism regulating $[Ca^{2+}]_i$ levels.

Working on an independent and apparently unrelated problem we had reported that in primary cultures of granule cells prepared from neonatal rat cerebellum GM1 could inhibit the translocation to the neuronal membrane of cytosolic protein kinase C elicited by the addition of glutamate to the neuronal culture[9]. Since the structure of GM1 includes a sphingosine molecule (Fig. 3) we decided to test whether a preincubation of the culture with GM1 could reduce the glutamate excitotoxicity *in vitro*. We could report that GM1 in a dose-related manner can inhibit the excitotoxicity elicited by glutamate[10]. This protection was maximized when the cells were preincubated with GM1 for about 60 minutes[11]. Moreover this protection could be related to the GM1 insertion in the neuronal membrane, for the increase in neuron GM1 content elicited by various GM1 concentrations correlated with the degree of GM1 protection against glutamate excitotoxicity[11].

These results prompted us to investigate whether by modifying the GM1 structure we could shorten the incubation time and enhance the protective action of GM1 against glutamate neurotoxicity. As a result of this investigation we discovered that among lysoganglioside derivatives of GM1 the N-dichloro derivative (LIGA 20, Fig. 3) possessed a protective action which was one order of magnitude greater than that of GM1[12]. Moreover this action not only was prompt and did not require a preincubation of the neuron with the protective agent, but also it lasted longer than that of GM1[12]. We then became interested in the mechanism whereby sphingoglyocolipids protect against the glutamate excitotoxicity. It became clear that *in vitro* the prevention of the protein kinase C translocation from cytosol to the neuronal membrane elicited by GM1 and LIGA 20 could not be dissociated from their protection against glutamate excitotoxicity[10]. Presumably the prevention of the phosphorylation of specific neuronal membrane proteins ($Na^+/Ca^{2+}$ exchanger?) mediated by the protein kinase C translocation, was a factor involved in the sphingoglycolipid protection from glutamate excitotoxicity. Moreover a direct measurement of glutamate channel gating in neurons pretreated with sphingoglycolipids failed to prevent the normal channel gating of glutamate[12]. This fact could also be verified by a direct visualization of $Ca^{2+}$ influx using a specific fluorescent probe[13]. However sphingoglycolipids attenuated the destabilization of $Na^+$ and $Ca^{2+}$ homeostasis elicited by a 20-minute exposure of the cell culture to 50 μM glutamate in absence of $Mg^{2+}$.[14] .

We then experimented with several rat models of stroke to verify whether also *in vivo* sphingoglycolipids could reduce the size of a cortical infarct elicited by a photochemical procedure[15]. In brief, this involves application of a cold white light to the exposed skull during the intravenous injection of rose bengal. This substance under the excitation of white light liberates oxygen singlets which have a damaging action on endothelial cells and produce a photothrombosis. Since sphingoglycolipids when given before the rose bengal do not prevent the oxygen singlets formation they fail to reduce the size of the primary lesion[15]. However GM1 and LIGA 20 can curtail the further development of the cortical infarct and reduce the necrosis occurring in the area penumbra that surrounds the cortical infarct[15]; they cause a 30% to 40% reduction of the infarct when the extent of the lesion is evaluated at seven days after the onset of the thrombosis. During the evaluation of the lesion we could document that an activation of a telencephalic protein kinase C occurring from two to 14 hours after the lesion is inhibited by a pretreatment with both LIGA 20, GM1 or dizocilpine[15]. Since this blocker of NMDA receptors was active in reducing protein kinase C activation we could infer that this process was triggered by glutamate[15]. Moreover if the lesion is applied bilaterally in the sensory motor cortex, at seven days after the lesion, the rats exhibit a cognitive deficit, that can be evaluated by using water maze tasks[16]. The rats pretreated with GM1 or LIGA 20 and receiving daily treatments with these drugs after the infarct, fail to evince a severe cognition deficit as detected by the water maze test. Actually their ability to learn new tasks compared with that of sham operated rats is significantly better than that of untreated rats[16].

A similar protection by LIGA 20 and GM1 was described by others[17-18] using a ligature of the medial cerebral artery to induce the brain damage.

We then compared the plasma and brain levels of GM1 and LIGA 20 in rats receiving the two drugs by mouth at various times before sacrifice. While GM1 virtually fails to reach the plasma or brain tissue when administered orally, the LIGA 20 reaches both plasma and brain by this route of administration[19]. Since the LIGA 20 levels measured in brain (about 1 μM) after oral administration are comparable to those that *in vitro* protect from glutamate excitotoxicity, we decided to study whether an oral pretreatment with LIGA 20 can reduce the size of the photochemical infarct and ameliorate the rat cognition deficit studied seven days after the infarct[16]. Also others[18] have verified that a pretreatment with oral LIGA 20 could protect the rats from the brain lesion induced by medial cerebral artery ligation. These authors reported that LIGA 20 could evince a protection when given orally before the production of the infarct[18]. We[19] and others[18] reported that the rate of LIGA 20 disposition *in vivo* is very slow

(T½ about 48 hr), while it concentrates in brain very rapidly after oral administration. This finding encouraged us to proceed with tests directed at evaluating whether there is a window of opportunity that allows to obtain a protection by injecting LIGA 20 after the induction of the experimental brain damage. The results obtained[16] allow us to conclude that an injection of LIGA 20 given after the induction of the experimental lesion can reduce the size of the infarct if the treatment is given within five hours after the injury.

**Dr. Quigley:** May I interrupt for a moment? Yesterday we had a discussion of whether we were actually rescuing cells or whether it was only a temporary delay in cell death. In your model, is this a permanent protection of the penumbra area cells? They do not ever die?

**Dr. Costa**: It is difficult to be categorical, but if a treatment with LIGA 20 is given before[15] or within five hours after thrombosis[16], there is a reduction of the infarct at seven days. We know that the infarct has reached maximal dimensions at 24 hours, hence we can suggest that the protection of neuronal death in a measurable volume of penumbra verified seven days later has probably resulted from a long-lasting protection, perhaps a permanent one. In fact this statement can be supported also with neuronal counts in the penumbra area which are higher in pretreated rats than in rats receiving the photothrombosis alone[15]. Moreover also from the functional standpoint the remarkable protection detected speaks in favor of a permanent protection from neuronal death. Using the model with bilateral lesions of the sensory motor area we could demonstrate a protection against the cognition deficit as measured with water maze tasks[16].

Let me conclude by stressing that we can only hypothesize that the protective action of sphingoglycolipids does not result from a blockade of glutamate receptors but from an antagonism of the destabilization of neuronal $[Ca^{2+}]_i$ homeostasis caused by the pathological and persistent activation of glutamate receptors permeable to $Ca^{2+}$.[12]. To understand better the mechanism of this protection we have studied the role of the inhibition of protein kinase C translocation in the protection and we found that this inhibition could not be dissociated from the protective action[20]. We suggest as a working hypothesis that phosphorylation of $Na^+/Ca^{2+}$ exchanger or of some proteins that are indirectly involved in the regulation of this exchanger may hinder the efficacy of this exchanger in extruding $[Ca^{2+}]_i$ from neurons. Inhibition of such phosphorylation might render the activity of $Na^+/Ca^{2+}$ exchanger more efficacious in $Ca^{2+}$ extrusion in the presence of high $Na^+$.

Now we are concentrating our efforts on the study of the role that the accumulation of intraneuronal $Na^+$ may have in hampering the $[Ca^{2+}]_i$ extrusion via the $Na^+/Ca^{2+}$ exchanger[21]. We know that sphingoglycolipids reduce simultaneously the destabilization of $[Na^+]_i$ and $[Ca^{2+}]_i$ elicited by a pathologically abusive stimulation of the receptor[14]. This indirectly indicates that the protective action of GM1 and LIGA 20 in glutamate excitotoxicity may be related to an action of these molecules on the $Na^+/Ca^{2+}$ exchanger function. We know that in brain there are different molecular forms of the $Na^+/Ca^{2+}$ exchangers and that in the retina has been described a specific isoform of the exchanger which can be found also in the brain. An obvious difference in the structure of various $Na^+/Ca^{2+}$ exchanger isoforms appears to be an amino acid deletion in the intraneuronal domain of this exchanger. Do these deletions possess a functional significance? Is the phosphorylation of the intracellular domain of the exchanger or the interaction of this domain with phosphorylated proteins (calmoduline?) changing to the $Na^+$ affinity of the $Na^+/Ca^{2+}$ exchanger? These and many other pertinent questions remain still unanswered.

**Dr. Siesjö**: This is a nice summary of a lot of things which you have done *in vitro*, and now also started doing *in vivo*. In your original hypothesis you assumed that gangliosides would block the translocation activation of PKC...

**Dr. Costa**: Will reduce the duration of the translocation.

**Dr. Siesjö**: Yes. but *in vivo* in full brain or global ischemia, several groups have shown that there is a translocation, but there is a deactivation of PKC, so that, I mean ...

**Dr. Costa**: Yes, the translocation is what is important. It is not important that the activity of the enzyme is reduced during translocation; what is important is that a protein kinase catalytic activity operates in a new milieu, and operates on substrates that were not available to the enzyme before. Our paper on the *in vivo* study of protein kinase activation during photochemical stroke appeared in the *Journal of Neuroscience*[15]. These data show that sphingoglycolipids inhibit protein kinase C activation (and presumably its translocation) but not the activation of early inducible genes, which may mediate the synaptic plasticity events associated with their protection against excitotoxicity *in vivo*.

**Dr. Siesjö**: I take it that your original hypothesis is now expressed in such a way that you say that it is the translocation which is the important part, and that it is a long-standing event which will change the characteristics of the membrane afterwards.

**Dr. Costa**: Right.

**Dr. Siesjö**: I have another question, and that relates to your stroke model. The model you used with rose bengal is an unconventional stroke model, because usually when you occlude a cerebral artery, like the middle cerebral artery, you do not get a very pronounced opening of the blood–brain barrier. With this photochemical lesion you get a pronounced opening of the barrier, and that occurs initially immediately when you apply the lesion to the tissue. So this is an unconventional way of inducing stroke...

**Dr. Costa**: I would not agree with you: when you open the skull and meninges you usually hamper the blood–brain barrier function, especially after you tie one of the main brain vessels.

**Dr. Siesjö**: No there are masses of articles published on the ability of tracers ...

**Dr. Costa**: I certainly disagree with this. It is enough that you cool off the brain that you change the blood–brain barrier properties.

**Dr. Siesjö**: Not for macromolecules. But anyhow, the point I am making ...

**Dr. Costa**: What do you mean for macromolecules?

**Dr. Siesjö**: I mean for proteins.

**Dr. Costa**: Ah, for proteins, then you do not talk anymore about the blood–brain barrier but of proteins entering the neuron via specific carriers. Perhaps you are considering the cellular barrier. I wanted to convince the audience that from a pharmacological viewpoint, sphingoglycolipids will enter the brain and act on the brain. The experiments on the protection by GM1 and LIGA 20 against brain lesions following ligature of the medial cerebral artery are now in the press[17,18]. I brought the attention of this group to the photothrombosis by rose bengal for two reasons. They use rose bengal as a diagnostic tool in the eye, and they apply light during the test. Perhaps the light they use may not trigger the oxygen singlet formation. And secondly, this model is closer to the clinical problems surrounding a stroke because you do not open the skull when you have a stroke, but you may have a thrombosis and rose bengal causes a thrombotic infarct. I know that conventionally the ligature of the medial cerebral artery is the most used, and GM1 and LIGA 20 protect also in this model[17,18]. I am a pharmacologist by training and by my professional life, and I am convinced that really the model including a ligation of blood vessels is not a good model if you want to study the action of a drug that crosses the blood–brain barrier by specific mechanisms, as might be the case of GM1 and LIGA 20. Indeed any lesion of the brain abolishes the blood–brain barrier if it causes ischemia.

**Dr. Siesjö**: I am predictably going to disagree with you, because I think, it is all right as long as you can show that the drug is acting both in the unconventional and in the conventional models of ...

**Dr. Costa**: There are publications on the beneficial effects of GM1 and LIGA 20 also in lesions caused by the ligation of cerebral arteries[17,18]. Also the involvement in GM1 protection of the translocation of protein kinase C has been published[15].

**Dr. Anderson**: Dr. Langer has a question first.

**Dr. Langer**: You clearly demonstrated that the GM1 mechanism of action of neuroprotection is different from blockade of NMDA receptors. Can you demonstrate that an antagonist of NMDA receptors acting at the channels, for instance, like MK 801, would be additive in its neuroprotection to GM1 or is it a synergistic effect, if you use proportionately low doses of each one?

**Dr. Costa**: The difficulty is the half-life of the MK 801 because in order to have the synergistic long term effect *in vivo* you would need two drugs that have a similar half-life. MK 801 has a half-life that is very short, three or four hours, and since the lesion is operative for 14 to 24 hours you need to repeat several times high doses of MK 801 (dizocilpine)... and if you do that you have to deal with the toxicity of dizocilpine. The data I presented indicate that the protection of MK 801 in this non-conventional model was the same as you can get with the gangliosides. You cannot obtain a better protection because the action of the free radicals is not blocked by GM 1 nor by dizocilpine.

**Dr. Langer**: Eliprodyl may be more appropriate because...

**Dr. Costa**: Huh?

**Dr. Langer**: Eliprodyl, our compound, that would be more appropriate because it has a longer half-life.

**Dr. Costa**: I will send you some LIGA 20 or GM1 for these tests.

**Dr. Anderson**: I would like to ask a question that may bring some relevance to glaucoma, and that is whether or not the glutamate receptors are excusively on the cell bodies or whether they also exist on the axons where you would not expect them because they should not have receptors. And secondly, since the protective mechanism is not acting directly on the receptor but by a mechanism further along, would axons also be protected by gangliosides in addition to the cell bodies being protected by gangliosides?

**Dr. Costa**: No, there are not many glutamate receptors in the axons. But, there is a neurotoxic activity of glutamate, on oligodendrocytes, leading to demyelinization as a result of a glutamate action on these glia cells. This action probably is not mediated by NMDA receptor for glutamate. These cells have an uptake of glutamate that can become important. In the presence of high levels of glutamate in interstitial fluids huge amounts of glutamate can be taken up in the oligodendrocytes and this amino acid will kill these cells by $Ca^{2+}$ independent mechanisms ... perhaps oxidative stress. *In vitro* this other mechanism of cell death triggered by glutamate can be inhibited by pretreatment with glutamate uptake blockers.

**Dr. Anderson**: Astroglia as well? The optic nerve head has astroglia, but no oligodendroglia.

**Dr. Costa**: Perhaps astroglia may not be sensitive; the experiments were done with oligodendrocytes. Moreover glutamate action on oligodendrocytes causes demyelinization. This process uncovers sodium channels, and when sodium enters in the neuron, it is extruded by the $Na^+/Ca^{2+}$ exchanger which exchanges the $Na^+$ for $Ca^{2+}$. Such a calcium influx may lead to a $Ca^{2+}$ dependent neuronal death. This theory is documented and proposed by the scientists of the Neurology Department at Yale University. Demyelinization is important in stroke, because in stroke there is not only a lesion of cell body but often there is a lesion of axons. I will try to answer your question about gangliosides in demyelinating axonal injuries. I may quote a clinical study published in the *New England Journal of Medicine* claiming ganglioside protection in spinal cord injury. There is now a multicenter study on spinal cord injury to definitively test whether gangliosides can ameliorate the consequences of spinal cord injuries. And I could not imagine another lesion that involves mostly axonal injury than a closed canal lesion of the spinal cord. Gangliosides appear to have also another protective action which I did not discuss. This is a capability to potentiate the action of neurotrophins and this action may be operative in the clinical use of gangliosides in stroke and in spinal cord injuries.

**Dr. Quigley**: I just want to ask briefly, what cells in the retina might be susceptible to glutamate toxicity?

**Dr. Costa**: I think, many. Two almost for sure: the bipolar cells receive a glutamatergic input, and also the ganglion cells receive glutamatergic synapses.

**Dr. Quigley**: Photoreceptors, do you think? Rods and cones, are any of them glutamate sensitive?

**Dr. Costa**: These cells transduce photons into current by a mechanism involving cyclic GMP and a specific phosphodiesterase, thus their function *per se* is not regulated by glutamate. But at least in fish they receive a glutamatergic input regulating dark and light adaptation which appears mediated by AMPA receptors.

## References


1. Rothstein J.D., Jin L., Dykes-Hoberg M., Kuncle R.W. Chronic inhibition of glutamate uptake produces a model of slow neurotoxicity. *Proc. Natl. Acad. Sci. USA* 90: 6591-6595, 1993.
2. Nanay Y., Smith C.P., Hediger A. The elusive transporters with a high affinity for glutamate. *TINS* 16: 365-370, 1993.
3. Weiler R. and Schultz K. Ionotropic non-N-methyl-D-aspartate agonists induce retraction of dendritic spinules from retinal horizontal cells. *Proc. Natl. Acad. Sci. USA* 90: 6533-6537, 1993.
4. Tanabe Y., Masu M., Ishii T., Shigamoto R., Nakanishi S. A family of metabotropic glutamate receptors. *Neuron* 8: 169-179, 1992.
5. Seeburg P.H. The molecular biology of mammalian glutamate receptor channels. *TINS* 16: 359-365, 1993.
6. Szekely A.M., Barbaccia M.D., Costa E. Activation of specific glutamate receptor subtypes increases cfos proto-oncogene expression in primary cultures of cerebellar granule cells. *Neuropharmacology* 26: 1779-1782, 1987.
7. Szekely A.M., Costa E., Grayson D.R. Transcriptional program coordination by N-methyl-D-aspartate sensitive glutamate receptor stimulation in primary cultures of cerebellar neurons. *Mol. Pharmacol.* 38: 624-633, 1990.
8. Connor J.A., Wadman W.J., Hackberger P.I., Wong P.K.S. Sustained dendritic gradients of $Ca^{2+}$ induced by excitatory amino acids in CA1 hippocampal neurons. *Science* 240: 649-653, 1988.
9. Vaccarino F., Guidotti A, Costa E. Ganglioside inhibition of glutamate-mediated protein kinase C translocation in primary cultures of cerebellar neurons. *Proc. Natl. Acad. Sci. USA* 84: 8707-8711, 1987.
10. Manev H., Costa E., Wroblewski J., Guidotti A. Abusive stimulation of excitatory amino acid receptors: a strategy to limit neurotoxicity. *FASEB* J. 4: 2789-2794, 1990.
11. Favaron M., Manev H., Alho H., Bertolino M., Ferret B., Guidotti A., Costa E. Gangliosides prevent glutamate and kainate neurotoxicity in primary neuronal cultures of neonatal rat cerebellum and cortex. *Proc. Natl. Acad. Sci. USA* 85: 7351-7355, 1988.
12. Manev H., Favaron M., Vicini S., Guidotti A., Costa E. Glutamate-induced neuronal death in primary cultures of cerebellar granule cells: protection by synthetic derivatives of endogenous sphingolipids. *J. Pharm. Exp. Ther.* 252: 419-427, 1990.
13. De Erausquin G., Manev H., Guidotti A., Costa E., Brooker G. Gangliosides normalize distorted single-cell intracellular free $Ca^{2+}$ dynamics after toxic doses of glutamate in cerebellar granule cells. *Proc. Natl. Acad. Sci. USA* 87: 8017-8021, 1990.
14. Costa E., Armstrong D.M., Guidotti A., Kharlamov A., Kiedrowski L., Manev H., Polo A., Wroblewski J.T. Gangliosides in the protection against glutamate excitotoxicity. *Progr. Brain Res.* 101: 357-373, 1993.
15. Kharlamov A., Guidotti A., Costa E., Hayes R., Armstrong A. Semisynthetic sphingolipids prevent protein kinase C translocation and neuronal damage in the perifocal area following a photochemically induced thrombotic brain cortical lesion. *J. Neurosci.* 13: 2483-2494, 1993.
16. Kharlamov A., Zivkovic I., Polo A., Armstrong D.M., Costa E., Guidotti A. A Lyso GM1 derivative (LIGA 20) given orally after cortical thrombosis reduces infarct size and associated cognition deficit. *Proc. Natl. Acad. Sci. USA* 91: (in press).
17. Simon R.P., Chen J., Graham S.H. GM1 ganglioside treatment of focal ischemia: a dose response and microdialysis study. *J. Pharm Exp. Ther.* 265: 24-29, 1993.
18. Seren M.S., Lazzaro A., Yang C.L., Canella R., Bassan M., Zanoni R., Manev H. Orally administered glycolipid derivative LIGA 20 reduces infarct volume and behavioral impairment after focal cerebral ischemia. *J. Pharm. Exp. Ther.* 268: 460-465, 1994.

19. Polo A., Kirschner G., Guidotti A., Costa E. Brain content of glycosphingolipids after oral administration of monosialoganglioside GH1 and LIGA 20 to rats. *Molec. Chem. Neuropath.* 21: 41-53, 1994.
20. Manev H., Guidotti A., Costa E. Protection by gangliosides against glutamate excitotoxicity. *Adv. Lipid Res.* 25: 269-287, 1993.
21. Kiedrowski L., Brooker G., Costa E., Wroblewski J.T. Glutamate impairs neuronal calcium extrusion while reducing sodium gradient. *Neuron* 12: 295-300, 1994.

# 12. OPTIC NERVE INJURY

BRUCE R. RANSOM, M.D., Ph.D.

**Dr. Caprioli**: Dr. Ransom has been working for some time on white matter lesions, white matter ischemia, and has used the optic nerve as a model, and he is going to share his experience and thoughts about that with us.

I have learned a lot thus far, and I am sure that that is going to continue.

I am going to give you a rather personalized and high-speed tour of the pathophysiology of white matter injury using the rat optic nerve as a model system. As a preliminary comment, I would admit that I am not at all sure that the details that I will tell you about today have any exact relevance for the pathophysiology of glaucoma. I would rather invite you to think about the things I am going to say as potentially important background information about the biology of optic nerve axons.

As a neurologist, my interest in studying white matter injury derives from an interest in understanding more about certain varieties of stroke. The majority of strokes involve both gray matter and white matter. A percentage of ischemic strokes involve white matter predominantly; these are often referred to as lacunar infarcts. At the outset, it seemed highly probable that the pathophysiology of axonal death is likely to be different than the pathophysiology of nerve cell body death simply because in the instance of neuron cell bodies and dendrites, where there is synaptic machinery, glutamate excitotoxicity is an important element in this pathophysiological cascade. In white matter, of course, there are no synapses, and therefore the pathophysiology is almost certain to be distinctive.

We have developed a model system for looking at this question using the rat optic nerve. I do not have to go into much detail about the anatomy of optic nerves to this group. The optic nerve, of course, is not a nerve at all but rather an extruded central white matter tract. In the rat, at least in the black hooded Long-Evans rat, there are about 100,000 myelinated axons in the optic nerve and this is a structure that is relatively simplified in comparison with gray matter. We basically only have axons, myelin, astrocytes and oligodendrocytes. There is no synaptic transmission. The presence of all of these axons gives us a convenient way to assess the function of the nerve by eliciting a supermaximal compound action potential. We do that in the following fashion.

We remove the rat optic nerve from the animal and put it in a typical tissue slice chamber on a small net. We perfuse it continuously with a physiological solution at 37°C, and I want to emphasize that everything I will show you today was done at 37°C; I think that is relatively important when translating from *in vitro* experimentation to what happens *in vivo*. We attach a stimulator to one end by way of a suction electrode and a recording apparatus to the other end, again using a suction electrode (Fig. 1A). The stimulus parameters are adjusted so that we can maximally activate the nerve. The presumption is that we are activating all of the axons that are viable, and recording the sum total of this activity at the other end. Through a couple of clever tricks and some computerization, it is possible to get a very quantitative measure of the functional integrity of the nerve in this particular manner (Stys *et al.*, *J Neurosci* 1992 12(2):430–439; Waxman *et al.*, *Brain Res* 1994, 644:197–204).

The anoxia itself is induced by simply changing over from a gas mixture which con-

*Optic Nerve in Glaucoma, pp. 181–198*
*edited by S.M. Drance*

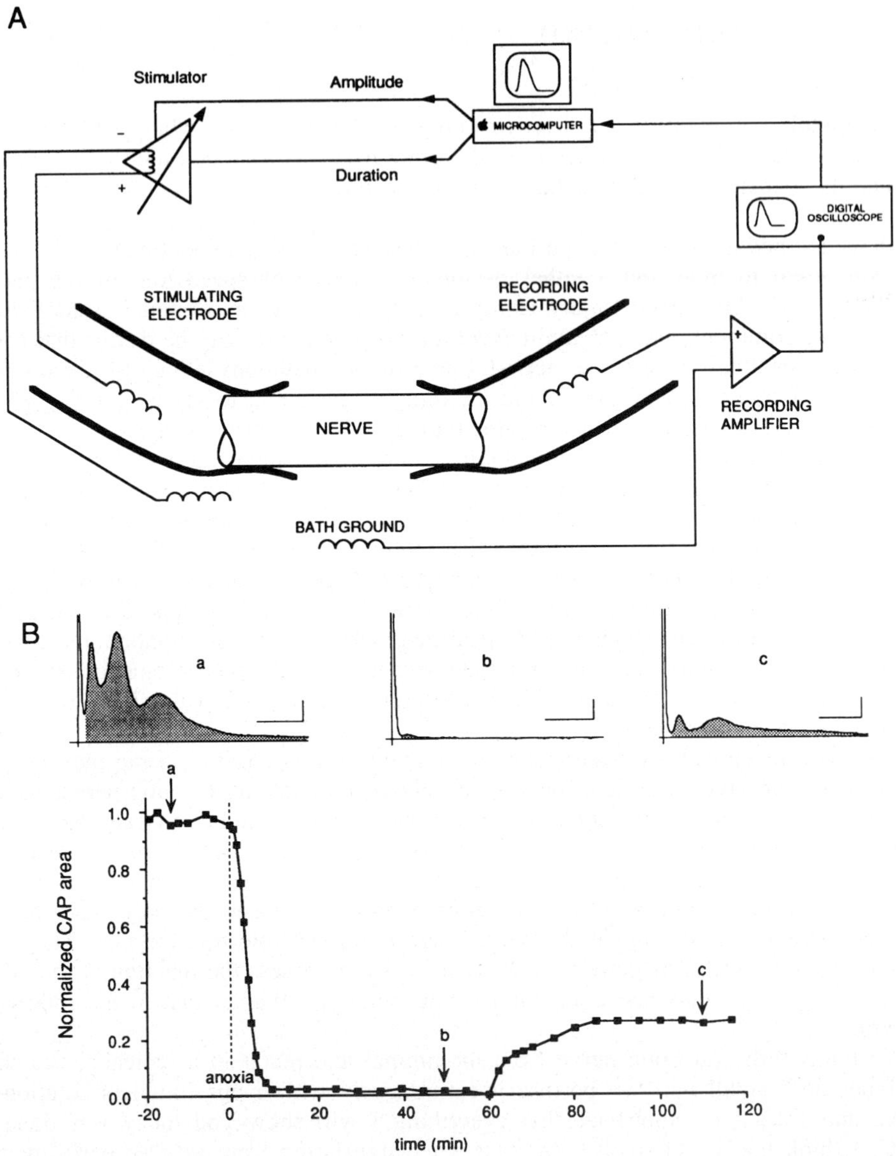


*Fig. 1.* Method of measuring rat optic nerve function before and after anoxia. A: Scheme of the recording arrangement. The rat optic nerve is stimulated via one suction electrode and the CAP is recorded from the other end of the nerve with a second suction electrode. Signals are amplified, digitized and transferred to a microcomputer for processing and storage. B: Effects of anoxia on WM function. The function of the optic nerve was monitored as the area under the CAP (a-c): this is shown graphically as percentage of the control CAP integral. Anoxia was begun at time zero. The CAP area rapidly declined becoming virtually zero after 10 minutes of anoxia (residual area was mostly stimulus artifact). A standard 60-minute period of anoxia was used in most experiments. After $O_2$ was reintroduced, the CAP area partially recovered. Postanoxic CAP measurements were routinely made 60 minutes after the end of anoxia since recovery always reached a plateau by this time. Specimen records of the CAP under control (a), anoxic (b), and postanoxic (c) conditions are shown. Calibration marks are 1 msec and 1 mV. (Reproduced with permission from: Ransom *et al.*, *Molecular and Cellular Approaches to the Treatment of Neurological Disease*, 1993, pp. 121–151. Raven Press, New York.)

tains 95% oxygen and 5% $CO_2$ to one which contains only nitrogen and 5% $CO_2$. We have measured oxygen tension at the level of the tissue and know that within a minute or two we get down very close to zero oxygen tension. The return of oxygen has a time course which is similar.

Before I go any further I want to recognize some of the colleagues that have worked with me, including Walter Carlini, Peter Davis, Peter Stys, Wolfgang Walz and Steve Waxman. Notably absent from this list is a current postdoc in the lab, Bob Fern, and I will get to some of the work he has been involved with at the end of the talk.

We started with a fairly straightforward list of questions that we needed to answer. First of all, we needed to find out whether or not anoxia had any effect whatsoever on white matter. That may sound surprising, but up until a few years ago there really was no rigorous white matter model where this question had been specifically asked.

Next we wanted to know whether or not an exposure to anoxia would result in some irreversible damage. We thought it would be important to look at ionic changes, because these are often an important first step in the cascade of events following disruption of energy metabolism, and such changes can reflect important changes in the capacity of nervous tissue to maintain normal transmembrane ion gradients. It also gives you a reflection of the metabolic condition of the tissue.

Finally, and perhaps most importantly, we wanted to get at the mechanisms of anoxic axonal injury. If there was irreversible injury, how did this come about? And this, we hoped, would give us insight into how to prevent or modify the injury. Or, in the words of Mark Twain, "first get your facts and then you can distort them at your leisure". We will do a little of that at the end.

Now this is perhaps the most important slide (Fig. 1B) that I will show you, and it is critical that before I go on, you understand exactly what is going on here. This is the typical supermaximal compound action potential that is elicited from an adult rat optic nerve. It is a boringly stereotypic event with three peaks which certainly represent three different speeds of conduction velocity in these axons. We look at the area under the curve, which gives us a quantitative measure of all of the axons contributing current to make the compound action potential. And for both intuitive as well as theoretical reasons, one can expect that each axon adds a small and linear amount of current to the signal here. So that as we lose axons, axons stop participating in the signal, then the signal gets smaller.

The answer to the first question, *i.e.* does anoxia cause dysfunction in white matter, is clear: anoxia does shut the axons down. You can see here that after a very brief period of anoxia, the signal is gone entirely. After we return the oxygen there is a partial return, but not a complete return of function (Fig. 1B). I am going to talk about this kind of data in other experiments, and what I am going to do is relate the data back to this control event, and we will normalize it to 1 or 100%. At the moment we apply anoxia there is a very rapid loss of function which eventually drops to zero. This event happens within four to seven minutes, indicating that dysfunction in mammalian central white matter has a time course that is quite similar to the dysfunction that arises in gray matter, maybe a little bit slower but certainly things go bad in a hurry.

After a period of 60 minutes of anoxia, you can see that the nerve has sustained irreversible injury since return of oxygen fails to cause a full return of function. All of the postanoxic recordings will be done one hour after the anoxic period, and at this point the residual amount of function remains stable for many hours. Not unexpectedly, the amount of irreversible injury is proportional to the period of anoxic exposure. It is important, and I will try to do this as I go along, to draw some comparisons with what happens in gray matter structures exposed to anoxia.

For brief periods of anoxia, brief at least as far as white matter is concerned, let us say periods of less than 20 minutes of complete anoxic exposure, the recovery from such an insult is nearly complete. After a period of 60 minutes of anoxia, you have lost about 65 to 70% of the normal compound action potential (*i.e.* about 35% recover). And it is not until about 90 minutes of anoxia that you reliably lose the compound action potential entirely. This tends to be a rather significant difference from what one sees in gray matter, at least as it has been studied *in vitro*. Ten to 20 minutes of anoxia in a synaptically active structure such as a piece of hippocampus in similar *in vitro* circumstances would certainly lead to irreversible and complete loss of synaptic function.

**Dr. Quigley**: Dr. Ransom, are you comparing this to the control tissue that had not also gone on for 60 minutes or 120 minutes or in each case is it being normalized to a control that was also kept in a jar for two hours.

**Dr. Ransom**: Yes, that is terribly important, and I appreciate you asking that question. The control compound action potential under circumstances where there are no manipulations, after an initial stabilization period, is absolutely rock solid for many many hours, so it is always referred back to the initial control.

**Dr. Drance**: Is that effect cumulative in any way? In other words, suppose you have a full recovery after 15 minutes and then you have a second one, does the second one recover as well?

**Dr. Ransom**: That is an interesting question and I think it relates to some of the things that we have heard previously in this meeting; that there may be a priming effect of a first insult. We have not done those experiments, but they would be very valuable to do.

**Dr. Caprioli**: What I would like to know is, when you talk about, let us say, 80% recovery, does that necessarily mean that 80% of the axons are firing full-tilt and 20% are not firing at all, or can that mean that 100% of the axons are firing suboptimally. In other words, are there sick cells in there or ....

**Dr. Ransom**: Sick sodium channels for instance. That is a good question and I do not have an absolutely precise answer. It turns out, as all of you know, optic nerve axons, and particularly those in the rodent, are very very tiny, and we are having to look at these in an aggregate fashion as opposed to one at a time. For theoretical reasons, and for some ultrastructural reasons that I will get to, it is probable that what we are talking about is a loss of function in 70% of the axons after 60 minutes of anoxia at 37 degrees, as opposed to a reduction of 70% in the functional currents being generated by *all* of the axons. If you lower sodium in the extracellular space in an effort to reduce the amplitude of an action potential, you can only lower it a small level before you get complete blockade, and that lowering of the sodium allows you to adjust the action potential down to about 60%, let us say, of its previous normal height, and at that point it is gone altogether. So I do not think that this represents a progressive loss of sodium channels.

**Dr. Siesjö**: I wonder, have you titrated the functional response of hypoxia in terms of oxygen tension. Is there a critical oxygen tension about or below which you get damage and above which you would not get any damage irrespective of the time of exposure.

**Dr. Ransom**: This is all going to be transcribed, so I am going to have a lot of experiments to do when I get home. No, we have not done that.

**Dr. Zeimer**: How do your facts apply to glaucoma. Could you tell us ahead of time how you think that will apply to glaucoma, so that I think while we listen to you talk we can try to distort it and apply it.

**Dr. Ransom**: I was trying to get out of trying to do that. I tell you what, let me put that off until the end of the talk, let us come back to that. I do not want to dodge that bullet entirely, but let us go on.

Now, I am going to talk almost exclusively about adult tissue, but I want to show you that there is something fascinating that goes on during development. In neonatal rat optic nerve the axons are totally unmyelinated and are very slowly conducting. The neonatal rat optic nerve could care less whether or not there is any oxygen around, so long as there is a little glucose in the bath, it is perfectly happy. Over the period of postnatal life from Day 10 to Day 20, this structure acquires its adult sensitivity to anoxic injury. For the first eight to 10 days of life, 60 minutes of anoxia is irrelevant to the rat optic nerve, complete function is either fully or partially maintained during anoxia itself, but certainly is present after the insult. Between Day 10 and 20, there is a steep development of the adult level of anoxic sensitivity. Now, there is an awful lot of things that happen between Day 10 and 20, and obviously this is an area which would be extremely interesting to pursue in greater depth, to begin to understand what biological alterations take place during this time. I will tell you that one of the striking things that happens between Day 10 and 20 is that every single optic nerve axon acquires a thick coat of myelin. At the end of the talk, if someone is interested, I will speculate, and it will clearly be speculation, on how this might wind up relating to the development of anoxic susceptibility.

Now we are back to adult tissue. Everyone has some sort of summary slide talking about the mechanisms of brain cell injury related to anoxia or some other sort of insult. I have tended to think about this as a two-stage process (Fig. 2). We are going to hear a lot more about some of the details here in subsequent talks this morning. I want to point out that there is fairly uniform agreement that anoxia is not good for neural tissue, that it leads rapidly to a decrease in ATP, and this quickly begets derangements of ionic gradients across membranes and a loss of excitability. There is also fairly uniform agreement that one of the critically regulated intracelluar ions, calcium, is deranged during this time, and that there is an increase in intracellular calcium that then sets in motion a second and very poorly understood set of events. I will not talk about this second stage, these calcium activated events, at all other than to point out that there is a long list of potential actors. There are a number of enzyme systems, for example, which are activated by increases in calcium; any one of them could wind up resulting in membrane destruction and a loss of critical membrane proteins such as pumps, sodium channels, other ion channels, etc. I am going to focus our attention on what happens in the first part of the paradigm (Fig. 2).

First, let us have a look at the ionic derangements that occur. Using ion-sensitive microelectrodes, it has been quite easy to look at changes in extracellular pH and extracellular potassium (Fig. 3). The extracellular potassium concentration is normally highly regulated in brain and in brain tissue *in vitro*. It is quite clearly in

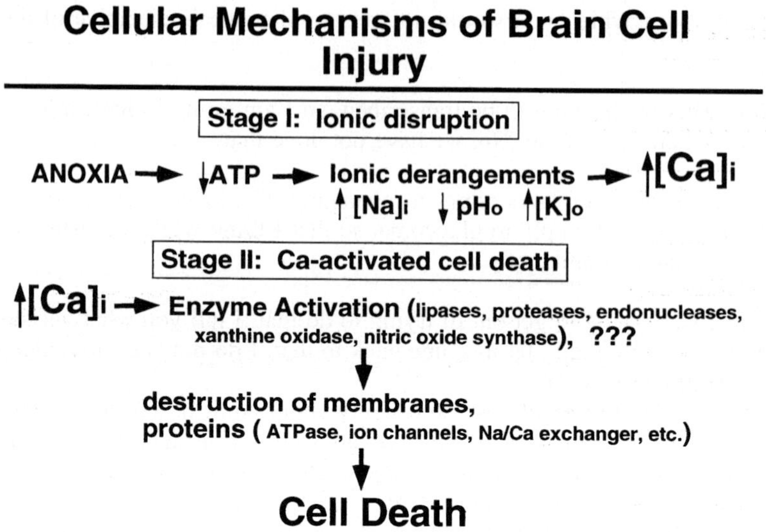


*Fig. 2.* Scheme of events associated with anoxic brain cell injury (see text).

equilibrium with the bath at a level of about 3 millimoles. When you start anoxia, within four or five minutes there is a slow creep in the level of extracellular potassium concentration, and then it rapidly goes up and it reaches a peak level in the neighborhood of 12 to 15 millimoles. Now, this is distinctly different than in gray matter, where generally the increase in extracellular potassium concentration with anoxia is much much higher, sometimes reaching levels of 60 to 100 millimoles.

At the same time that this change in potassium is taking place, there is an acid shift in the extracellular space, and this acid shift is proportional to the amount of glucose in the bath. If you have more glucose present, you have more substrate for anaerobic metabolism, and the acid shift is strikingly greater. Now, I would like to emphasize that these changes *per se* are probably not involved in irreversible injury to the optic nerve. You can expose it for extended periods of time to strikingly high levels of potassium; this results in dysfunction but no lasting irreversible injury. The same is true for high levels of lactic acid. These changes do reflect a switch from aerobic metabolism to anaerobic metabolism, and they do reflect changes in the capacity of the optic nerve, all of its elements, to maintain ion gradients. This level of increase in potassium will cause a complete loss of excitability and certainly depolarize membranes.

I do not have time to talk about where these ions are coming from. I simply want to say in passing that the only place they could be coming from in the optic nerve is from glial cells or from axons. We have evidence indicating that astrocytes are striking contributors to this increase in extracellular potassium concentration and to the export of protons to the extracellular space, so this is not exclusively an axonal property.

Now let us get back to the question of how these ionic derangements are translated to an increase in intracellular calcium concentration. As a comparison I will simply mention, and again you are going to hear much more about this in the com-

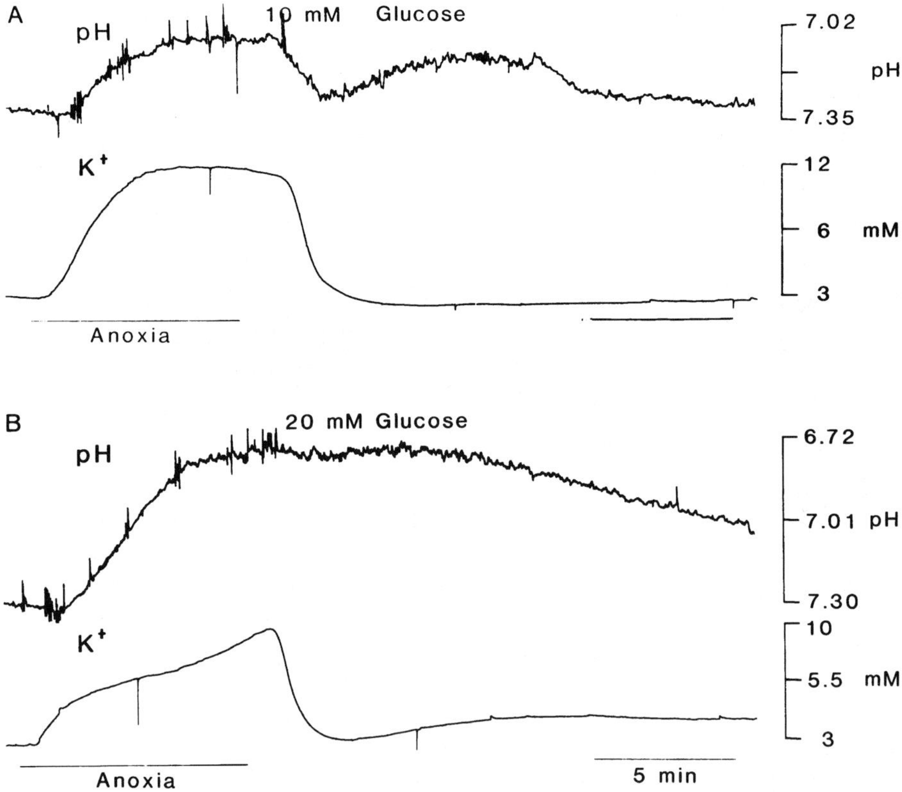


*Fig. 3.* The effects of anoxia on $pH_0$ and $[K^+]_0$ in the rat optic nerve. Separate ion selective microelectrodes, placed within 100 μM of one another, were used to measure $pH_0$ and $[K^+]_0$ in an adult rat optic nerve. The nerve was bathed in 10 mM glucose. The period of anoxia is shown by the bar. Under these circumstances, anoxia causes an acid shift within two to three minutes which averages approximately 0.3 pH units. Simultaneously, there is an increase in $[K^+]_0$ that averaged approximately 10-12 mM. These ionic abnormalities were gradually corrected in the post-anoxic period. The abrupt vertical deflections in the $pH_0$ recordings are artifacts related to vapor condensation on the electrodes. (Reproduced with permission from: Ransom *et al.*, *J Cerebral Blood Flow Metab*, 1992, 12:593–602.)

ing lectures, that in gray matter it is pretty well established that some of the events that are important include the release of excitotoxins, which activate channels that are partially permeable to calcium, and, perhaps to a lesser extent, activation of voltage-gated calcium channels. Now to first decide whether or not these early anoxic events result in a critical increase in intracellular calcium concentration, we did a very simple-minded experiment. We asked, “Does the development of irreversible injury in optic nerve axons depend on the presence of extracellular calcium?” and the answer is that it does.

Optic nerves exposed to anoxia in the absence of calcium showed almost complete CAP recovery (Fig. 4). This kind of interaction with calcium is graded. Intermediate levels of calcium (*i.e.* between 0 and 2 mM) during anoxia, give intermediate levels of CAP recovery (Fig. 4B). Moreover, the period of time the nerve was exposed to normal 2 mM calcium during anoxia determined outcome (Fig. 4C). If

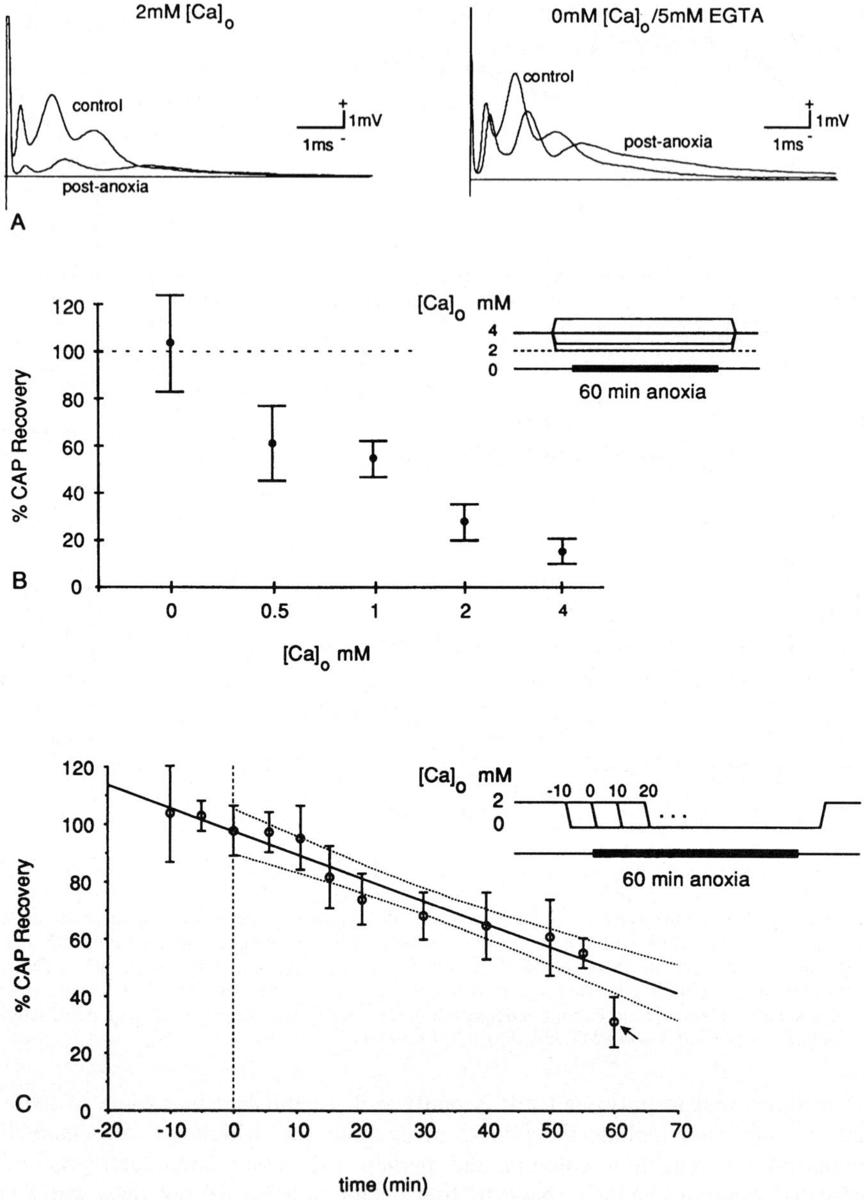


*Fig. 4.* Effect of perfusate [$Ca^{2+}$] on CAP recovery from 60 minutes of anoxia. A: CAPs before ("control") and 60 minutes after anoxia in 2.0 mM [$Ca^{2+}$] or zero [$Ca^{2+}$]/5 mM EGTA are shown. CAP recovery from anoxia is enhanced in the zero $Ca^{2+}$ solution. B: Average (± S.D.) percentage of CAP recovery after a standard 60-minute period of anoxia as a function of perfusate [$Ca^{2+}$] during anoxia. Test solutions were begun 10 minutes before anoxia onset and continued until 10 minutes after the end of anoxia (see inset). The percentage of recovery of the CAP gradually diminished as perfusate [$Ca^{2+}$] increased from 0 to 4 mM. All points were significantly different from the normal [$Ca^{2+}$] of 2 mM ($p<0.005$). C: Effect of duration of $Ca^{2+}$ exposure during anoxia on degree of CAP recovery. The graph shows percentage of CAP recovery (measured 60 minutes after re-oxygenation) as a function of the time at which the perfusion solution containing zero [$Ca^{2+}$]/5 mM EGTA was begun in relationship to the 60-minute anoxic interval. The x-axis denotes the number of minutes after the start of anoxia when the zero [$Ca^{2+}$] solution entered the chamber,

bath calcium was only available for the last 30 minutes of anoxia the outcome was better than if it had been present from the beginning.

Now, the nominal interpretation of this result is that calcium is moving from some extracellular compartment to some intracellular compartment. Two questions come to mind. First of all, which compartment is it moving into? Clearly it could be axonal, and in fact, intuitively, that would make the most sense. But it could also be into a glial compartment, particularly into the oligodendrocyte. Function would reasonably be lost if there was a loss of myelination, or at least functional myelination, so that saltatory conduction could no longer take place. The second question is, how does the calcium get in?

Now, I can only give you indirect evidence with regard to the first question, of which compartment experiences the calcium increase. And I will do that using a few ultrastructural observations that we have made. In a normal rat optic nerve, you see myelinated axons and occasional astrocytes, and a fairly well organized and tight extracellular space. After 60 minutes of anoxia, there is a grave disruption of this picture. The axoplasm especially of large axons, is now shriveled up and huddled in one corner of its normal location. Space appears between the axolemma itself and the inner lamella of myelin. Some smaller axons look relatively intact. There is partial disruption of the extracellular space. Ultrastructural cytoarchitecture, *i.e.* the microtubules and the neurofilaments, are severely damaged in axons after 60 minutes of anoxia. Likewise, the mitochondria, which are normally beautifully preserved in well fixed tissue, are swollen up with a complete disruption of the crystae. We use these kinds of observation to at least indirectly suggest that the calcium is probably moving into an axonal compartment. There has been a lot of work inducing calcium to move into axons, and whenever you do that under very controlled experiments elsewhere, you find that you get exactly this kind of picture, but I admit that this is certainly indirect.

Next question, How does the calcium move from the extracellular space into the cytoplasmic compartment? It came up in the last talk whether or not there might be transmitter-activated channels on axons. And this is probably a question that needs to be answered on an area by area basis. I can certainly tell you that in our studies on the rat optic nerve, there are no glutamate-gated ion channels on these axons. And in fact, we have applied industrial strength glutamate and aspartate to these axons for extended periods of time and absolutely nothing happens. So we are crossing this off the list as a possible way by which calcium might enter axons during anoxia. What about voltage-gated calcium channels? Clearly this is something of concern to people studying nerve cell bodies where there are plenty of voltage-gated calcium channels; in the rat optic nerve there appear to be none. We have tried a variety of calcium channel blockers, and they are without benefit to the nerve under these conditions of anoxic exposure. So that left us with two possibilities. One of them more theoretical than anything else, that perhaps calcium goes through another channel during anoxia. What we call the "sodium channel" is not permeable to sodium

---

←
and the y-axis represents the average (± S.D.) percentage of CAP recovery. Thus, time = -10 minutes corresponds to a switch to zero [$Ca^{2+}$] 10 minutes before the start of anoxia. Inset illustrates relationship between timing of solutions and anoxia. When zero [$Ca^{2+}$] was begun prior to anoxia, the area under the CAP regained 100% of its control amplitude. As the change to zero [$Ca^{2+}$] solution was delayed with respect to the start of the anoxic period, progressively less recovery was observed.

alone; rather there is a permeability ratio, so that it mainly lets in sodium but it can let in an occasional calcium ion as well. For reasons that I will not go into in detail, this is a very unlikely explanation.

That left us with a single actor, the sodium-calcium exchanger. Now, some of you may not be familiar with sodium-calcium exchange, so I am going to spend a moment talking to you about this. This is a ubiquitous protein transporter that is found in almost every cell that has been studied. Its job is primarily to regulate calcium down to nanomolar, high nanomolar levels, in cells, with the remaining calcium regulation primarily the job of the calcium ATPase. The sodium–calcium exchanger works by the energy stored in the sodium gradient. It does not break down ATP. The sodium gradient would normally favor the inward movement of sodium, and as sodium moves down its gradient it is coupled to outward movement of calcium. You will notice that the stoichiometry of this reaction is that three sodiums go in, and one calcium comes out; this is true for many transporters but not for all that have been studied. That means for every net cycle of this particular machine, a net positive charge comes in. This transporter therefore is sensitive to the membrane potential. If you depolarize a cell that contains this transporter you discourage the further movement of sodium down its gradient, because now there is less of an electrochemical gradient for that to happen. It is terribly important to add one final point: This transporter has absolutely no preference about whether or not it moves calcium out of the cell or into the cell, it will work in either direction. All it cares about are the thermodynamics of the situation in which it finds itself. If you increase intracellular sodium concentration and depolarize the cell, then it is perfectly happy to rapidly move calcium from outside to inside, and sodium from inside to outside. Now, if this is in fact what is going on during anoxia in the rat optic nerve, it suggests a couple of simple and fairly straightforward experiments.

Anything you can do to block the increase in intracellular sodium ought to be protective, and we looked at that in two ways. First, tetrodotoxin was used to block voltage-gated sodium channels and to see whether or not block of sodium movement into axons might be protective. With increasing concentrations of tetrodotoxin, we got increasing levels of improvement. So certainly this is consistent with the idea that sodium might be moving through voltage-gated sodium channels and increasing its intracellular concentration on that basis.

I do not have time to talk about the exact nature of the sodium channels that are engaged in allowing sodium entry during anoxa, but these are likely to be slightly atypical sodium channels, which do not completely inactivate. We have fairly convincing evidence that rat optic nerve axons do, in fact, possess non-inactivating sodium channels. These channels would remain open even when the membrane potential was persistently depolarized, as would be the case in these axons during anoxia.

The other experiment you can do is to simply remove sodium during the anoxic period. The sodium-calcium exchange requires a certain basal level of intracellular sodium concentration in order to function. And that level is in the neighborhood of about 20 to 25 millimoles. By removing sodium you deplete intracellular sodium and block exchange operation. When sodium is replaced by either lithium or choline, this results in a dramatic improvement in recovery from 60 minutes of anoxia.

Now, the final thing that you certainly want to see is that if you block reverse sodium-calcium exchange, this is also protective. And we have used three drugs to try to do this. Two are derivatives of amiloride called benzamil and dichlorobenzamil, and the other is a drug that is frequently used as a stabilizer of cardiac rhythms called bepridil. At low concentrations these drugs are rather specific inhibitors of sodium-calcium exchange. All of them, applied during anoxia, partially protect the rat optic nerve against anoxic injury.

I would like to summarize this sequence of pathophysiological steps in a schematic diagram (Fig. 5). Under normal circumstances, where there is plenty of oxygen and plenty of glucose, there is sufficient ATP and the sodium pump works quite normally to maintain ion gradients. That means that intracellular sodium is regulated to a low level, whereas there is plenty in the extracellular space, and intracellular potassium concentration is regulated to a high level, whereas there is very little in the extracelluar space. If you decide to "operate" the optic nerve for sending messages (*i.e.* action potentials), that is fine, because the sodium that comes in through the voltage-gated sodium channels is rapidly removed by this pump, which is fully energized. Under these conditions, the sodium-calcium exchanger is running in its forward mode; it is busy removing calcium from the cell, regulating it down to these high nanomolar concentrations.

**Dr. Siesjö**: If the axon has to remove calcium all the time, by what routes would calcium enter to create the need to remove it continuously by the exchanger?

**Dr. Ransom**: I do not know, I am not sure exactly what the basal needs are for the axon. My suspicion is that these axons have a very unfavorable surface to volume ratio, they have got relatively small volumes for their surface, so even a small amount of calcium leak, say, for example, through the sodium channel during activity, might wind up being a problem for the axon and necessitating the presence of machinery such as this sodium-calcium exchanger. But really that is speculation, and I can not give you a specific answer to that question.

**Dr. Choi**: Is there any evidence for internal calcium stores in these axons, do they have calciosomes? That might be another way that calcium could increase intercellularly.

**Dr. Ransom**: Yes, that is another good question, it may be fun to try to deplete intracellular stores and repeat some of these experiments in the absence of calcium and see what the outcome is.

**Dr. Choi**: But do they have these stores?

**Dr. Ransom**: There are some submembranous cisterns, and these in fact could be calcium stores. There is certainly not a lot of endoplasmic reticulum in these axons.

**Dr. Costa**: There could be one other calcium source in the axons. Mitochondria could be a source of calcium storage in the axon.

**Dr. Ransom**: That is true, and there are some mitochondria, for sure.

**Dr. Quigley**: Is this something that also would apply to unmyelinated axon since the area we are interested in in glaucoma is an area of unmyelinated axons , just barely "un" like a one-sided node of Ranvier.

**Dr. Ransom**: Yes, I think it would, certainly.

Under circumstances where you do not have any oxygen and are forced to rely on an increasingly chancy distribution system for glucose alone, certainly the ATP levels fall, and now at this point the pump can no longer do its job adequately and you get a breakdown in transmembrane ion gradients. Under these circumstances, when sodium comes in through activated voltage channels, and as depolarization ensues, which will certainly happen, there is no possibility of quickly removing it by way of the sodium pump. Those are the circumstances that favor reverse sodium-calcium exchange, and if anyone is interested I will show you some thermodynamic reasons why this happens rather quickly and for relatively small amounts of depolarization. In any event, we believe that reverse sodium-calcium exchange loads these axons with calcium during anoxia (Fig. 5).

So, taking you back to a very quick comparison of white matter and gray matter, I simply wanted to point out that in white matter the steps that appear to be mediated by NMDA receptors and voltage-gated calcium channels are not operative, and the calcium loading appears to go by way of reverse sodium-calcium exchange, which is conditioned by progressive membrane depolarization due to energy failure and an increase in intracellular sodium concentration.

Based on this sort of pathophysiological schema, one could make a list of things that ought to protect the axons from destruction. Certainly if you can do something to reduce sodium influx during anoxia, that is a good idea. We have done this using TTX (see above), and this provides protection. We tried some interesting compounds that are sitting on most people's pharmacological shelf, including local anesthetics and anticonvulsants, all of these things are known to block use-dependent sodium channels or sodium channels in general, and in fact, all of them have some benefit in protecting against anoxic injury. It would be terrific to come up with a sodium-calcium exchange inhibitor which blocked only reverse exchange. And since this transporter has been cloned it seems reasonable to think that the stage is set for further developments which might allow the development of a molecule that could selectively block reverse sodium-calcium exchange. That would be a terrific drug.

And then there are a variety of other things that are certainly on the horizon. For example, the local anesthetic drug QX134 a quaternary compound, has the property of being selectively effective in blocking non-inactivating sodium channels, the exact channels most likely involved in sodium loading during anoxia. The application of QX314 in relatively small concentrations that actually do not do very much to the compound action potential, so you can imagine giving this to an individual and having it result in absolutely no change in nervous system function, causes dramatic improvement in function after 60 minutes of anoxia.

Before I conclude I will tell you a new wrinkle in this whole story that involves neurotransmitters. This is new, presently unpublished work.

Bob Fern, a postdoctoral fellow, stumbled upon the observation that in white matter the application of the neurotransmitter substance GABA, which is the major inhibitory neurotransmitter substance in the central nervous system of mammals, is protective against anoxic injury. This particular GABA effect is present at very low concentrations 1 μM, and disappeared at higher concentrations of GABA, suggesting to us that it may be acting at a receptor that eventually desensitizes. Curiously, it is not acting at the most well known GABA receptor, *i.e.* the GABA-a receptor that mediates inhibition by way of a chloride flux, but appears to be acting at a GABA-b receptor. Thus the specific GABA-a agonist, THIPP, has no benefit, but the specific

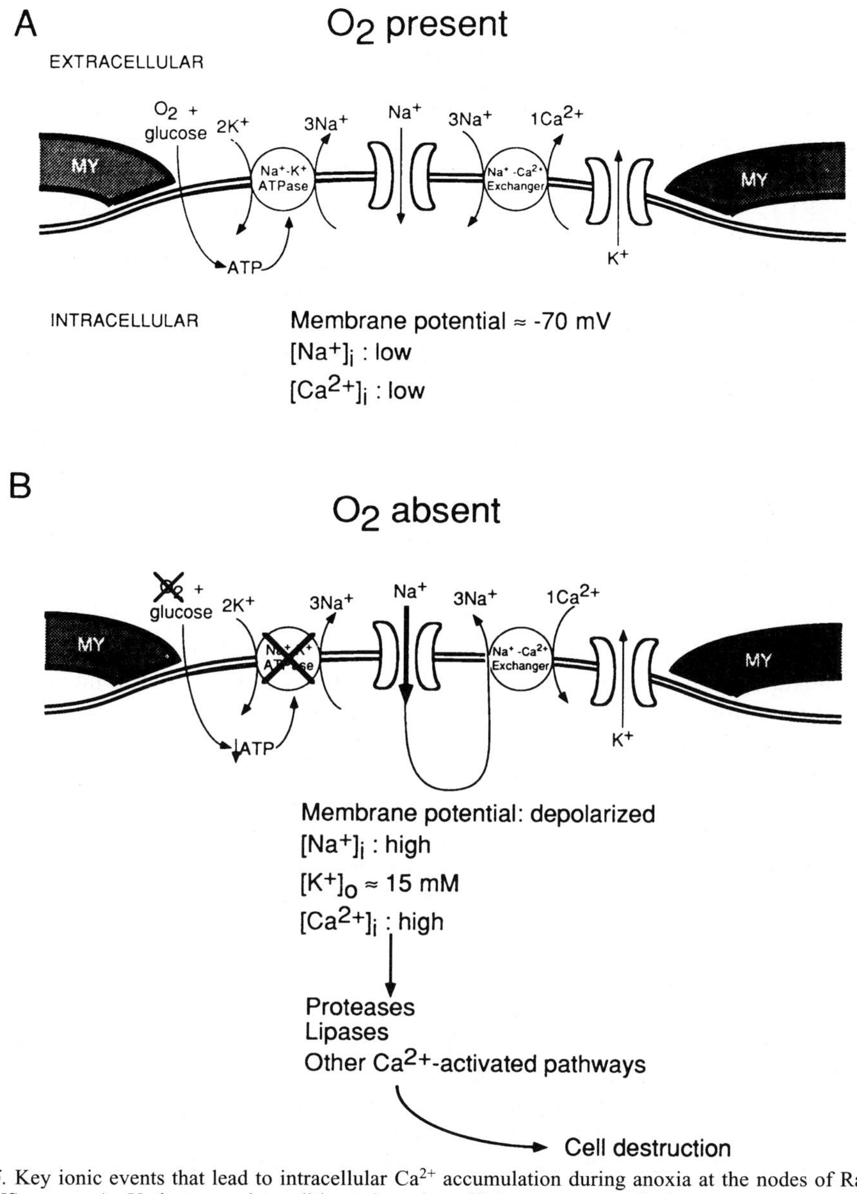


*Fig. 5.* Key ionic events that lead to intracellular $Ca^{2+}$ accumulation during anoxia at the nodes of Ranvier of CNS axons. A: Under normal conditions there is sufficient oxygen and glucose present to generate enough ATP to operate the necessary ion pumps that are critical to maintaining excitability. If $[Na^+]_i$ increases due to action potentials, this increase is easily compensated by enhanced $Na^+$ pump activity. The steep $Na^+$ gradient produced by the $Na^+$ pump in conjunction with high negative membrane potential, drives the high capacity $Na^+$–$Ca^2$ exchanger in the forward direction, which helps to maintain low $[Ca^{2+}]_i$. There is reason to believe that both the $Na^+$ pump and the $Na^+$–$Ca^{2+}$ exchanger might be preferentially located at the nodes because this is where activity-dependent ion fluxes occur in myelinated axons. B: In the absence of oxygen the generation of ATP is seriously reduced because it is now exclusively coming from glycolysis. The shortfall of ATP (the extent of which depends on glucose availability) causes ion gradients to deteriorate, and the speed of deterioration is augmented by action potential activity, which increases the workload on the $Na^+$ pump. As the transmembrane $Na^+$ gradient falls and the membrane depolarizes, the $Na^+$–$Ca^{2+}$ exchanger is driven to work in reverse and begins loading the axon with $Ca^{2+}$. The ultimate destruction of cellular integrity is probably mediated by $Ca^{2+}$-activated destructive enzymes such as proteases and lipases (see Fig. 1), but these final steps have yet to be clarified.

GABA-b agonist, baclofen, is strikingly protective. GABA is normally present in the rat optic nerve and our experiments suggest the possibility that anoxia might be releasing endogenous stores of GABA, and that the GABA from the nerve acts in an "autoprotective" fashion to preserve function or to reduce the amount of irreversible injury. This idea was strengthened by the observation that a blocker of GABA re-uptake, nipecotic acid increased recovery from anoxia.

GABA-b receptors are known to be connected to G proteins and to complex second messenger systems, and we did a few experiments to see whether or not that might be the case here. The protective effect of GABA created by the application of 1 mM GABA, is blocked by pertussis toxin, which would block G protein systems. The steps that might happen afterward could be fairly complex, but we decided to test a few compounds and discovered that the protein kinase C system mimicked the benefit that we saw with the direct application of GABA, suggesting perhaps that GABA was acting at a GABA-b receptor and this was resulting in a G protein step leading to activation of protein kinase C. Finally, if you block protein kinase C by the application of H7, then the benefit of GABA is entirely lost. Anoxia, we suspect, causes a release of endogenous GABA stores, and these released GABA stores activate protein kinase C via a G protein. Exactly how this sequence produces protection is presently unclear.

I will stop at this point and thank you for your attention.

**Dr. Caprioli**: Bruce, you promised Ran Zeimer that we were going to tie this together with glaucomatous damage, and perhaps I could just intervene a little bit in that regard. I think that if we are going to consider ischemic or anoxic damage at all as a possible process in glaucoma, this would be a highly localized process with repeated small insults that may result in what appears to be a chronic degenerative disease rather than a large infarct of the type that you are studying. So there are a couple of questions that arise from that hypothesis, if you will. And one of these is to follow up Harry's question about the machinery that you find at the nodes of Ranvier, and you seem to think that they would also exist proximal to the myelinated sheath, proximal to the cell body as well. At the level of the lamina and prelaminar area.

**Dr. Ransom**: Yes, right, and you might have suspected that I have some experimental data up my sleeve to support that notion; I truly do not. The reasoning is based on the observation that the primary players in this pathophysiological sequence, including the sodium-calcium exchanger, are all present in axonal membranes. So really, it is an argument based only on inferences and nothing experimental. Is it testable? Yes, I think that there are going to be wonderful probes for the sodium-calcium exchanger that will come out of the cloning of this protein, and it will be possible to develop monoclonal antibodies and molecular probes for looking at this.

**Dr. Caprioli**: You indicated that there are no glutamate receptors that you can find, at least, you presented evidence that there are not any receptors in the myelinated portion of the nerve. Now, these receptors are in high concentration in the cell body, of course, and presumably some of them might float down the cell membrane, and I wonder if there have been any studies to indicate the density of such receptors as a function of distance from the cell body, you know, toward the lamina, for instance.

**Dr. Ransom**: That is a fascinating thought, and clearly there are some instances where there appears to be a mismatch between the presence of receptors and the presence of machinery for the normal use of those receptors. An example would be the dorsal root ganglion cell body. Although there are no inhibitory synapses directly on that structure, it makes GABA receptors for translocation to its presynaptic terminals, and yet there are a few on the cell body. Now, in this particular instance, our studies are confined to the myelinated portion of the axon, and we can not find evidence of any glutamate receptors. But I do not know the answer to your specific question and it is worth considering further.

The only other thing I would add is, that as I am learning more about cell biology, I am discovering that the capacity of a cell to manufacture something and send it to an exactly correct address is pretty darn good, and it would not be a surprise to me if there was a really very specific and abrupt termination of the insertion of these receptors right at the axon hillock, with no extension into the axonal membrane.

**Dr. Siesjö**: As you know, I belong to your fan club, I have read a lot of your articles, but I am going to raise a question about how we can translate the *in vitro* experiments to *in vivo* conditions. And of course, the reason is that if you suspend a nerve in an artificial solution, and I think a calcium concentration of 1.3 mM or whatever you have, then you have an unlimited source of calcium, when the nerve is anoxic for, say, 60 minutes under those conditions there is the possibility to load the axon with calcium because you supply more calcium all the time. *In vivo,* of course, the amount of calcium available is very restricted, because it is that confined to the extracellular fluid, and there you need transport across the blood–brain barrier, to get even more calcium. So the question is, how do you think these results can apply to *in vivo* conditions where you have a very limited source of calcium. Have you, for example, measured the influx of calcium, the total amount of calcium, flowing into the nerve during, say, 60 minutes of anoxia?

**Dr. Ransom**: No, we have not done that. I know Dennis has done some nice studies using calcium-45 as a marker for total calcium accumulation, and you could do studies like that in this system. But let me come back really to the essence of your question. I agree with you. The truth of the matter is that during a stroke, the availability of calcium is quite limited. It is the calcium that resides in the extracellular space that is immediately able to enter cells. Additional calcium can enter cells only by diffusing into the anoxic region from adjoining areas that are not anoxic. In our studies the calcium has to diffuse in from the bath to the nerve, this distance may be shorter than in most *in vivo* situations. It may be that the way to translate what I am talking about here to the intact situation is to make very careful measurements about the concentration of calcium in the extracellular space of white matter regions of the brain during anoxia, and then just simply duplicate that level of calcium in our bath. The single piece of data that is missing right at the moment from carrying out such experiments is to know exactly what the extracellular calcium concentration is in the extracellular space of white matter. People have primarily looked at gray matter regions where calcium falls very quickly to levels which are very low, let us say a tenth of a millimole.

**Dr. Quigley**: If we were going to duplicate the semiphysiologic condition of an optic nerve, we would be sitting there conducting impulses all the time. In your *in vitro* circumstance, are you artificially producing those impulses during the 60 minutes of anoxia, which would simulate the metabolic demands of transmission.

**Dr. Ransom**: Yes, I understand your point entirely, and it is a point well taken. It comes back to Joe's point, of trying to juxtapose this kind of information *vis à vis* a situation of injury such as you might find in glaucoma. To do this, you are going to be thinking more on microscopic terms, you are going to be thinking about tiny fascicles of nerves, as opposed to something that goes on with the whole nerve. Under these circumstances, it is a far easier thing to juxtapose what I have been telling you about to global ischemia, where there is suddenly no blood to the whole brain. Under those circumstances, potassium accumulates and completely abolishes excitability. So the nerve may be trying to work, it may be trying to send signals from the retina back to the brain, but it can not do that. The excitability is abolished by this breakdown of ion gradients, and that is true really for any area in the brain that has an anoxic insult of this sort.

It would be interesting to model more closely the circumstances that are relevant to glaucoma. One might do that experimentally by isolating small fascicles and intermittently stimulate them while exposing them to reduced levels of oxygen; this ought to be possible.

**Dr. Quigley**: With also intermittent low levels of oxygen, rather than total anoxia.

**Dr. Ransom**: That is right.

**Dr. Langer**: Your data indicate that there are GABA-b receptors and a transporter for GABA which is functional because it inhibited with nipecotic acid. Where are these sites located, the GABA-b receptor and the uptake system?

**Dr. Ransom**: We do not have all this information right at the moment. The GABA uptake system is clearly located in a variety of places. There is solid evidence that it is located in astrocytes. There is a high affinity GABA-specific uptake system in astrocytes that can accumulate GABA against a very steep concentration gradient, and so I suppose that is the primary site for the GABA uptake mechanism. As far as the receptors are concerned, I would argue, just intuitively at this point, that the GABA-b receptors are probably located on the axons. Is there any evidence for that? Yes; in the neonatal rat optic nerve it is very clear that you can apply GABA and get a dose response curve in terms of changes in the functional excitability of the nerve. And it has a classic pharmacology. Unfortunately, those are GABA-a receptors. We know virtually nothing about the distribution of GABA-b receptors in this structure, that is going to take some further work.

**Dr. Anderson**: In an effort to make this relevant to the structure that we are all looking at here, certainly there are a lot of astrocytes that are in that region, and the GABA receptors that you talked about might be there. How about the GABA stores that are necessary for this mechanism, is there a GABA store that might be present in this region? Is GABA manufactured locally at the synapse in the lateral geniculate body? Or is GABA manufactured in the cell body and transported along the axon, so that the axon might be in the process of transporting this down the axon to an end terminal, and therefore this would constitute a store. Where is the store of GABA?

**Dr. Ransom**: I am going to take a flyer in answering that, but I should quickly say that there are neurochemists in the audience and they may have very specific information about GABA. Let me say that GABA is not just involved as a synaptic transmitter, but it is a molecule that winds up in lots of metabolic pathways. So you can take an astrocyte from any region that you want, or in a dish, and find GABA in that astrocyte. So there is probably no problem coming up with a store of GABA. Astrocytes have it in them, and probably neural elements outside of synaptic regions have it in them as well, so I would not think that that is a particular problem.

**Dr. Langer**: The GABA-b receptors are the same type of receptor that are located on the terminal, and they modulate transmitter release through a negative feedback mechanism, but they are functional and they are in the terminal and they are consequently transported down the axon. The question is whether during transport down the axon you can demonstrate any functional role, because what we know is that they are functionally active in modulating transmitter release when they are located in the membrane of the nerve terminal that releases GABA.

**Dr. Ransom**: I think that is helpful, it means that they are moving down, they are passing through these axonal areas, and if a few decorate nodes of Ranvier or other sites in the axon, that would not be a terrible surprise.

**Dr. Hoffman**: One question I have is about the mechanism by which the neonatal axons are resistant to anoxia. It was not clear to me exactly what the mechanism was. Presumably there are potassium channels as well as sodium channels distributed continuously along the unmyelinated portion of the neonatal axon, is that correct?

**Dr. Ransom**: It is correct that there are both sodium channels and potassium channels distributed along the unmyelinated neonatal axon.

**Dr. Hoffman**: I guess my question is, is that more analogous to the initial portion of the unmyelinated optic nerve prior to acquiring a myelin sheath and after it goes through the lamina in terms of its susceptibility to anoxia, or do you think there is a fundamental change that occurs in the neuron during development, where it becomes more sensitive. Or do you think it is a local phenomenon having to do with surface to volume ratios and the distribution of channels.

**Dr. Ransom**: Paul, if you have any specific ideas as to why the neonate acquired adult levels of anoxic susceptibility, it was not from me that you got that information. I do not have that answer. I said that I had a speculation, and it is this: The density of sodium channels in unmyelinated axons is extraordinarily low. It is surprising to discover that a tenth of a sodium channel every square μm is enough to run a perfectly healthy action potential down one of these tiny unmyelinated axons. The density of sodium channels at nodes of Ranvier in adults is extraordinarily high, it is a thousand per square micra, so there is a 10,000-fold difference in the density of sodium channels if you compare nodes of Ranvier to these unmyelinated axons. Now, I have explained that accumulation of intracellular sodium is critical to the development of circumstances for reverse sodium-calcium exchange. During myelination, you get a topographic redistribution of sodium channels, all the sodium channels that had been distributed uniformly along the unmyelinated nerve wind up being consolidated at the node of Ranvier. This is an ideal circumstance for rapid local reversal of the sodium gradient followed by calcium loading, and I think that may be one of the things that happens to confer increased anoxic susceptibility.

**Dr. Hoffman**: So I guess my question is, in the unmyelinated portion of the axon prior to the lamina, is the density of sodium channels low as it is in the developing system or is it a little bit higher in the adult?

**Dr. Ransom**: I do not know the answer to that.

**Dr. Hoffman**: So if it were low, then that portion of the axon may be relatively resistant to anoxia (Dr. Ransom: Absolutely.), which is quite relevant to the discussion of glaucoma.

**Dr. Costa**: In order to make a point relative to the eye, one is to consider another GABA receptor and that is the GABA-c receptor, which is specific for the eye and is made by two subunits, RO1 and RO2. This behaves abnormally, it is not inhibited by bicuculline, is not augemented by benzodiazepine, so one should consider, in the optic nerve, that there there is also this type of GABA receptor. This receptor opens a chloride channel. This is another class of receptor and was cloned by the people at Johns Hopkins. The two subunits are present in the brain, but very scarce, very abundant in the retina, and also Miledi has done some work on this. You know, Miledi found that the GABA receptor in the retina could not be modulated by benzodiazepine, and I think this receptor could be explored.

**Dr. Ransom**: It would be very interesting to have a look for the presence of GABA-c receptors in the optic nerve.

# 13. NEURONAL DEATH

BO K. SIESJÖ, M.D.

**Dr. Caprioli:** I would like to introduce Dr. Siesjö, who is Professor and Chairman of the Laboratory for Experimental Brain Research, University of Lund, Sweden, and he will share his expertise in the role of calcium-mediated neuronal death with us.

Let me explain to you my background. I am an MD, but I have not seen a patient for 25 years. I am thus doing full-time research. The Laboratory for Experimental Brain Research consists of about 25 scientists, organized into two groups. My own group works with calcium-related, and acidosis-related brain damage, and we have an interest in free radical pathology. Tadeusz Wieloch's group is working with the stimulus–response–metabolism coupling and the signal transduction pathway in ischemia and other conditions; he and his collaborators are specifically interested in regulation of protein synthesis and gene expression as well as in the role of kinases and phosphatases.

Our laboratory is interested in cell death in the brain. To study mechanisms of cell damage we employ different models, encompassing global ischemia, forebrain ischemia, focal ischemia, hypoglycemic coma, and status epilepticus. Many years ago, I was stimulated by the calcium hypothesis of cell death. As many of you know, this is a relatively time-honored hypothesis. It was launched about 20 years ago by Fleckenstein who was interested in cardiac cell death in ischemia, and by Wrogemann and Pena, as well as by Salpeter, who were interested in cell death in muscle dystrophy (for literature, see Siesjö[1]). These authors even discussed agonist-related cell death. At that time, though, it was not glutamate but acetylcholine which was the villain in the discussions. My own contribution was to suggest that selective neuronal vulnerability in ischemia/hypoxia, hypoglycemia, and status epilepticus was calcium-related, reflecting the high density of calcium channels in the apical dendrites of burst-firing neurons with an innate epileptogenic proclivity[2].

Dr. Bray discussed yesterday the possibility that you who work on the eye may have to take an interest in the classification of death. Wyllie *et al.*[3] have classified cell death in two categories, necrosis and apoptosis. Generally, those who are interested in ischemic tissue damage believe that cell death is of the necrotic type. The major reason why apoptosis has been discussed at all is that following a brief period of transient ischemia, it may take two or three days before some of the cells die, and they may resume function in between, so the possibility has been raised that apoptosis, or programmed cell death, may be involved. The evidence was originally against that, because there was neither the morphological criteria nor the effect of transcriptional or translational inhibitors on the cell death, which you should expect if apoptosis was involved. However, this is an unresolved issue, and recent results demonstrate that the characteristic DNA laddering of apoptosis is observed after transient ischemia[4].

In spite of that, I will discuss necrosis and the factors which may lead to necrotic cell death. All of you know that cells feed on glucose and that they use oxygen to produce ATP. From this simple graph you can distinguish two types of insults which would lead to ATP failure and to cell death (Fig. 1). One would be hypoxia or ischemia, which block pyruvate oxidation at the pyruvate dehydrogenase (PDH) step, thereby leading to energy failure. The second one would be hypoglycemic coma,

*Optic Nerve in Glaucoma, pp. 199–222*
*edited by S.M. Drance*

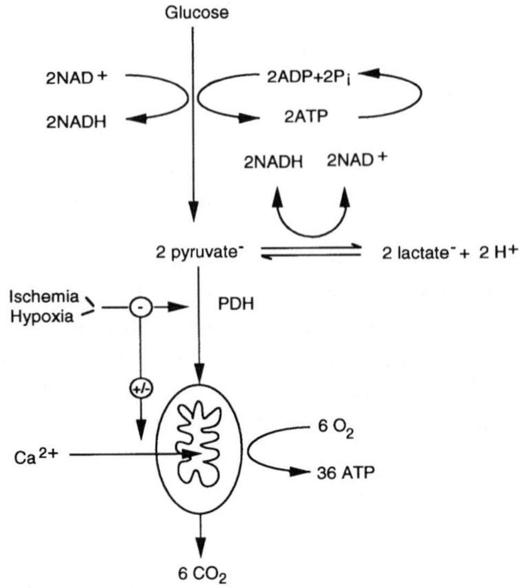


*Fig. 1.* Schematic diagram illustrating the stoichiometry of ATP production during anaerobic and aerobic metabolism of glusose. Ischemia and hypoxia reduce or block pyruvate oxidation by pyruvate dehydrogenase (PDH), leading to reduction of pyruvate to lactate. The latter reaction actually consumes $H^+$. However, if the ATP formed during glycolysis is consumed as soon as it is formed the production of 2 lactate⁻ leads to the release of 2 $H^+$. If the mitochondria retain a membrane potential, they will sequester much of the excess calcium entering; however, if they are de-energized (with collapse of their membrane potential), they will release their calcium content. (Reproduced with permission from Siesjö[5].)

which deprives the cell of its major substrate, thereby depleting the energy stores. There is a fundamental difference between hypoglycemia and ischemia, which is interesting. Thus, hypoglycemic coma will not lead to the production of lactate, with the simultaneous appearance of hydrogen ions, but it will lead to energy failure and to all the other bad things which ischemia or hypoxia will do. So it is useful to study both models.

I have to show one of those slides that Bruce Ransom indicated many of us would be showing, but it seems essential that we resort to some kind of basic scheme when discussing the loss of calcium homeostasis which occurs in ischemia and hypoxia, and in hypoglycemic coma (Fig. 2). One of our basic assumptions is that the severity of the calcium-induced cell damage is proportional both to the magnitude and to the duration of the rise in the free cytosolic concentration $[Ca^{2+}]_i$. Second, this rise must be a function of the pump-leak, a relationship which applies both to the plasma membrane and to intracellular membranes.

If we look at the plasma membrane, then influx of calcium would occur through voltage- and agonist-operated calcium channels. Efflux occurs by ATP-driven transport, and as you have already heard, by 3 $Na^+/Ca^{2+}$ exchange. The pump-leak relationship at the level of intracellular membranes may be illustrated by the endoplasmic reticulum. Here, we have release of calcium in response to agonist activation of surface receptors coupled to phospholipase C, and production of inositol trisphosphate ($IP_3$). Resequestration of calcium occurs at the expense of ATP. You have already heard from Dr. Costa that when the free cytosolic calcium concentration increases, and when diglycerides are formed, you can translocate and activate C kinase with an ensuing phosphorylation of proteins. This is just one example of a calcium-triggered mem-

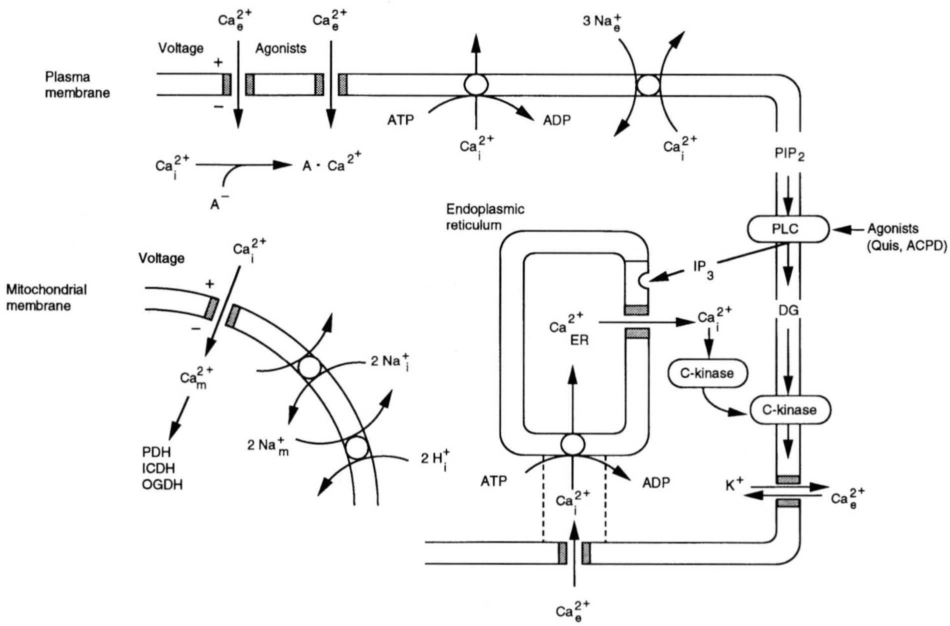


*Fig. 2.* Schematic diagram illustrating regulation of cytosolic calcium concentration $[Ca^{2+}]_i$. Influx across the plasma membrane occurs via voltage- and agonist-operated calcium channels, while $Ca^{2+}$ is extruded from the cell by ATP-driven transport or $Ca^{2+}/2Na^+$ exchange. Calcium is sequestered by mitochondria, endoplasmic reticulum (ER), and so called calciosomes (not shown) at the expense of respiratory energy or ATP, and it is bound by proteins, lipids, and other molecules ($A^-$ in the figure). Release of $Ca^{2+}$ from the ER occurs in response to agonist activation of receptors coupled to phospholipase C, and the formation of inositol trisphosphate ($IP_s$) from phosphatidyl inositol biphosphate ($PIP_2$). A rise in $[Ca^{2+}]_i$ can cause translocation of protein kinase C (PKC) to membranes where the kinase may be activated by diglycerides formed during $PIP_2$ hydrolysis.. Since PKC modulates cation channels, the PLC-$IP_3$-PKC pathway exerts feedback control of membrane potential and calcium influx.

brane perturbation which could lead to a change, sometimes a sustained one, in the activity of ion translocators, receptors, and ion channels.

I wish to emphasize the fact that although mitochondria normally may not sequester a lot of calcium, because calcium is a messenger across the mitochondrial membrane and a regulator of mitochondrial enzymes, the mitochondria represent an important buffer store, and if you deprive the tissue of ATP and of oxygen, then the cells can no longer use this buffer. Hence the free cytosolic calcium concentration may rise to high levels.

Now, let us discuss pathways of influx of calcium through the plasma membrane (Fig. 3). Presynaptically, we have at least two voltage-sensitive channels, the N and the P type, and postsynaptically we have, as Dr. Costa has discussed, the NMDA and the AMPA receptors, which gate channels wich are permeable to sodium and potassium, and in the case of the NMDA receptor also to calcium. As Dr. Costa also mentioned, magnesium would normally block the NMDA receptor-gated channel. In order to get a calcium influx through this channel, what you need is release of transmitter activating both receptors. When the AMPA receptor is activated sodium will enter the cell. That will depolarize the membrane; as a result of this magnesium pops out of the channel and calcium can enter. But depolarization, of course, will also lead to postsynaptic influx of calcium through the L and T types of voltage-sensitive calcium channels.

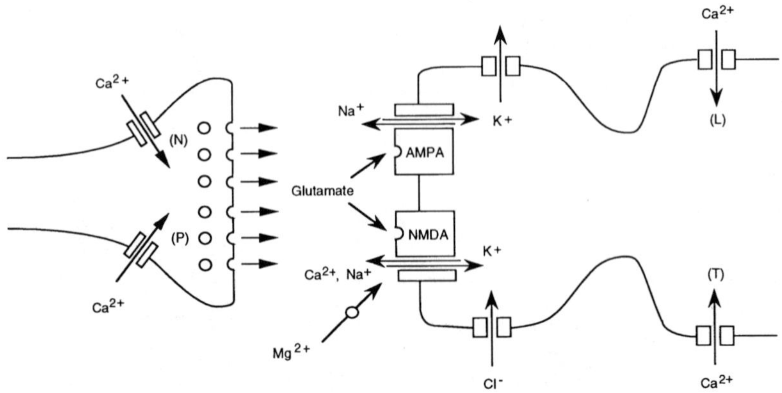


*Fig. 3.* Schematic diagram illustrating presynaptic and postsynaptic ion channels, with emphasis on voltage-sensitive (VSCC) and agonist-operated (AOCC) calcium channels. Presynaptically, the VSCC involved in transmitter release are assumed to be of the N and P types, whereas the L and T types are assumed to be localized to dendrites. It is further assumed that unspecific channels exist which are permeable to calcium (US). Release of the excitatory transmitter glutamate (Glu) is shown to activate two types of receptors, selectively sensitive to amino-3-hydroxy-5-methyl-4-isoazole proprionic acid (AMPA) and to N-methyl-D-aspartate (NMDA), respectively. The AMPA receptor gates a channel that is permeable to monovalent cations ($Na^+$, $K^+$, and $H^+$) whereas the NMDA-gated channel also is permeable to $Ca^{2+}$. Normally, this channel is blocked by $Mg^{2+}$, but the block is voltage-dependent. By leading to depolarization, AMPA receptor activation and $Na^+$ influx relieve the block, allowing $Ca^{2+}$ to enter. Depolarization also occurs by entry of $Na^+$ via voltage-sensitive $Na^+$ channels, some of which are slowly inactivating (IA). Depolarization also allows $Ca^{2+}$ to enter via VSCC of the L, T, P, and N types. Inhibition is assumed to be mediated by activation of $K^+$ and $Cl^-$ conductances, localized to both pre- and postsynaptic membranes. (Modified from *Annals of Emergency Medicine* 1993;22:959-969.)

Depolarization will also activate presynaptic (and postsynaptic ?) channels of the N and P types. In other words, transmitter release can open up multiple pathways for calcium entry into the cell.

Let me discuss one problem which is controversial in the literature. If you read the literature on calcium metabolism of isolated neurons, some people maintain that there is no close relationship between the rise in the free cytosolic calcium concentration and cell death. Tymiansky and collaborators[6] approached this problem and found that, yes, that was a problem because they could not find a clear relationship between the increase in free cytosolic calcium concentration during exposure of glutamate, and cell death. What they did was to expose cells to a prolonged glutamate transient, and recorded the increase in intracellular calcium. During continuous glutamate exposure, $[Ca^{2+}]_i$ showed a peak increase and then returned to a steady state level which was higher than normal. After various periods, there was deregulation with a further increase in calcium concentration, which heralded cell death. What they now did was to vary the extracellular calcium concentration and, thereby, the rate of calcium influx. They then found that there was a close correlation between calcium influx and cell death.

In summary, when there is a low extracellular calcium concentration and a low influx of calcium into the cell, it takes a longer time before deregulation occurs. If extracellular calcium was increased, though, there was very quick deregulation. These authors also concluded from their experiments that it really matters whether calcium enters through voltage-sensitive calcium channels or through glutamate-gated channels. They considered the possibility that when calcium enters through some of the

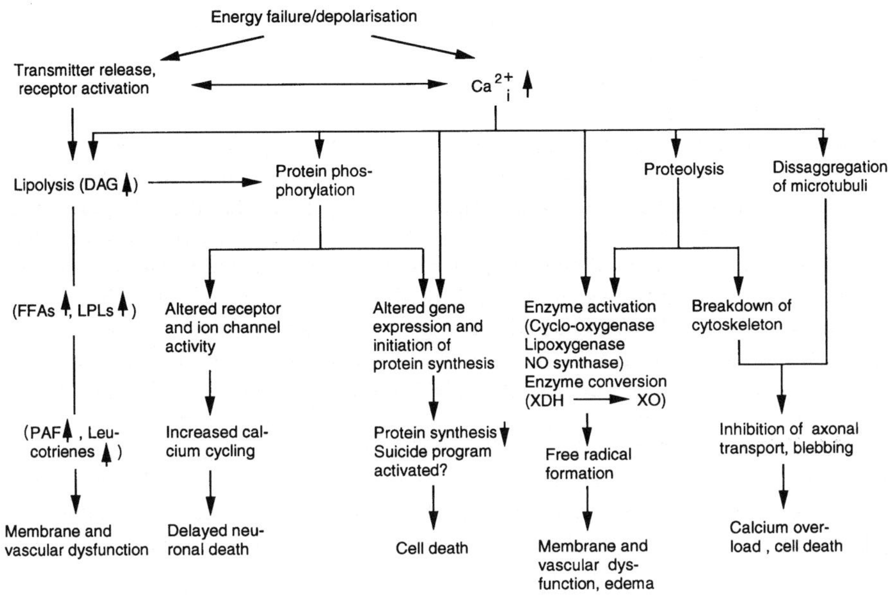


*Fig. 4* . Schematic diagram illustrating the primary effects of depolarization and receptor activation and secondary effects of an increased intracellular calcium concentration $[Ca^{2+}]_i$. The major adverse effects of a massive rise in $[Ca^{2+}]_i$ involve lipolysis, altered protein phosphorylation, proteolysis, and disassembly of microtubuli. Lipolysis leads to production of diacylglycerides (DAG), lysophospholipids (LPL), free fatty acids (FFA), and platelet activating factor (PAF). An altered protein phosphorylation is envisaged to influence protein synthesis and to lead to an altered gene transcription, possibly with activation of a latent suicide program. A rise in $[Ca^{2+}]_i$ also activates enzymes (*e.g.* cyclo-oxygenase, lipoxygenase and NO synthase) which lead to the production of free radicals; calcium-activated proteolysis could act similarly by converting xanthine dehydrogenase (XDH) to xanthine oxidase (XO). (Modified from *Annals of Emergency Medicine*, 1993;22:959-969.)

channels the calcium will be bound or sequestered and very little of it will contribute to cell damage by activation of the neurotoxic cascades. When, on the other hand, calcium enters by other pathways, it may activate those very cascades. Therefore, when one considers the free cytosolic concentration, the important thing may be where you are in the cell and by what routes calcium has entered.

Let me summarize current hypotheses about how calcium can lead to cell death (Fig. 4). We start from the premise that energy failure and depolarization lead to transmitter release, receptor activation, and a rise in the free cytosolic calcium concentration. There are four major sequences which are being discussed as contributing to the final cell death. One is the activation of lipolytic enzymes, with an ensuing accumulation of free fatty acids and of diglycerides. The free fatty acids themselves or the powerful leukotrienes and the thromboxane formed further down in the sequence can lead to membrane damage. Second the increase in calcium concentration, and the increase in the diglyceride concentrations, will affect protein phosphorylation which can then lead to an altered receptor or ion channel function, or it can lead to an altered gene expression, perhaps also to a long-lasting decrease in protein synthesis. Possibly, but this is of course uncertain, the responses discussed can activate a suicide program in the cells. Third, there is a pathway going from calcium to free radical formation which I will come back to. Fourth, probably one of the most important calcium-related events would be proteolysis and disaggregation of microtubuli, which would lead to a breakdown of the cytoskeleton and inhibition of axonal transport, perhaps also to blebbing of the plasma membrane.

I now wish to address a problem which I think anyone of you would be bothered by when you try to read the literature. There are two apparent paradoxes in the literature. One is that NMDA receptor antagonists, whether they are competitive or non-competitive, essentially fail to ameliorate brain damage due to dense global or forebrain ischemia, if you keep the temperature constant. But they do reduce infarct size to approximately 50% of control when you give them in ischemia due to MCA occlusion. The other problem is that AMPA receptor antagonists ameliorate damage due to both forebrain or global ischemia, and to MCA occlusion. In other words, we have the paradox that so-called excitotoxic damage, secondary to glutamate release, cannot be ameliorated by NMDA antagonists if the insult is dense, brief ischemia with long recovery, but it can be ameliorated by AMPA receptor antagonists, and to some extent by flunarizine and nicardipine which, at least in some central neurons, are fairly good blockers of the T type of voltage-sensitive calcium channels. I should also like to mention to you that there are now interesting results with a blocker of the N type of calcium channel, in that the omega conopeptide SNX111 can reduce the damage following forebrain ischemia in gerbils and rats, even when you give it many hours after the ischemia.

We are talking now about brief ischemia, a long maturation period, and damage which comes after two or three days, and about drugs which can be given six, 12, and up to 24 hours afterwards and still ameliorate the damage. That, of course, makes it absolutely necessary for us to try to see what are the differences in the ischemic types. In global or forebrain ischemia, we have dense ischemia which is always transient. If it is short-lasting, we encounter only selective neuronal necrosis, which is often conspicuously delayed. If the ischemia is more long-lasting the damage is more dense, and laminar necrosis or infarction is encountered. In focal ischemia, we have a completely different pathophysiology. A dense core of ischemic tissue (the "focus") has usually the same fate as ischemic tissue in global or forebrain ischemia. However, this core is surrounded by a "penumbra" zone, and that penumbra zone has a less dense ischemia, containing cells which are at risk in the sense that they can survive for a couple of hours[7] (for a review, see Siesjö[5,8]). This is the area where drugs like NMDA and AMPA receptor antagonists probably act. I will start by discussing dense forebrain or global ischemia.

Let me show a graph, illustrating events during ischemia of two minutes duration. We observe that if the ischemia is dense, there is very rapid energy failure, as exemplified by the extensive breakdown of phosphocreatine (Fig. 5). ATP is upheld for some time but it is then rapidly hydrolysed, and lactate content increases gradually. At the time when ATP is around 30% or 40%, there is a massive release of potassium from cells and a marked cellular uptake of calcium, and of sodium plus chloride. These are extracellular recordings. However, as clearly shown by Silver and Erecinska[9], who succeeded in putting calcium microelectrodes into CA1 cells of the hippocampus during ischemia, the intracellular calcium concentration increased precipitously. In their experiments, there was an increase of the free cytosolic concentration to approximately 30-40 micromolar, from a normal concentration of about 100 nanomolar. Indeed, the cells are flooded with calcium in ischemia.

Silver and Erecinska also found that if they used ketamine or MK-801, they could delay this increase in the free cytosolic concentration. And now we return to the paradox. In the presence of these NMDA antagonists, the free cytosolic concentration is in-

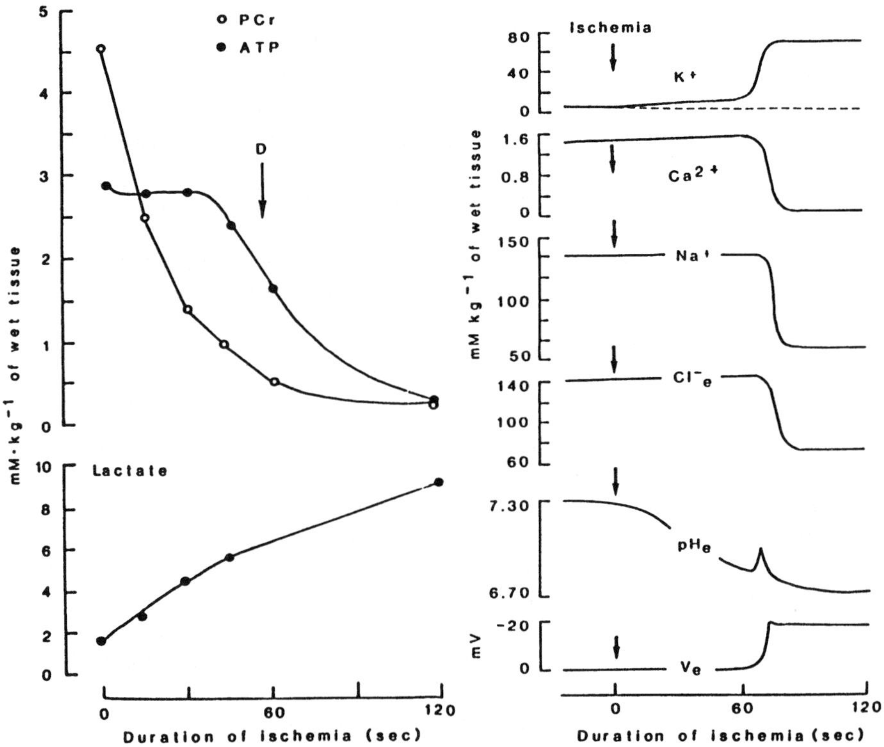


*Fig. 5.* Graphs depicting the coupling of energy failure and ionic fluxes during ischemia. *Left:* Tissue concentrations and phosphocreatine (PCr), adenosine triphosphate (ATP), and lactate during the first 120 seconds of complete ischemia. D= depolarization. *Right:* Changes in extracellular concentrations of $K^+$, $Ca^{++}$, $Na^+$, $Cl^-$, ($Cl^-_e$), and pH ($pH_e$) and in DC potential ($V_e$). Note that $K^+$ increases when the ATP concentration is greater than 90% of control values, and that ion homeostasis is lost when ATP has decreased to below 50% of control values.

creased very slowly, yet the cells are not protected by this drug in this particular type of ischemia. That clearly demands an explanation.

Focal ischemia, as I have said, is different since we have a densely ischemic core and a perifocal penumbra zone which is less densely ischemic. It has been shown that in the core the potassium is leaving the cells and calcium is entering, and that is the end of the tissue unless you can reperfuse it. But in the penumbra zone, several groups have now shown that there are irregularly occurring potassium and calcium transients (*e.g.* ref. 10). The suggestion has been made that in this energetically compromised tissue, you encounter calcium transients with are sufficiently prolonged to lead to a gradual recruitment of damaged cells and, thus, a gradual extension of the focus into the penumbra zone.

There is a phenomenon as you probably all know, called spreading depression. In the rat, spreading depression can be elicited just by putting KCl on the surface of the dura. During spreading depression there is a decrease in extracellular calcium. The cells take up calcium, and $Ca^{2+}_e$ decreases dramatically, each time there is spreading depression travelling across the neocortical surface. Yet, Nedergaard and Hansen[11] showed that you can elicit spreading depressions and load the cells transiently with calcium for five hours without incurring cell damage. It can be shown that just by restricting the energy production in the tissue, for example by lowering the plasma glucose from 4.5 to 2.1, 1.8 or 1.3 mM you can markedly increase the duration of the calcium transients[12]. This suggests that in an energetically compromised tissue we encounter calcium transients which are sufficiently prolonged to lead to progressive cell damage. However, it remains to be established that induced spreading depressions give rise to neuronal cell damage in an energy-compromised situation .

**Dr. Anderson:** I am, of course, thinking about glaucoma while hearing about the models that you have, and the relevance to us. The thing that occurs to me here is that we might be dealing with not a total ischemia or lack of ischemia, but something that is in between. And this penumbra zone might be the one that more mimics what we are interested in, so we will be interested and paying attention to that. But it also occurs to me, and I want to ask this question, how much of this difference is related to the fact that instead of having total lack of blood flow, as in the more involved area, there is kind of a marginally adequate blood flow, and how much of what is happening here is an overflow of toxic products from the more densely affected zone. Because we do not have, I suppose, in glaucoma, the densely affected zone to flood in the products, we have only the partial ischemia, and so with regard to the events that you are describing in this penumbra, it would be interesting for me to know how much of that was due to marginal perfusion and how much of that was due to an overflow of toxic products from the adjacent region of absent blood flow.

**Dr. Siesjö:** That is, of course, an extremely relevant question and we have been concerned with the problem .

**Dr. Zeimer:** Can I add something to that so that you can address both? (**Dr. Siesjö:** Absolutely.) The other issue is, if we believe that the damage is at the level of the lamina cribrosa, we are dealing with an area where there are only axons. Now, from the process that you described, which one(s) do you think are present along an axon, as opposed to in the cell body itself?

**Dr. Siesjö:** I think that Bruce Ransom actually addressed some of these questions. But let me respond to Dr. Anderson´s question. I think the penumbra zone is probably a relatively good model for incomplete energy failure as it occurs in hypoxia or incomplete ischemia or in hypoglycemia. The reason why spreading depressions or ischemic depolarizations occur is that we have the ischemic core, and the core will serve as the "source" in terms of eliciting spreading depressions. So essentially what the core will do is to elicit glutamate- and potassium-induced transients which will travel across the tissue, and these are considered potentially dangerous in a partly energy-compromised tissue. We attempted to address this issue, not only by restricting energy production by moderate hypoglycemia (plasma glucose 1-2 mM), but also by inducing tissue hypoxia without or with unilateral carotid artery occlusion, and by occluding both carotid arteries in otherwise normal animals[13]. Although none of these procedures are suppposed to reduce tissue ATP concentrations, they all restrict the capacity of the tissue to generate ATP in response to a metabolic challenge. In support of this contention are the prolonged, sometimes greatly prolonged, calcium transients accompanying induced spreading depressions. Yet, although animals with this restricted capacity of ATP generation had very long depolarization

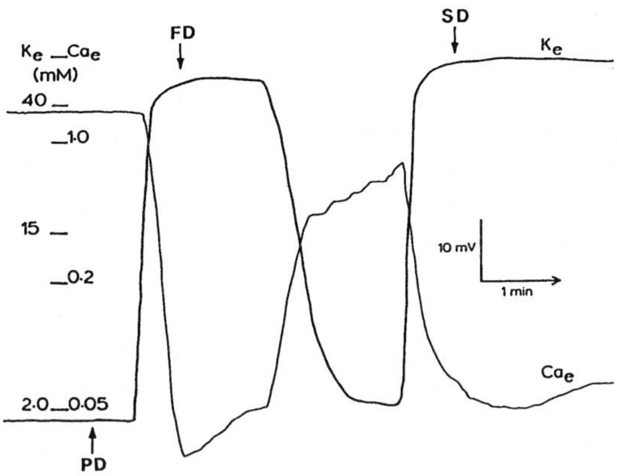


*Fig. 6.* Changes in extracellular potassium ($K_e$) and calcium ($Ca_e$) activity in severe hypoglycemia, at about the timed of onset of isoelectricity. The measurements were made using triple-barreled, double-ion-sensitive microelectrodes to record both ions at the same point simultaneously. $K_e$ starts to increase first and reaches a peak at an average of 48 + 11.5 $Ca_e$ to 0.18 + 0.28 mM. This sequence of ion changes resembles a cortical spreading depression. Both ions show partial normalization followed by a second more permanent change.

times, sometimes giving a total duration of calcium transients exceeding 40 minutes, cell damage was infrequently encountered. The results suggest that in focal ischemia, cells in the penumbra zone probably succumb because of their proximity to dying cells. Dr. Anderson's question is thus extremely relevant. We believe that the "toxic" products released encompass excitatory amino acids, reactive oxygen species (including $H_2O_2$ and $\cdot O_2^-$), and pro-oxidative iron[13].

This leads to the question: what is really happening in tissues which are destined to incur cell damage in response to ischemic or hypoglycemic insults? I wish to exemplify the pathophysiological events by taking the example of hypoglycemic coma. These are tracings of extracellular potassium and calcium concentrations (Fig. 6). If you give insulin to an animal, and wait until the plasma glucose concentration is close to 1 mM, there is a sudden release of potassium into the extracellular fluid and a decrease in the extracellular calcium concentration. Sometimes there is an abortive recovery, but then there is a sustained rise in the extracellular potassium and a decrease in the extracellular calcium concentration. Obviously, the energy-deprived cells release potassium and take up calcium, as they do in ischemia. But this is not a situation of complete energy failure since the tissue still has about 30% of the ATP stores. Why is there such a complete breakdown of calcium homeostasis? I wish to emphasize a point which I find extremely important. That is that if you lose cell calcium homeostasis, it can be due to one of two things: ATP failure or an increase in the calcium conductance of the membrane. To disrupt $Ca^{2+}$ homeostasis you can either decrease the pump or increase the leak, or you can do both.

As we observe, there is an initial ionic transient in hypoglycemic coma. We found that this occurs as a spreading depression, affecting one hemisphere before the other one. What we then could do was to measure ATP and phosphocreatinine in the undepolarized hemisphere, this was 10 to 30 seconds before the depolarization came, and compare the data to postdepolarization values. We observe that the energy state is upheld before depolarization occurs. The data showed that the energy state is upheld at normal values before depolarization and is then suddenly disrupted. What it probably means is that the ion conductances are suddenly activated, and when they are activated the tissue is quickly running out of its energy stores, because the leak is so large that the pump cannot restore the ionic gradients. Therefore, when we discuss loss of calcium homeostasis, it is not only the decrease in blood flow or oxygen tension and the decrease in the ATP which matters but also the activation of ion conductances. Essentially, one may encounter states where the pump cannot manage the leak.

Let me continue discussing ischemia of brief duration where reflow is optimal. Then, we encounter primarily neuronal damage, which is restricted to the selectively vulnerable regions, and is of the delayed type. It can be delayed up to three days in the CA1 sector of the hippocampus. We see the same type of selective vulnerability, but not with an identical distribution, in hypoxia and hypogycemic coma and status epilepticus[14]. Therefore, we can make the assumption that this is a non-vascular lesion, *i.e.* primarily a lesion affecting neurons, and that the microvessels are not damaged. It is an interesting fact that this damage to the tissue is extremely temperature sensitive as shown by many groups, and pioneered by the Miami group[15]. What you observe in this graph is cell damage due to ischemia of five, 10, and 15 minutes duration at 35°, 37° and 39° (Fig. 7). As the graph shows, one can decrease the number of necrotic CA1 cells by induced hypothermia and increase the damage by induced hyperthermia. This is seven days of recovery and the same results were obtained with two weeks of recovery. Clearly, if temperature is increased damage is aggravated. This means that temperature has a very pronounced effect on this kind of delayed neuronal death.

Is this because temperature affects glutamate release, as suggested by the Miami group? The response to this question is not obvious. If you put a calcium electrode in the extracellular fluid, and induce ischemia at 37° and 33°, you observe that at 33°, there is a small delay in the loss of calcium homeostasis, but calcium enters cells at the same rate as it does at 37°C, and $Ca^{2+}_e$ falls to the same, low value[16]. Thus, even though hypothermia reduces glutamate release this may not be the reason why the tissue is protected. Probably, temperature affects postsynaptic membranes or intracellular events in the signal transduction pathway. Dr. Costa, just to mention this, hypothermia which is protective, is known to prevent the deactivation of PKC in the ischemic brain.

How can we explain the delayed damage? The suggestion has been made that we are dealing with a transient insult which gives a long-lasting change in cell calcium homeostasis. Dienel's work[17] showed that after ischemia and 24 hours recovery, the rate of incorporation of $^{45}Ca^{2+}$ was increased, but the total calcium concentration as measured with atomic absorption spectroscopy techniques or with PIXE techniques across the hippocampal layers, is not increased[18]. So let us make the assumption that something has gone wrong with pre- or postsynaptic function which will predispose the cells to this delayed death. We have assumed that transient ischemia gives a long-lasting change in cell calcium metabolism (*e.g.* Siesjö[19]). For example, glutamate release after the ischemia may be enhanced because of a change in the presynaptic membrane functions, or the postsynaptic receptors or ion channels may have been upregulated. What we will then have is increased $Na^+$ influx which, by leading to depolarization, can lead to calcium influx through a number of pathways. We may then also explain why it is not efficacious to give a blocker of the NMDA-gated channels or a blocker of voltage-sensitive calcium channels. This could be be-

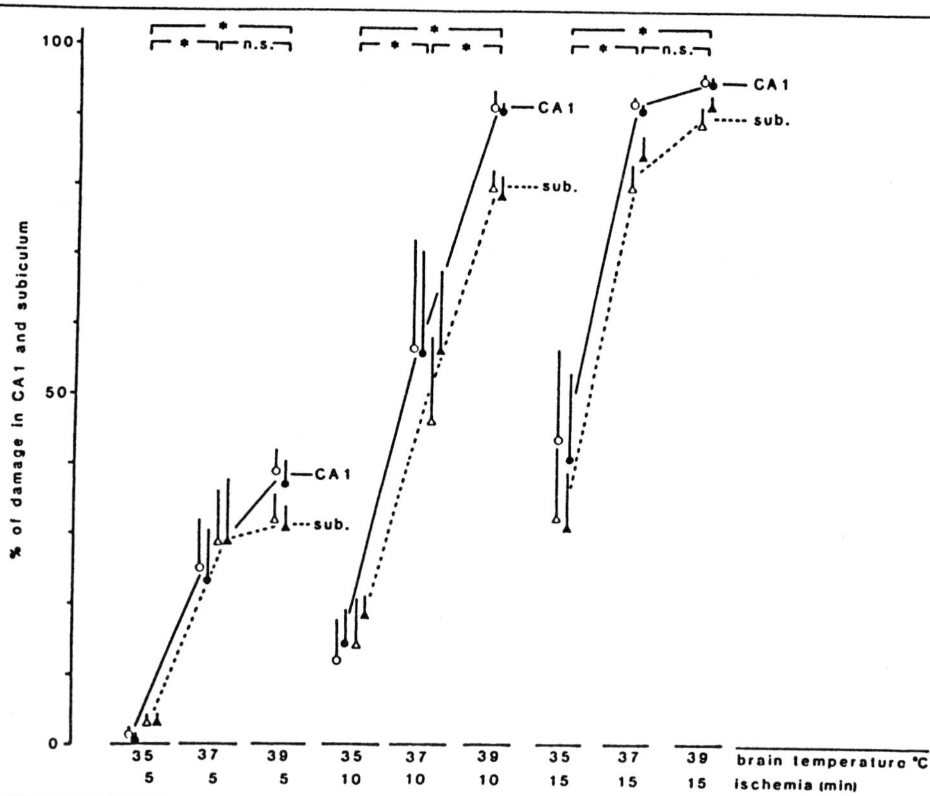


*Fig. 7.* Influence of temperature on ischemia-induced neuronal necrosis in the hippocampus (CA1 sector and subiculum). Quantitative calculation of percentage of damaged neurons was performed bilaterally in each animal. There was no statistically significant difference between right and left hemispheres. Values are mean + SE. Statistics were analyzed by analysis of variance, followed by Scheffé F test. n.s.=not significant; sub=subiculum. (Reproduced with permission from Minamisawa *et al.*: *Annals of Neurology* 1990;28: 26–33.)

cause there are so many pathways by which calcium can enter, that blocking one of them will be ineffective. However, it is clear that one can ameliorate damage by blockers of the N type of calcium channels or of the AMPA receptors. Such antagonists would block the whole event upstream, *i.e.*, they would reduce $Na^+$ influx and the associated depolarization. This is one possible explanation for why you can have an effect of an AMPA receptor blocker but not of NMDA receptor blockers.

However, it is not absolutely certain that we are dealing with membrane events at the level of the plasma membrane. A Japanese group[20] induced ischemia in the gerbil for two and a half to three and a half days; that is before the CA1 cells are morphologically dead. The authors patch-clamped CA1 cells in the hippocampal slices and found that if they stimulated the input to the CA1 cells tetanically, the cells depolarized. Usually, the depolarization was irreversible and the cells died. APV, a competitive NMDA antagonist, could not prevent these irreversible depolarizations. Furthermore, the authors could induce this irreversible depolarizaton by injecting $IP_3$, and they could prevent it by injecting a calcium blocker, BAPTA. The upshot of this: that, possibly, the sustained change in the calcium metabolism after a transient insult involves abnormal $Ca^{2+}$ fluxes across internal membranes, which may involve $IP_3$ receptors or some other response element involved in intracellular calcium signalling.

But what about the molecular mechanisms? It has been shown, in the gerbil and in the rat, that if we subject animals to ischemia, and then induce recovery, there is a very slow recovery of overall protein synthesis; however, protein synthesis only returns in those regions where cells are going to recover but not in the regions where dense neuronal damage is incurred after a delay[21,22]. So it seems that the delayed cell death is proceeded by failure of resumption of protein synthesis. It is an established fact, though, that the post-ischemic brain will synthesize heat-shock and stress proteins, and that they will express messenger RNAs for growth factors[23,24]. Even a non-lethal insult will, of course, lead to the expression of the immediate early genes and to other changes in the cascades we are looking at, including the expression of messenger RNAs for growth factors. One concept which is now being discussed is that following irreversible insults cells fail to express messenger RNAs for the proteins which may be needed for the recovery of the cells, or fail to synthesize the proteins encoded, *e.g.* the growth factors. This concept will probably be discussed a lot in the future.

Another possible mechanism by which calcium could act would of course be to trigger free radical formation. All of us know that free radicals are normally formed in cells, the superoxide radical being the most prominent one (*e.g.* see ref. 25). Furthermore, cells produce hydrogen peroxide, a precursor of free radicals. That is allright, because cells possess an efficient enzymatic and non-enzymatic defense system. The bad thing would be if superoxide radicals could react with hydrogen peroxide to yield hydroxyl radicals (·OH). Normally they cannot, because the reaction between $\cdot O_2^-$ and $H_2O_2$ is extremely slow. However, the reaction can be catalyzed by iron, so if iron can be decompartmentalized and split off from its protein bindings, this could possibly start a free radical reaction sequence. We know that calcium can trigger several reactions which will lead to free radical production. For example, it has been proposed that calcium can lead to a conversion of xanthine dehydrogenase to xanthine oxidase by limited proteolysis. We also know that calcium activates phospholipases and, thereby leading to production of arachidonic acid, and to accumulation of its products and that it activates nitric oxide synthase. All these sequences, thus triggered, lead to production of free radicals. And if iron is delocalized, free radical damage could become a prominent pathogenetic mechanism.

We now have good evidence that forebrain ischemia leading to delayed neuronal damage can be ameliorated by diffusable free radical scavengers such as PBN[26] and dimethylthiourea[27]. The effects are observed in the subiculum, in the CA1 sector proper, in the caudoputamen, and the neocortex. This means that even when we have only neuronal damage in the brain following a moderate insult, we can ameliorate it by a free radical scavenger. Dennis Choi may discuss the comparable data obtained in *in vitro* systems.

It seems appropriate to discuss also ischemia of longer duration, and ischemia induced under suboptimal conditions like hyperthermia, or pre-ischemic hyperglycemia. The assumption has been made that when ischemia is increasing in duration more neurons are recruited, meaning that damage is increasing with time. Secondary to this, and when neuronal damage becomes very massive, one observes glial cell and vascular damage, which may be secondary to the neuronal damage. Parallel to this, though, is primary vascular damage, which takes longer to develop but which ultimately leads to infarction[28]. I show a slide which is intended to remind you of the fact that hyperglycemia leads to accentuated damage, as does hyperthermia. The question we are raising is whether these conditions affect neurons directly or whether they also affect vessels, and, thereby, the capillary circulation.

I think all of you know that if we induce complete ischemia, then the amount of lactate formed depends on the pre-ischemic plasma glucose concentration (see ref. 29). So hypoglycemic animals form less lactate, hyperglycemic ones more. If there is incomplete ischemia, then glucose-infused animals can accumulate massive amounts of lactate, just because the trickle of flow continuously provides substrate for anaerobic glycolysis. We know that this is not good, because hyperglycemia accentuates damage. We also know that both the extracellular pH and the intracellular pH will fall to lower values in the hyperglycemic animals than in the normoglycemic ones. This acid transient may last about 60 minutes, but after that period both metabolic state and acid-base metabolism appear normalized.

Following a long period of ischemia in hyperglycemic subjects and recovery for only, say, 60 or 90 minutes, then massive edema develops and the end result is infarction. If you have a brief period of ischemia, 10 or 15 minutes, then specific gravity measurements reveal a transient post-ischemic edema in both normoglycemic and hyperglycemic animals. In the hyperglycemic ones, however, seizures appear after about 18 to 26 hours and the animals go into status epilepticus, dying with grossly swollen brains. Evidently hyperglycemia induced 24 hours previously leads to this catastrophic end result. We know that it is the acidosis which makes the trick, because what we can do is to induce exaggerated acidosis, not only by inducing pre-ischemic hyperglycemia, but also by taking normoglycemic animals and making them grossly hypercapnic[30]. If the $pCO_2$ is high enough then pH during ischemia is reduced to the same level as observed in hyperglycemic animals. As you see from this graph, the animals which are hypercapnic have much more damage in the caudoputamen, CA1, and in the neocortex. So acidosis of this degree is obviously bad. The damage has little to do with the hyperglycemia *per se*, it must be the acidosis. What we have to explain, though, is why hyperglycemic animals do not develop seizures.

And then we come to a problem which Dr. Choi has already pointed out and one which I think we have to address in the future. The problems concern the relationship between calcium metabolism and acidosis. It has been reported from several laboratories that if one measures the NMDA currents in cells as a function of pH, the NMDA currents decrease at low pH, and at a pH of about six, very little current is carried by these channels. Dennis Choi's laboratory and also Sapolsky's laboratory have shown that if you expose neurons to glutamate at different extracellular pH and estimate cell damage by measuring LDH release, then it is clear that a reduction of extracellular pH to 6.9 and 6.4 will progressively improve recovery. Similar results are obtained in cells exposed to anoxia. In other words, acidosis is protective *in vitro*. It has also been shown that $^{45}Ca^{2+}$ enters much more slowly during acid conditions, and that the increase in free cytosolic concentration is less pronounced. Our own results have shown that if we make cells acid, then glutamate exposure leads to a smaller peak increase in calcium concentration[31].

The controversy is reinforced by recent *in vivo* experiments. When we put an extracellular calcium electrode into the brain, and induce ischemia, we find that hyperglycemia and hypercapnia retard calcium influx, exactly as MK-801 does[33]. The results obtained in hypercapnia make it likely that hyperglycemia slows down

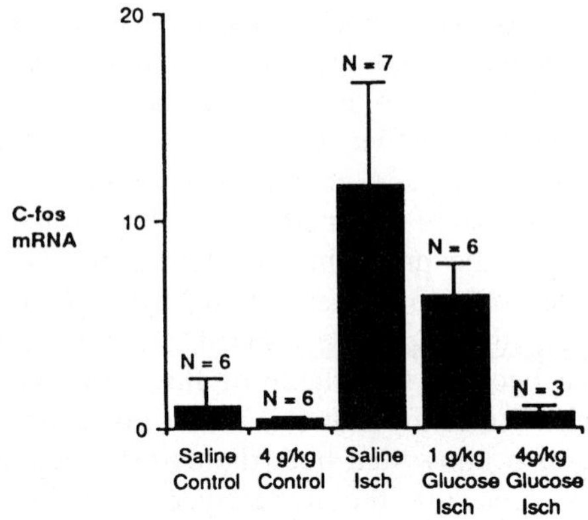


*Fig. 8.* Brain c-fos mRNA levels following transient ischemia, and the effect of pre-ischemic glucose administration. All values were expressed relative to the lowest brain level of mRNA among control, saline-treated animals. Isch = ischemic animals. All values expressed as mean ± SD. (Reproduced with permission from Combs *et al.*[32].)

calcium influx by inducing acidosis and those obtained with MK-801 that acidosis acts by inhibiting calcium influx via NMDA-gated calcium channels. Clearly *in vitro*, cells are protected by the acidosis, but *in vivo*, the damage is aggravated. This is something which we have to explain in the future, when discussing calcium-related damage. It could be that the low pH *in vivo* acts on other cells than the neurons, and that this is detrimental in the long run. For example, it could act on astrocytes or endothelial cells. However, what speaks against this contention is that enhanced acidosis seems to aggravate damage to neurons even when gial cells or endothelial cells seem to have escaped damage[30,34]. Although acidosis blocks influx of calcium into cells having NMDA receptors, it could be detrimental. One reason could be that acidosis exaggerates free radical damage by shifting the following reaction to the right (see ref. 29).

$$\cdot O_2^- + H^+ \rightleftharpoons H\cdot O_2^- \ (1) \qquad pK' = 4.7$$

where the anion superoxide radical is converted to a more pro-oxidant, more lipid soluble free radical species. Alternatively, low pH can rip off iron from its bindings in transferrin, so it now comes loose and can be chelated by low molecular weight compounds to yield pro-oxidant iron species which trigger free radical damage.

It has recently been made likely that the delayed cell death following transient ischemia has an element of apoptosis, as evidenced by a characteristic laddering of DNA[4]. In non-neuronal cells, an endogenous endonuclease has been identified which seems responsible for internucleosomal cleavage of DNA, and for apoptotic cell death; interestingly, this endonuclease (DNase II) is activated by a dercrease in pH below 6.5[35,36]. On the basis of these results, and of EM evidence of chromatin condensation in hyperglycemic animals subjected to ischemia, we have speculated that exaggerated acidosis during ischemic insults leads to DNA fragmentation and apoptotic cell death[37].

Figure 8 I picked out because of the discussion we had yesterday. This is from

Combs *et al.*[32], and from a recent article where the authors looked at normal and hyperglycemic animals exposed to transient ischemia.In this article they reported results on the expression of c-fos messenger RNA following ischemia. If ischemia was induced in control animals, there was expression of c-fos messenger RNA. This is the expected result, following an insult. However, what is interesting was that when the authors loaded these animals with glucose in increasing concentrations, they suppressed the expression of messenger RNA. Perhaps we are dealing with a block in the defense response of the cell, where messenger RNAs are expressed for stress proteins and growth factors, or to an inhibition of the synthesis of the protein products of these messenger RNAs. Clearly, I think we now have a better background when trying to interpret calcium-related damage, and its relationship to free radical damage, and we begin to understand acidosis-related damage. Thank you for your attention.

**Dr. Langer:** In your scheme of events, if you follow the cascade starting with enhanced glutamate release, it would appear that if there were pharmacologic intervention presynaptically through the adenosine receptors that inhibit glutamate release, it might theoretically be of therapeutic interest. Is that the case, or would this effect be marginal and not sufficient to prevent a massive release of glutamate in ischemia?

**Dr. Siesjö:** Firstly, I would like to stress the fact that if you have very dense ischemia, the uptake of calcium by cells is very rapid, and is very difficult to influence by drugs. But by working with very precise techniques, and close temperature control, you can establish that MK-801 and acidosis really retard the influx of calcium into cells and transforms that into a two-stage process, where it may take five or six minutes for the extracellular calcium to be taken up by cells. Since neither MK-801 nor acidosis ameliorate damage, it does not seem to matter that you can somewhat reduce postsynaptic calcium influx through NMDA-gated channels. I also wish to recall that hypothermia, which is protective, reduces glutamate release without having a major effect on calcium influx into the cell[16]. It is tempting to conclude that the protective effect of hypothermia is exerted downstream to the influx of calcium, and that its influence on glutamate release is an epiphenomenon.

The situation may be different in the post-ischemic period, in which critical depolarization could be responsible for the ultimate (delayed) neuronal damage. Here, it may be advantageous to either reduce presynaptic glutamate release, or its effect on postsynaptic glutamate receptors. In support, there is evidence now that the AMPA receptor blocker NBQX and the N type of calcium channel blocker, SNX111, ameliorate damage even if you give them many many hours after the ischemia. The situation is also completely different if we have marginal ischemia as in the penumbra zone of a focal ischemic lesion. Let us say that the blood flow is less than 50% of control, and that repeated depolarization waves will hit the tissue, each one leading to a calcium transient. In this situation, drugs acting an glutamate release and on the NMDA or AMPA receptors, are probably very good, because they can block these depolarization events. This is probably because we are now dealing with calcium influx at higher membrane potentials than when you have a very dense ischemia. In such situations, adenosine would do good because it can prevent presynaptic depolarization and calcium influx, apart from increasing blood flow.

**Dr. Hoffman:** You showed that the mRNA level is increased for early immediate genes and for growth factors. Do you know which cells are synthesizing those?

**Dr. Siesjö:** Good question. They are definitely neurons but some of these cells are ones which are perhaps not involved in the ischemic process or, at least, they are not susceptible to ischemic damage. You see marked expression in dentate granular cells, and some expression also in the CA1 and cortical neurons, but the density there is not that impressive. In general, this is an area where we need to know much more, particularly at the single cell level. In pursuing this problem we have to remember that, following brief periods of ischemia, the number of cortical neurons dying is relatively small.

**Dr. Ransom:** How about glial cells?

**Dr. Siesjö:** Glial cell damage is virtually lacking following brief periods of ischemia, or following hypoglycemic coma or status epilepticus. In these conditions neuronal damage is dominating. You have to go up to longer periods of ischemia or add preischemic hyperglycemia or hyperthermia to see glial and endothelial cell damage.

**Dr. Costa:** I was wondering if you are not giving enough value to the fact that many AMPA kinate receptors are calcium permeable, and you know, in your scheme this was the concept of one and a half to two years ago, but now with the messenger RNA editing and the presence of glutamine instead of arginine, it is only gliar-2 that is not permeable to calcium. And most of the receptors' structure, they may have one or the other one, either the kinate KA1, KA2, and gliar-2 represents 40% of the AMPA receptors that are expressed, we cannot remember that they may not all be homomeric, therefore calcium is entering. Moreover, you did not give enough credit to the fact that metabotropic receptor cannot increase calcium release, you know, just by being metabotropic, and that may have also a value. So it is not surprising that a blocker of AMPA receptor may be beneficial, also because it limits the entry of calcium.

**Dr. Siesjö:** The reason why I did not put too much emphasis on the change of subunit composition of AMPA receptors was that the results of Pelligrino-Giampietro *et al.*[38] have not yet been confirmed; in fact, two laboratories have obtained nonconfirmatory results. In principle, though, I agree that ischemia could make AMPA-receptor-gated channels permeable to $Ca^{2+}$.

**Dr. Costa:** This I know, I am not talking about the transformation, the one Pelligrino-Giampietro mentioned, I am talking about your systems, your scheme that would imply that every AMPA receptor is a homomeric with gliar-2.

**Dr. Siesjö:** I agree, and I will take this into account, because we may clearly have a conversion from one subunit to the other, making AMPA receptors permeable to calcium. Another reason why I did not stress it, is that you do have an effect also of drugs which act in a nonspecific way on sodium and calcium entry. Some effects have also been reported with flunarizine which supposedly acts on the T type of calcium channels, and on channels which probably also carry sodium into the cell. My general feeling is that, if you want to reduce post-ischemic ionic fluxes and protect the tissue from repeated calcium transients, you should try to block sodium influx. That can be achieved by blocking AMPA-receptor-gated channel or other $Na^{+}$-carrying channels.

**Dr. Caprioli:** In order to shorten the discussion, ..... These details are very very fascinating and relevant to many broad areas of stroke, but we might want to concentrate on our glaucoma problem, and for these details you have many symposia. Can we discuss anything about glaucoma that may be relevant to this, any people that have questions?

**Dr. Costa:** But I think it is important to understand how it is made, our receptors in the eye. You know, this is what is lacking and I think this is very very important for you people of glaucoma to collaborate with somebody that helps you to define the receptors in the eye. This is essential. We can not predict, for instance, for the GABA, it was predicted that it was like GABA-a, but the fact the benzodiazepine does not give any disturbance in the visual, many people wonder if benzodiazepines really are modulating all the GABA-a receptor, why do we not have disturbance in vision when we give benzodiazepines? And then came the evidence that they are GABA-c receptors, not GABA-a receptor, with two new subunits. These may well apply to the eye for the other receptors.

**Dr. Siesjö:** Could I respond to your challenge by saying that, if we believe that axonal damage in glaucoma is caused by calcium overload and calcium-related damage, perhaps by enhancing proteolysis, then what we should take an interest in is the relationship between the pump and leak. And if the pump normally is the sodium/calcium exchanger, as Bruce Ransom has so beatifully described here, then one should perhaps discuss the possibility that kinking or trauma or compression of the axons could lead to an upregulation of the leak pathways. And perhaps by depolarization to a reversal of the sodium/calcium exchanger. So it is conceivable that trauma could lead to a long-lasting calcium overload of moderate degree, which in the long run leads to cell damage. Obviously one of the crucial things for you to try to find out is whether or not these axons show depolarization of a moderate degree.

**Dr. Anderson:** The other thing I might bring up for discussion is the fact that we seem to be dealing not with an acute total ischemic event such as is described here. Now, obviously, you have to study the extreme in order to know the moderate; we may be dealing with a lower grade of chronic ischemia and changes that would come and go. Moreover, the drugs that we must use to treat this condition and try to avoid the damage, if we are going to use that approach, is something that we have to give on a chronic basis. In an acute situation you may give a drug which has beneficial effect in this tissue, and for the moment will impair other functions. Obviously, when you give a drug which is going to change the function of neurons you are upsetting the normal physiology in addition to upsetting the pathophysiology or trying to overcome it, and some of these things, it strikes me, would have profound effects on the neural function of the organism.

**Dr. Siesjö:** Yes, there are groups now working with more chronic ischemia[39]. In the rat, a simple way to induce chronic ischemia is to ligate both carotid arteries. If you do that for three or four hours nothing happens, *i.e.* there is no cell death; if you do it for two or three weeks, you find that now in certain areas of the brain are cells that are knocked out of the population. And this is a low grade ischemia because blood flow is somewhere between 40 and 70% of control. But that is sufficient, if it is sustained over weeks, it leads to cell death.

**Dr. Anderson:** And can you administer agents which will help that and reduce the ischemic harm without at the same time impairing the neural function of the organism?

**Dr. Siesjö:** I do not think this has been done in a really systematic way. Anecdotally I think there are some data showing that you can give a free radical scavenger over a long period and prevent some of this damage.

**Dr. Caprioli:** To follow up on your important question that you initially raised about the penumbra, it seems that there are two possibilities. One that you suggested that cells may be sick for a prolonged period of time, but we are talking about a magnitude of time which is quite different from even the longest experiments that we have here, so-called chronic ischemia. And so I would like to first suggest another possibility, and that is that there may be acute events for very small numbers of cells at a time, which are recurrent over a patient's lifetime, and secondly that leads to the question, is it possible for neurons to be sort of sick or dysfunctional for a prolonged period of time. I mean, it would seem that they would either survive or die, but they would not be sick for years, let us say, and in glaucoma, of course, this is a very slowly progressive, chronic disease which occurs over decades.

**Dr. Siesjö:** I do not think there are any experimental models for that. But let me just emphasize that if you have a more low-grade ischemia, as you very often have in the penumbra zone, then I think there are two events which are of clear interest for the pathology incurred. One is the damage affecting the neurons, whether it is the cell body or an axon, and the second thing is what is affecting the microcirculation. The reason why I say so is that you can decrease the stroke size in experimental MCA occlusion by giving free radical scavengers which cannot cross the barrier. For example, one can give SOD and catalase, conjugated to polyethyleneglycol and still decrease the size of the infarct. I believe there is an inflammatory reaction in the endothelial cells, affecting the microvessels in tissues which have a marginal decrease in oxygenation and blood flow.

**Dr. Flammer:** I think we do have a model in medicine. In pituitary tumors we can have huge scotomas over months and even years and still they are reversible.

**Dr. Drance:** But surely we have an ideal model in glaucoma, because in fact so many of the visual disturbances have a very dense, absolute nucleus and are surrounded by areas that fluctuate and recover and then get worse again. I would have thought we had a singularly good model in glaucoma to in fact try and see what the effects on the penumbra are clinically.

**Dr. Anderson:** Of course, this is dependent on the assumption that we are dealing with an ischemic problem. We do have evidence of being able to improve the function, so we have some dysfunctional cells, but certain things can be done, including, for example, simply administering carbon dioxide, which will allow the neurons to function as reflected in vision improving....

**Dr. Siesjö:** Is that right?

**Dr. Anderson:** Transiently, yes. Carbon dioxide can be given, and Dr. Lutz Pillunat has some evidence that certain areas of relative reduction in vision can have relative improvement in vision when that happens, back toward the normal. Now, obviously, there are certain absolute defects that are gone because the neurons have died, but there is evidence for what Joe Caprioli has suggested, namely, that there are certain numbers of neurons which are not functioning but are alive.

**Dr. Siesjö:** Can I ask you a question, because I am ignorant about this area. We know from trauma research that the trauma may lead to a rupture of axons, and this will lead to axonal dissolution and other events, although there is not ischemia initially, and although there is no initial failure of ATP production. So this is just mechanical trauma to the axons probably damaging cytoskeletal elements by calcium-related mechanisms. Do you see retraction balls or cytoskeletal abnormalities in optic nerves?

**Dr. Quigley:** Were you referring to histopathologic retraction? Yes, you see transected axons in human glaucoma. Raybeck showed it with silver stains, you can show it with electron microscopy. I think that Dr. Flammer has raised one of the fundamental questions that I always like to pose to our students, which is, what is the fundamental difference between compression of the optic nerve by a tumor at the pituitary area and glaucoma? And the fundamental difference that I would express from what we see clinically is that it is almost routine for a person who has a pituitary tumor removed, for visual function to go from not being able to see the vision chart, to returning almost to 20-20 vision. I will give somebody an automobile if they showed me a glaucoma patient who has ever had that dramatic an improvement, having lost it and demonstrated repeatedly that it has been lost, and then it comes back. So that the degree of reversibility that occurs in a glaucoma patient is almost negligible. A recent study in which patients were treated with moderate pressure elevations with either laser or medicines has visual field data that show a very slight, 1 decibel improvement over 250 patients when their pressures were reduced. So there is a phase of reversibility, there are some cells that are dysfunctional but can be made to improve some. But there is a dramatic difference between what a tumor is doing to the optic nerve and what glaucoma is doing to the optic nerve. So if we understand that difference, I think we will know a lot about this pathophysiology.

**Dr. Ransom:** I can not help but respond to what has just come up. As I understand it, and correct me if I understand this incorrectly, when glaucoma proceeds to a point where there is visual field loss, and it is no longer fluctuating, is it not associated with a reduction in the number of ganglion cells? So of course, there would not be any return of function if you suddenly did something to relieve that condition, because the ganglion cells are no longer able of repopulating the retina. I would add...

**Dr. Anderson:** Yes there is a population of ganglion cells that are gone, but there is another population of cells, evidently, that are not functioning but can be made to function again that are in an intermediate state, because some relative visual loss can recover.

**Dr. Ransom:** Exactly, I think that is precisely correct. But this comes back to the point that transaction, or pressure, or other kinds of injuries might have an effect on axons that eventually proceeds to a state where the cell body becomes involved in the insult and finally disappears. The relevance of discussing in detail the calcium-mediated cell death is that it is not limited just to anoxia. We tend to think about it almost exclusively in that context, but that is certainly not the case. This is a final common pathway for any kind of injury to the cell, whether it is due to mechanical injury, or whether it is due to anoxia; and I think that there could not be a finer example of a multifactorial process than the thing that you brought us here to discuss, the business of glaucoma.

**Dr. Hoffman:** I think Harry´s point is well taken, but I should point out that there are a number of patients who have pituitary tumors who, when their compression is relieved, do not get better, clearly showing that if you compress an axon long enough, it is not reverisble. The point is, the point of a pituitary tumor is that there is reversibility in situation where you can measure normal function. So I do not think that it takes you any further to deciding whether or not glaucoma is on the basis of compression or ischemia. It is obvious that compression can give you a reversible block of function, and it is also true that compression, prolonged enough, can give you loss of axons, and in fact, in papilledema, we normally think of papilledema as relatively benign for the optic nerve unless it is prolonged and then we can start knocking out fibers, and presumably all you need to do in the retina in terms of retinal ganglion cell loss is to injure the axon enough so you made it discontinuous, and then the cell dies through apoptosis.

**Dr. Quigley:** Well, let us follow up on that. A patient who has a pituitary tumor who has profound visual field loss, loss of central vision, loss of color vision, can be predicted to improve if they still have visible nerve fiber layer intact heading toward the fovea. And when the nerve fiber there is gone, as Dr. Ransom is suggesting, obviously that is the patient who is not going to get better. And you and I, Neal, do this all the time, sit there and look at a patient with a pituitary tumor, and can predict fairly accurately whether that patient is going to improve or not. There is not a phase of glaucoma in which the patient has intact looking nerve fiber layer and profound glaucomatous visual field loss. Does not happen. If it does, I would like to see lots of examples. Dr. Anderson just said that there was this, a group of axons or a group of nerve fibers that are in a reversible stage; I propose to you, they are small minority of the optic nerve, in typical open-angle glaucoma at any one point in time. And, so does that express that the insult is exactly the same as the insult from a pituitary tumor, but it is happening to little microbundles at a time, or does it mean that there is a fundamental difference in the mechanism of injury. And Paul, you are right, I do not know whether tumor compression is anoxic or mechanical anymore than I know whether glaucoma is mechanical or anoxic, but to understand the difference one understands...

**Dr. Hoffmann:** I think Joe´s point in the very beginning is really relevant, and that is, you really do not know whether or not you are looking at a lesion which is restricted to selected populations of axons at any one time, and that cumulatively you do get the irreversible loss, but the pathological process is going on in those axons that are being affected.

**Dr. Siesjö:** I was very impressed yesterday by the discussion of axonal transport secondary to compression of the nerve fibers. I attended a session two or three years ago where we had four eminent calcium experts present. I recalled the scheme showing all of the bad things that calcium can do and asked them to speculate by identifying the most crucial change occurring after calcium overload, *i.e.* the event which will kill the cell in the long run. All of them said proteolysis, and all of them implied that interruption of axoplasmic transport and of the traffic from the periphery up to the cell body and from the cell body out to the periphery is extremely important for cell survival. So I will speculate, if I may, that if you compress the axon for a sufficiently long period and interrupt the axonal transport that way, perhaps you have a dying back which is irreversible, but if you compress it for a shorter period and if the compression is not complete like, perhaps, in some of your tumor cases then you may have a resumption of function. Wild speculation.

**Dr. Hoffman:** Well, there are toxic models where you can actually selectively block various phases of axonal transport. One of the most striking ones is there is a model, there is a toxin called IDPN, and if you give it systemically, you can selectively block the transport of the neurofilaments. You get this giant ballooning of axons in the proximal internodal region, and the distal part of the axon actually becomes atrophic. And they are sort of depleted of neurofilaments, yet they continue to conduct. The conduction velocity obviously goes down, but they continue to conduct, fast transport continues, and there are other toxic models as well where you can show that you can selectively dissect out portions of the transport system. And that is for slow transport, you can impair neurofilament transport and you can do things like that. But as soon as you put in agonist which affect tubulin, and microtubules, like colchicine, it is essentially like a chemical axotomy, the same as cutting the axon in terms of that it does distally, you get distal degeneration. So I think that it is true that if you block critical portions of the transport system, you kill axons distally, and in the case of the CNS, when you kill the axon distally, you eventually kill the cell body.

**Dr. Flammer**: The problem is that this occurs only in patients who have optic nerve heads which still look quite good, and therefore we do not call them glaucoma patients. But, we do not know whether these patietns will have glaucoma, what we call glaucoma, in 20 years. If you take patients with huge vasospasm that have big visual field defects that are reversible in half an hour, but the optic nerve head looks good, therefore we can say that it is not a type of disease. But as the number of......in glaucoma patients is increased, we can speculate that these young people who have reversible damage, may end up, or some of them may end up, with irreversible damage in 10 or 20 years.

**Dr. Drance:** I just wanted to add briefly that we keep on talking about visual field defects, and we are doing white on white measurements. There are many other tests which are more appropriate, and, for instance, I can tell you for sure that we have a number of patients in whom there is a dramatic improvement in the color vision in spite of the fact that the visual field does not change, and I am sure in order for that to happen they must have some functioning axons or ganglion cells that are capable may be of modulation. I think we need to relook at out parameters.

**Dr. Siesjö:** Could I ask you a question about dark adaptation, how is that affected in your glaucoma patients? Is it affected?

**Dr. Drance:** It is affected markedly.

**Dr. Quigley:** Scotopic function is one of the major things that is injured early in the disease, and is useful even as a screening tool.

**Dr. Siesjö:** Right, because if you start lowering the oxygen tension of volunteers, and baloonists, the first function which is affected is the dark adaptation.

**Dr. Caprioli:** I think we all agree that there is some element of reversibility, and I think we are arguing about the amount, and I think that is probably not going to lead anywhere useful. Harry, do you have one last point you would like to make?

**Dr. Quigley:** I wondered whether there was any selectivity as far as cell size in the anoxic models that Dr. Siesjö has been telling us about. In the central nervous system, are bigger cells or smaller cells more or less likely to be killed through the anoxic system?

**Dr. Siesjö:** No, the cells dying could be small, they could be medium-sized, or they can be, like the Purkinje cells, very large. Cells dying in a selectively vulnerable area, like the CA1 area or the hilus of the dentate gyrus, may coexist with cells which have survived although they may be 50 or 100 µm away. Factors contributing to selective vulnerability include the functional type of cells, the type of receptor they possess, and their innervation. I previously showed one slide which showed that some cells were knocked out of the population of dentate hilar cells after a brief ischemic period. It turns out that these are somatostatin-containing cells, but in other areas they could be GABAergic cells. Very likely, cells which have a dense innervation with fibers releasing excitatory amino acids and/or a high density of receptors and ion channels, allowing calcium influx, are vulnerable to insults.

**Dr. Quigley:** Not necessarily the number of inputs, but the type of inputs, is what you are suggesting.

**Dr. Siesjö:** The type of input, yes. Some people also speculate that vulnerability depends on whether or not the cells have calcium binding proteins in high or low concentrations, but there are probably lots of other factors. For example, the activity of PKC, and the density of $IP_3$ receptors, have been correlated to vulnerability

**Dr. Caprioli**: Well, I wish we could press on with this good discussion, but I think we need to go on to the next presentation.

## References

1. Siesjö B K (1988) Historical overview. Calcium, ischemia, and death of brain cells. *Ann NY Acad Sci* 522:638-661
2. Siesjö B K (1981) Cell damage in the brain: A speculative synthesis. *J Cerebral Blood Flow Metabol* 1:155-185
3. Wyllie A, Kerr J, Currie A (1981) Cell death: The significance of apoptosis. *Int Rev Cytol* 68:251-307
4. MacManus J P, Buchan A M, Hill I E, Rasquinha I, Preston E (1993) Global ischemia can cause DNA fragmentation indicative of apoptosis in rat brain. *Neurosci Letters* 164:89-92
5. Siesjö B K (1992) Pathophysiology and treatment of focal cerebral ischemia. I. Pathophysiology. *J Neurosurg* 77:169-184

6. Tymianski M, Charlton M P, Carlen P L, Tator C H (1993) Source specificity of early calcium neurotoxicity in cultured embryonic spinal neurons. *J Neurosci* 13: 2085-2104
7. Astrup J, Siesjö B K, Symon L (1981) Thresholds in cerebral ischemia – The ischemic penumbra. *Stroke* 12: 723-725
8. Siesjö B K (1992) Pathophysiology and treatment of focal cerebral ischemia. II. Mechanisms of damage and treatment. *J Neurosurg* 77:337-354
9. Silver I A, Erecinska M (1992) Ion homeostasis in rat brain in vivo: intra- and extracellular $Ca^{2+}$ and $H^{+}$ in the hippocampus during recovery from short-term, transient ischemia. *J Cerebral Blood Flow Metabol* 12:759-772
10. Nedergaard M, Hansen A J (1993) Characterization of cortical depolarizations evoked in focal cerebral ischemia. *J Cerebral Blood Flow Metabol* 13:568-574
11. Nedergaard M, Hansen A J (1988) Spreading depression is not associated with neuronal injury in the normal brain. *Brain Res* 449:395-398
12. Gidö G, Katsura K, Kristián T, Siesjö B K (1993) Influence of plasma glucose concentration on rat brain extracellular calcium transients during spreading depression. *J Cerebral Blood Flow Metabol* 13:179-182
13. Gidö G, Kristián T, Siesjö B (1994) Induced spreading depressions in energy-compromised neocortical tissue: calcium transients and histopathological correlates. *Neurobiol Dis* 1:31-41
14. Auer R N, Siesjö B K (1988) Biological differences between ischemia, hypoglycemia and epilepsy. *Ann Neurol* 24: 699-707
15. Ginsberg M, Sternau L, Globus M Y-T, Dietrich W, Busto R (1992) Therapeutic modulation of brain temperature: relevance to ischemic brain injury. *Cerebral Brain Metabol Rev* 4:189-225
16. Kristián T, Katsura K, Siesjö B K (1992) The influence of moderate hypothermia on cellular calcium uptake in complete ischaemia: implications for the excitotoxic hypothesis. *Acta Physiol Scand* 146:531-532
17. Dienel G A (1984) Regional accumulation of calcium in postischemic rat brain. *J Neurochem* 43:913-925
18. Martins E, Inamura K, Themner K, Malmqvist K G, Siesjö B K (1988) Accumulation of calcium and loss of potassium in the hippocampus following transient cerebral ischemia: A proton microprobe study. *J Cerebral Blood Flow Metabol* 8:531-538
19. Siesjö B K (1993) Basic mechanisms of traumatic brain damage. *Ann Emergency Med* 22:959-969
20. Tsubokawa H, Oguro K, Robinson H P C, Masuzawa T, Kirino T, Kawai N (1992) Abnormal $Ca^{2+}$ homeostasis before cell death revealed by whole cell recording of ischemic CA1 hippocampal neurons. *Neuroscience* 49: 807-817
21. Hossmann K-A (1993) Disturbances of cerebral protein synthesis and ischemic cell death. In: *Neurobiology of Ischemic Brain Damage* (Kogure K, Hossmann K-A, Siesjö B K, eds), pp 161-177. Amsterdam: Elsevier Science Publishers B.V.
22. Wieloch T, Bergstedt K, Hu B R (1993) Protein phosphorylation and the regulation of mRNA translation following cerebral ischemia. In: *Neurobiology of Ischemic Brain Damage* (Kogure K, Hossmann K-A, Siesjö B K, eds), pp 179-191. Amsterdam: Elsevier Science Publishers B.V.
23. Nowak T S, Osborne O C, Suga S (1993) Stress protein and proto-oncogene expression as indicators of neuronal pathophysiology after ischemia. In: *Neurobiology of Ischemic Brain Damage* (Kogure K, Hossmann K-A, Siesjö B K, eds), pp 195-208. Amsterdam: Elsevier Science Publishers B.V.
24. Lindvall O, Ernfors P, Bengtzon J, Kokaia Z, Smith M-L, Siesjö B K, Persson H (1992) Differential regulation of mRNAs for nerve growth factor, brain-derived neurotrophic factor and neurotrophin-3 in the adult rat brain following cerebral ischemia and hypoglycemic coma. *Proc Natl Acad Sci USA* 89:648-652
25. Halliwell B (1992) Reactive oxygen species and the central nervous system. *J Neurochem* 59:1609-1623
26. Oliver C, Starke-Reed P, Stadtman E, Liu G, Carney J, Floyd R (1990) Oxidative damage to brain proteins, loss of glutamine synthetase activity, and production of free radicals during ischemia/reperfusion-induced injury to gerbil brain. *Proc Natl Acad Sci USA* 87:5144-5147
27. Pahlmark K, Folbergrová J, Smith M-L, Siesjö B K (1993) Effects of dimethylthiourea on selective neuronal vulnerability in forebrain ischemia in rats. *Stroke* 24:731-737
28. Siesjö B K, Katsura K, Pahlmark K, Smith M-L (1992) The multiple causes of ischemic brain damage: a speculative synthesis. In: *Pharmacology of Cerebral Ischemia* (Krieglstein J, Oberpilcher H, eds), pp 511-525. Stuttgart: Wissenschaftliche Verlagsgesellschaft
29. Siesjö B K, Katsura K, Mellergård P, Ekholm A, Lundgren J, Smith M-L (1993) Acidosis-related brain damage. In: *Neurobiology of Ischemic Brain Damage* (Kogure K, Hossmann K-A, Siesjö B K, eds), pp 23-48, Progr Brain Res vol 96. Amsterdam: Elsevier Science Publishers B.V.
30. Katsura K, Kristián T, Smith M-L, Siesjö B (1994) Acidosis induced by hypercapnia exaggerates ischemic brain damage. *J Cerebral Blood Flow Metabol* 14:243-250
31. Ou Yang Y-B, Mellergård P, Kristián T, Kristiánova V, Siesjö B (1994) Influence of acid-base changes on intracellular calcium concentration of neurons in primary culture. *Exp Brain Res* 101:265-271
32. Combs D J, Demsey R J, Donaldson D, Kindy M S (1992) Hyperglycemia suppresses c-fos mRNA expression following transient cerebral ischemia in gerbils. *J Cerebral Blood Flow Metabol* 12:169-172
33. Kristián T, Katsura K, Gidö G, Siesjö B K (1994) The influence of pH on cellular calcium influx during ischemia. *Brain Res* 641:295-302

34. Kristián T, Gidö G, Siesjö B (1995) The influence of acidosis on hypoglycemic brain damage. *J Cerebral Blood Flow Metabol* 15:78-87
35. Barry M, Eastman A (1993) Identification of deoxyribonuclease II as an endonuclease involved in apoptosis. *Arch Biochem Biophys* 300: 440-450
36. Barry M, Reynolds J, Eastman A (1993) Etoposide-induced apoptosis in human HL-60 cells is associated with intracellular acidification. *Cancer Res* 53: 2349-2357
37. Siesjö B, Katsura K, Kristián T (1995) Acidosis-related damage. In: *Advances in Neurology* (Siesjö B, Wieloch T, eds). New York, Raven Press
38. Pelligrino-Giampietro D, Zukin R, Bennett M, Cho S, Pulsinelli W (1992) Switch in glutamate receptor subunit gene expression in CA1 subfield of hippocampus following global ischemia in rats. *Proc Natl Acad Sci USA* 89:10499-10503
39. Tsuchiya M, Sako K, Yura S, Yonemasu Y (1992) Cerebral blood flow and histopathological changes following permanent bilateral carotid artery ligation in Wistar rats. *Exp Brain Res* 89:87-92

# 14. EXCITOTOXICITY

DENNIS W. CHOI, M.D., Ph.D.

**Dr. Caprioli**: It is my pleasure to introduce Dr. Dennis Choi, who is Professor and Chairman of Neurology at Washington University in St. Louis, and he is going to share his extensive experience with excitotoxins in the central nervous system.

I thought I would start with a bit of a general discussion about excitotoxicity and why some of you might be interested in this subject. The topic, of course, has just been very elegantly introduced by Mimo Costa. The term excitotoxicity was coined by John Olney, now more than two decades ago. He discovered that glutamate could kill central neurons, and realized, I think first, that this could be an important principle of disease. Glutamate is an excitatory transmitter, and certainly the ensuing years have taught us how important an excitatory transmitter glutamate is. Glutamate, by activating receptors (under most conditions by overactivating receptors) can kill central neurons, including retinal neurons. Olney coined the term "excitotoxicity" to put together, excitatory neurotransmission and cytotoxicity.

There are really three possible reasons why people in the glaucoma field might be interested in excitotoxicity (besides the very dull possibility that there is actually no reason to be interested in excitotoxicity). The first is that excitotoxicity might have a primary role in glaucoma pathogenesis. That is obviously a very remote possibility. I have been trying to pick up a little bit around the edges of this meeting; it seems that since many things are possible, this is possible. It seems conceivable that the primary pathology is at the level of cells, at the level of retina, in particular ganglion cells, and that subsequent pathologies are sequelae of that primary cellular pathology. In other words, stating it as a neurologist, I would say that glaucoma was a neuronopathy, rather than a neuropathy. You could imagine that some disturbance in the glutamate system itself or in closely related systems could produce overactivation of glutamate receptors as a primary reason for the neuronopathy. Nothing that I have heard so far would exclude this, although I would be the first to say that there appears to be no particular evidence for it.

The second reason why people in the glaucoma field may be interested in excitotoxicity is the concept of exacerbators, sort of an "afterburner" on injury. This is a theme that has emerged vigorously in neurology right now; we are looking at a variety of different kinds of injury, particularly acute injuries. But it has also come up as speculation in regard to a number of neurodegenerative diseases. One could certainly think of glaucoma as a neurodegenerative disease. Many of the questions, the very excellent discussion that was just going on, echoes the issues and discussions that arise when a group of neuroscientists get together and start talking about Parkinson's disease or Alzheimer's disease. The same fundamental questions of kinetics come up. Are the cells that are being lost in Huntington's disease, for example, being lost like blinking lights, just once in a while, or are all the neurons a little sick and chronically petering out over the 19-year course of the disease? These questions are common to glaucoma and to neurodegenerative diseases? The same considerations that have caused people in neurology to be interested in excitotoxicity as a secondary exacerbating factor might apply here. Many observations suggest that you can do a lot of nasty things to central nervous system tissue, and then trigger an excitotoxic component on top of that. You

*Optic Nerve in Glaucoma, pp. 223–232*
*edited by S.M. Drance*

can identify the excitotoxic component most convincingly by blocking it pharmacologically, blocking glutamate receptors, and seeing that you ameliorate the cell deaths. You can do this, as Dr. Siesjö nicely reviewed, with a number of energy depletion insults, like taking away the oxygen or taking away the glucose, or you can take away the magnesium and cause cells to fire. Perhaps of some special interest to people here are the trauma models which we touched on briefly in this discussion. Even *in vitro* you can take a set of neurons and you can transsect them mechanically, just take a stylette and scrape it through a neuronal cell culture. And what happens is a progressive degeneration away from that tear, not associated with any compromise of energy. pH and glucose and oxygen are all normal, but there is a propagation of that insult, rippling out in space, and you can show that the progression is due to excitotoxins, since if you block the glutamate receptors, the amount of cell death is much reduced and remains relatively restricted to the immediate vicinity of the tear.

So this idea of exacerbation: doing something unpleasant to a neuron, for example, depleting its energy stores, and causing it to become unhappy, depolarize and dump glutamate on its neighbors, eventually killing its neighbors. The idea has appeared in many many different settings. At least speculatively it might appear in a consideration of glaucoma mechanisms.

One animal model, before I leave this topic, that you might be interested in that has emerged recently has been the mitochondrial impairment models. The best work on that has been done using a compound, actually a human neurotoxin, 3-nitropropionic acid (3-NPA), which is responsible for a sugar cane poisoning in China. People eat mildewed sugar cane containing 3-NPA and they develop a subacute neurological illness associated with brain damage. Flint Beal at the Mass General has been studying this compound. If you inject animals with it, what develops is a chronically, relatively slow onset, excitotoxic damage that is quite selective.

So whatever the ultimate cause of glaucoma is, if you imagine that the retina is a glutamate syncytium, which it is, lots of glutamate, lots of glutamatergic synapses, why not imagine that some of the same rules which seem to be recurring in brain and in spinal cord might apply to retina. The sick retina might begin to overactivate glutamate receptors, and this overactivation might not be benign. So there might be some additional injury mediated by glutamate receptors on top of whatever causes glaucoma.

**Dr. Quigley**: I just wanted to ask very quickly if a cell process in a culture retracts on being exposed to an excitotoxin? Is that possible even though that process does not have receptors for the glutamate system on it? Is there some direct effect, or must the process or the cell exposed to the excitotoxin have receptors for the chemical itself?

**Dr. Anderson**: I will add to the question, please, must there be a source of glutamate?

**Dr. Quigley**: Always presuming that the glutamate was there. The question is, if you dump glutamate on a random neuron or a random neural process, is that damaging to it even without a receptor? I mean, assuming you are not dumping a bathtubful.

**Dr. Anderson**: I add my question to yours with respect to the optic nerve. Is there a source of glutamate in the optic nerve head that would cause an injury?

**Dr. Choi**: I do not believe so. I think if one starts to think about either possibilities one or two, one is working with more of an idea that ganglion cell injury is involved. In possibility two, you can easily imagine that the primary site of pathology is the nerve head or even distal to that, the optic tract or something, but that indirectly the ganglion cells become sick, and that the sick ganglion cells start hurting each other.

**Dr. Quigley**: How about anybody else? They also hurt an immediately adjacent amacrine cell or the bipolar cell...

**Dr. Choi**: I think that is entirely possible, I do not know much about the retina but I will give you a good example, of excitotoxic injury and the "bad neighborhood effect". When you start getting cell death you create an area which is not so good. The very fact that in ischemia there is astrocyte death, means that not only neurons are injured. Non-neuronal cells, including astrocytes, have also died. And if you block glutamate receptors, so that takes out the excitotoxic component, you reduce the overall size of the infarct by about half in most people's hands. That means that you also reduce the astrocyte death by about half also.

**Dr. Siesjö**: Dennis, did not Mark Matson show that in order to get cells to grow in tissue culture you need an optimal concentration of glutamate. If you have too little, too much, whatever...

**Dr. Choi**: I would say Robert Balasz probably has done the best work in that area with cerebellar granular cells. While that is true under certain circumstances, it would probably be best not viewed as a generalizable principle.

**Dr. Ransom**: Dennis, this is a very nice thing to do, to bring together a lot of the things that have been discussed. Now, to come back to the idea that you do not necessarily have to be talking about nerve cell bodies, I would say two things. Number one, glutamate is a metabolic component of the cytosol of lots of cells, and there is glutamate present at high concentrations in the nerve itself, you do not have to go to the cell body, it can be released by non-synaptic type mechanisms. So glutamate is there, that is absolutely certain.

**Dr. Choi**: But excitotoxicity is not.

**Dr. Ransom**: Well, not conventional excitotoxicity, but I think you would be the first person to agree that in this particular instance we are talking about something that may not necessarily be straightforward abrupt excitotoxicity. I would add, to answer Dr. Quigley's question, that you do not even necessarily have to have a receptor for these excitotoxins on the axons. You could imagine a sequence of events that is triggered through adjacent cells. To focus exclusively on the axons is to miss out on a whole lot of what is going on in the optic nerve, including in the optic nerve head. There are plenty of glial cells there, and I guarantee that there are glutamate receptors on those astrocytes. No one has ever ruled out the possibility that you could get release irritated or prompted by either mechanical events or by low levels of hypoxia or anoxia, which would result in glutamate coming out, activating the receptors on astrocytes, and over long periods of time. It is the kinetic process that is critical here, over long periods of time you could produce a type of pathophysiology that is unique to this particular area.

**Dr. Kaufman**: There was a study that was presented at the recent ARVO meeting, by Evan Dryer from Boston, where he showed elevated levels of, I believe, glutamate in the vitreous from glaucoma patients, and I think in the vitreous of laser-induced glaucoma. I think some of those may actually have been your animals, Harry. Do we have any idea where that is coming from? What the source of that glutamate is in that model? There are three or four times elevated glutamate levels in the vitreous.

**Dr. Quigley**: We discussed it with Evan as to whether or not it is worth attempting to measure glutamate levels postmortem or, at the time that we sacrifice monkeys that have had experimentally induced ganglion cell damage. What I have been trying to get at is a hypothesis that we could then go test when we look histologically at tissue. If a component of the glaucoma process is that as a ganglion cell dies, from whatever the initial mechanism it died from, if it also kills off somebody else in the neighborhood, then we should see loss of cells in the retina that are not just ganglion cells. Now there are other reasons to think other cells might die, by trans-synaptic degeneration, or by some other mechanism, so, some of us are actively looking right now at cells other than ganglion cells dying in the retina, and we have the possibility of counting. I think you have given us another reason for looking in great detail at the bipolar cell layer and the photoreceptor cell layer and the glia that live in the nerve fiber layer next to ganglion cells.

**Dr. Anderson**: If there is a loss of bipolar cells, for example, they are not in large number because we have not in passing recognized that as a loss in histopathological specimens. Now you are going to count and see whether you can detect it quantitatively, but qualitatively there has not been a recognition of neighborhood loss of cells.

**Dr. Quigley**: But that does not necessarily rule this out as a contributing feature, though, Doug. I mean, I might look at 20 glaucoma eyes and show you that statistically those 20 glaucoma eyes have the same number of bipolars as 28 matched normal eyes. That shows that every glaucoma eye does not have a huge excitotoxic neighborhood effect. It does not show that 20 or 15% did not have local excitotoxic effects that were contributory and it got lost in the statistics. You know, you can not rule out some, but if you say, is it a big effect, is it the whole effect, is it a major portion, it does not look like it is right now.

**Dr. Anderson**: Now, to explain for a moment the finding that you brought up, Paul, that was presented at ARVO. I thought that part of the explanation for that observation could be that the nerve fiber layer is reduced and the ganglion cell layer is reduced and therefore there is no longer a thick tissue layer between the area where glutamate is a transmitter and it is produced and the vitreous, so that there is a greater diffusion. Thus, the observation may not have to do with the pathologic process, but as a consequence of the fact that there is less tissue between the outer retinal layers and the vitreous. Nobody knows. That was an explanation that occurred to me as I was looking at the data. How do you explain this?

**Dr. Kaufman**: But to go along with that explanation, if that is correct, once you do get higher levels because of some damage to some ganglion cells or other tissues in the area, you then have a higher level which could itself produce more cell death, and you have kind of a vicious downward spiral, so they are not mutually exclusive mechanisms at all.

**Dr. Epstein**: Can I ask what I am sure is a very naive question. This excitotoxicity is a receptor-mediated phenomenon, and I do not understand, are there other examples of a situation where you will saturate a receptor and you get a toxic effect. I neither understand what advantage to the organism would be to have this kind of thing. I can understand I think what Harry was saying, that glutamate just diffuses into the cytoplasm that you get a toxic effect, but why would you have a saturated receptor-mediated toxic effect.

**Dr. Choi**: First of all, you do not have to saturate the receptors, it depends on conditions. Second, it is not unique to the glutamate system, there are other transmitter systems where you can get cell death by activating receptors. Third, why? That is a great question. I think there are two broad possibilities. One is that it somehow is useful to the nervous system. As you know, death is very much part of the life of a nervous system, in constructing a nervous system, large number of neurons are sculpted away, and although most of that has been ascribed to apoptosis, it is conceivable that excitotoxicity plays a role there. Second is that it is just simply a sequela and a casualty of having fast synaptic transmission. There are lots of examples, for example the immune system. If you want to walk on two feet, you get back pain. You want to crawl out of the ocean, you get oxygen free radical injury and if you want to think faster than a worm you have excitotoxicity. Maybe that is the way it goes.

**Dr. Anderson**: Well, I wonder about another thing, in response to this. It occurs to me that excitotoxicity might be a prolonged stimulation of a receptor. Usually when you have a transmission in which you have a glutamate stimulating a post-synaptic receptor. A response occurs and there are clean-up mechanisms for getting rid of the glutamate. Here we are talking about glutamate staying on the receptor for a prolonged time and therefore maintaining the intracellular calcium for a long time, instead of as a transient that induces the transmitted response. That was what I thought was a potential explanation for toxicity in what is otherwise a physiologic mechanism.

**Dr. Choi**: Yes, I did not think we were asking a question about mechanism, which we can talk about a little bit later, but just really why should we be at risk for excitotoxicity at all.

Just to mention one other model of relevance. Marmor, I think, was the first to show that in retina *per se* you can demonstrate an excitotoxic component to hypoxic injury. He and his colleagues produced a model of retinal hypoxia, I believe, by increasing intraocular pressure until it exceeded the retinal artery pressure. They achieved retinal damage that way and measured it by looking at the ERP. That damage could be ameliorated by using an NMDA antagonist. So there is some reason to think that the kind of things that Dr. Siesjö was talking about in brain also apply specifically to retina.

The third and I think best reason for people interested in glaucoma to care at all about excitotoxicity is that, even if it has no specific relevance to the pathophysiology of glaucomatous neuronopathy or neuropathy, as a model, as a defined sequence of cytopathology leading to death, definition of the mechanisms underly-

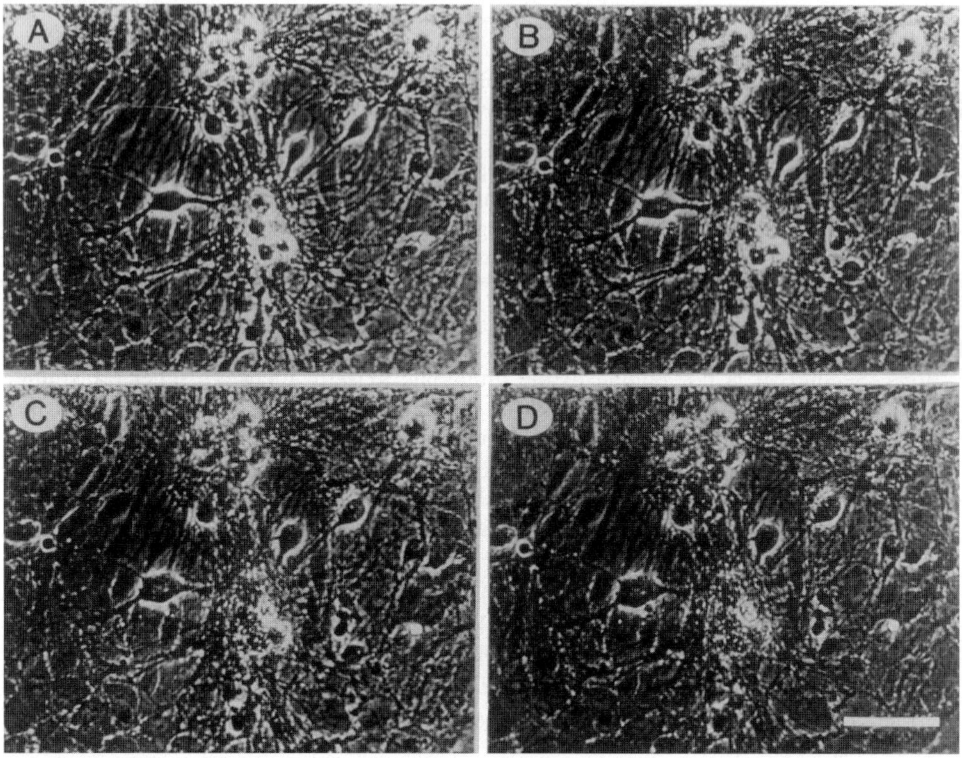


*Fig. 1.* Acute time course of glutamate neurotoxicity. Serial phase contrast micrographs showing a field of cortical cells before (A), immediately after (B), 10 minutes after (C), and 25 minutes after (D) exposure to a single 90 second pulse of 1 mM glutamate. The dish was maintained on the stage of the physiology microscope, and the field was continuously observed after glutamate was delivered by pressure ejection from a puffer pipette placed in the middle of the field. Bar: 50 μM. (Reproduced with permission from: Choi *et al.*, *The Journal of Neuroscience*, February 1987, 7(2): 357-368.)

ing excitotoxicity may teach us something about glaucoma. This is a very real possibility. I drew up a metaphor at a meeting that Dr. Siesjö and I attended several years ago, a Dahlem conference, and we talked about a death funnel. The idea is simply that, while there are probably an infinite number of different insults which you can deliver to a cell, there may not be an infinite number of final ways a cell dies. Now, this is speculation, although it has considerable support. There may be convergence in injury. You may start with a million different specific insults, and you can call one glaucoma, we can call another one hypoxia, but ultimately, when you get down to it, when you get downstream, there may be relatively limited defined things that are going wrong. Some strong candidates for what might be down in the funnel include: disturbances in calcium homeostasis, disturbances in free radicals, or disruptions of cytoskeleton. These same themes emerge over and over again in different kinds of cell injuries under widely different conditions. If one takes a slice through the funnel, longitudinally, by studying the excitotoxic process and defining it, one could learn something valuable to approaching glaucoma, even something useful in terms of potential therapeutics, without ever getting one's hands on the cause of glaucoma.

Those are the three reasons that I would think that people here might be interested in regarding the excitotoxic process. With that as an introduction, I am going to try to give you a bit of a general outline, or summary, of some of the current thoughts that my colleagues and I have about the mechanisms underlying excitotoxicity.

So the model system that my colleagues and I have been working with to study excitotoxicity is shown in Figure 1. These are cortical cell cultures, neocortex placed in culture a couple of days, standard Nissl stain, you can see the neurons and they are lying on top of an astrocyte bed. If you put glutamate in the dish for a few minutes and wash it out, and come back the next day, the neurons but not the glia are totally destroyed, it is really a very dramatic phenomenon, and very absolute, death is clearly death. And you can look at this with higher time resolution. This is a phase contrast micrograph of cortical neurons in life, you can see the cell bodies here, and if you bring a pipette down in the field and you inject glutamate, what happens is that very visibly, in real time, the cells begin to swell. And this is what John Olney first saw when he started to talk about excitotoxicity. Ten minutes later you can see the changes are very obvious, this is just 90 seconds later. And by 20 minutes, I will point out that this original clump of neurons, bright cell bodies here, have become virtually invisible. They are still there, but they are huge, they are large and swollen, and they are phase dark, suggesting that the inside of the cells is no longer so different from the outside of the cells. What we think has happened is that by bathing these cells with glutamate, we have activated the glutamate receptor-linked channels, and a lot of sodium has rushed into the cells, taking with it chloride and water, salt water. Essentially these cells have swelled up, blown up with salt water. This is a pretty nasty phenomenon, but it is not necessarily the lethal event. What appears to be the lethal event is a delayed degeneration, so the cells blow up like a balloon and then over a period of time, over a period of hours they go on and degenerate. One can trigger this kind of injury quite rapidly, and this shows how rapidly. If you ask, how many minutes does one have to stimulate glutamate receptors to get cell death (we measure cell death by measuring lactate dehydrogenase efflux in the bathing media), you can see that up to about a minute it is reasonably benign. Some numbers of cells are dying, but most of them are not. But when you get around two or three minutes, most of the neurons in the dish are lethally injured and go on to degenerate over the next hours. Notice that this degeneration correlates pretty well with a second index, which is a large amount of $^{45}Ca$ which moves from the bathing medium into the cells. We have focused on these $^{45}Ca$ movements, and we find that they give a pretty good prediction of whether or not cells are going to die under a variety of conditions. There is a mass movement of calcium right from the bathing medium into the neurons that is a reasonable correlate and predictor of whether or not they are going to die. For example, if one takes the calcium out of the bathing medium, interestingly the cells blow up like a balloon, but then they recover, they no longer go on to die. So we have come to the notion that the bulk movement of calcium rushing into the cell is a key trigger for this kind of cell death. We have taken to calling this kind of cell death *rapidly triggered excitotoxicity* to emphasize that two to three minutes worth of continuous stimulation is all that is required to send these cells on their way. Now, of course, that is grossly unphysiologic, as someone pointed out the other day, signalling glutamate is present for brief fractions of a second, at synapses, so normally a cell would not see sustained glutamate concentrations. But we are doing something pathological, something which likely happens under conditions of acute injury.

Dr. Costa nicely discussed in detail what is known about glutamate receptors at this time. Just to refresh, AMPA kainate receptors open sodium channels, NMDA

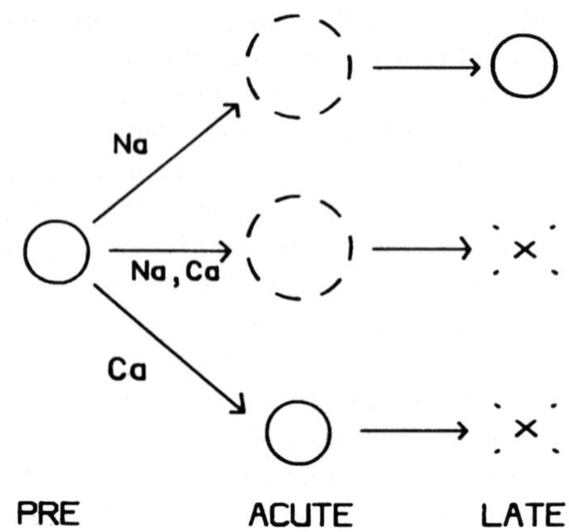


*Fig. 2.* Two components of rapidly triggered excitotoxicity.

receptors open channels permeable to calcium, and a whole series of metabotropic receptors are linked to inositol metabolism, cyclic AMP and the like. So, based on these fundamental characteristics, you can envision that the NMDA receptor might play a special role in rapidly triggered excitotoxicity, and that is in fact the case. If you block the NMDA receptor selectively with a drug like D-APV, you can bring down cell death and also bring down $^{45}$Ca. This is simply NMDA receptor blockade at this point out here, AMPA kainate receptors are still functional, so glutamate can still excite the neurons, glutamate can still cause the cells to blow up like balloons by causing salt water to rush in, but glutamate no longer triggers the delayed calcium-dependent cell death, suggesting that NMDA receptors are required for this kind of excitotoxicity. This is summarized in Figure 2.

Under physiological conditions neurons blow up like balloons and go on and degenerate, a process separable into the blowing up like a balloon, which is mediated by NMDA as well as AMPA kainate receptors but is not intrinsically lethal to many cells, and a more lethal component critically dependent on calcium in the extracellular space accompanied by movement of calcium into the cells mediated by NMDA receptors, lacking in acute morphological concomitants, but resulting in the delayed cell degeneration. So that is a thumbnail sketch of rapidly triggered excitotoxicity.

There is another form of excitotoxicity which we have taken to calling slowly triggered excitotoxicity, and at least in cell cultures we have learned that if we selectively stimulate AMPA kainate receptors we can destroy all the neurons just as easily. But in order to do so we have to stimulate the receptors for a prolonged time, many hours.

With 24-hour exposure, 10 μM concentrations of either kainate or AMPA can induce widespread death of cultured cortical neurons. This slowly triggered, AMPA/kainate receptor-mediated excitotoxicity may also be initiated by excessive $Ca^{2+}$ influx. Most channels gated by AMPA or kainate receptors have limited $Ca^{2+}$ permeability, but $Ca^{2+}$ influx can occur indirectly, for example through voltage-gated $Ca^{2+}$ channels activated by the $Na^{+}$ influx and membrane depolarization associated with AMPA/kainate receptor stimulation. Other indirect pathways for $Ca^{2+}$ entry may include reverse operation of the $Na^{+}$-$Ca^{2+}$ exchanger, membrane stretch-activated conductances, or leak conductances activated by cell swelling. In addition, recent studies by Iino and colleagues as well as Miller and colleagues, have indicated that some AMPA receptors may gate channels permeable to $Ca^{2+}$, possibly reflecting a molecular composition lacking the Glu-R2/Glu-RB subunit. A minority of our cortical neurons may possess large numbers of AMPA receptor-gated $Ca^{2+}$ channels, and perhaps as a direct result, are especially vulnerable to damage mediated by AMPA receptor overactivation.

The chain of events triggered by overexposure to glutamate: glutamate neurotoxicity can be modelled as a three-stage process: induction, amplification, and expression. First, the prolonged availability of extracelluar glutamate is transduced by neuronal membrane receptors into potentially lethal intracellular derangements, in particular, intracellular $Ca^{2+}$ overload.

Second, modulatory events amplify these derangements, increasing their intensity and promoting the involvement of other neurons. Following the induction of glutamate toxicity, a multiplicity of events may act to further amplify resultant internal derangements, especially local elevations in $[Ca^{2+}]_i$ (Choi DW: Methods for antagonizing glutamate neurotoxicity. *Cerebrovasc Brain Metabol Rev* 2:105-147, 1990). These amplification events may include:

1. Additional influx of extracelluar $Ca^{2+}$ through voltage-gated $Ca^{2+}$ channels, reverse operation of the $Na^+$-$Ca^{2+}$ exchanger, $Ca^{2+}$-activated $Ca^{2+}$ channels, or stretch-activated cation channels.
2. The release of $Ca^{2+}$ from intracellular stores, for example mediated by elevations in $IP_3$.
3. The activation of key enzyme families - including C kinases and calmodulin-regulated enzymes- and genes, that together may lead to a lasting enhancement of certain processes relevant to excitotoxicity, including $Ca^{2+}$-dependent glutamate release from nerve terminals, post-synaptic receptor responsiveness to glutamate, and $Ca^{2+}$ influx through voltage-gated channels. The activation of phospholipase $A_2$ and nitric oxide synthase increases formation of the intercellular messengers arachidonic acid and nitric oxide, that can induce pro-excitotoxic changes in the glutamate system. Once formed in post-synaptic neurons, these messengers can diffuse freely across lipid membranes to affect neighboring neurons and glia.
4. Glutamate efflux from injured neurons, which may induce further excitotoxic injury, a positive feedback loop that might both intensify existing injury, and help propagate excitotoxic injury onto neurons spared by the initial insult.

The net contribution of these amplification steps to neuronal death may be a function of the strength of initial induction events. Following intense activation of NMDA receptors, enough $Ca^{2+}$ may enter neurons directly through NMDA receptor-gated channels to produce lethal effects without subsequent amplification. Amplification may therefore be more important to slowly triggered excitoxicity than to rapidly triggered excitotoxicity.

Finally, these derangements, perhaps especially the sustained elevations in $[Ca^{2+}]_i$, trigger the cytotoxic cascades responsible for subsequent delayed neuronal disintegration, the expression of cell death. Many specific $Ca^{2+}$-triggered destructive events may be common to rapidly triggered excitotoxicity and slowly triggered excitotoxicity. One important class of expression cascades may be the unleashing of $Ca^{2+}$-activated catabolic enzymes, such as the $Ca^+$- activated neutral protease, calpain. Elevated cystolic $Ca^{2+}$ also activates phospholipases capable of breaking down cell membranes and liberating arachidonic acid, and endonucleases capable of breaking down genomic DNA.

Another important class of expression cascades may involve oxygen free radicals. These reactive molecules can initiate many destructive processes including lipid peroxidation. Once formed, they may promote further excitotoxic injury by promoting glutamate release. 21-Aminosteroid inhibitors of lipid peroxidation can reduce the death associated with both rapidly triggered and slowly triggered excitotoxicity on cortical neurons. Free radical production might be linked to loss of cellular $Ca^{2+}$ homeostasis in several ways, including: 1) $Ca^{2+}$ activation of phospholipase $A_2$, leading to the liberation of arachidonic acid which upon further metabolism leads to free radical production; 2) $Ca^{2+}$ triggering the conversion of xanthine dehydrogenase to xanthine oxidase, a right enzymatic source of free radicals; and 3) stimulation of NMDA receptors leading to the activation of nitric oxide synthase and the release of nitric oxide, which in turn can react with superoxide to form peroxynitrite and promote the production of hydroxyl radicals. Dawson and colleagues in Snyder's laboratory at Johns Hopkins found that pharmacological inhibition of nitric oxide synthase, or removal of the nitric oxide precursor, arginine, from the culture medium, reduced rapidly triggered excitotoxicity in rat cortical cultures.

# 15. HEAT SHOCK PROTEIN

JOSEPH CAPRIOLI, M.D.

This morning we have learned a lot about potential mechanisms, but unfortunately its relevance to glaucoma is speculative. One of our challenges is to bridge those two areas and see if we can develop information about mechanisms which may be more relevant to glaucoma. I am afraid that is going to be a little time away, and we have a lot of work to do in order to get there.

In terms of hypotheses about glaucomatous damage, I think it would be foolish to make a single hypothesis at this point. We do have perhaps hypoxic factors, perhaps mechanical factors, maybe there are some intrinsic genetic retinal ganglion cell factors which are important, and other risk factors, and all of these may be operating to a greater or lesser extent, even in individual patients. In an individual patient pressure may be the predominant factor causing damage, and in another it may be vascular, and in another one there may be some retinal ganglion cell susceptibility, perhaps even excitotoxicity which is playing a role. But one thing we need to keep in mind is that any hypothesis must allow for the very slow and chronic progression of the disease that we know occurs. Dr. Costa mentioned this morning about amyotrophic lateral sclerosis, and this is an interesting disease because it is a chronic neurodegenerative disease, and there is new evidence that glutamate receptors may play a role in that disease.

With this vague introduction, I would like to talk about some preliminary work that we have done in the laboratory with retinal ganglion cell cultures. We have been interested in looking at heat shock protein. In contradistinction to the other speakers that have been up here this morning, I am not an expert in this field, but I will share with you the little that I do know.

But first let me talk a little bit about the system that we are using. These are retinal ganglion cells in culture, and our idea was to develop some information about basic mechanisms of damage, and this is going to make Ran Zeimer very unhappy, but whether or not any of this work has any relevance to glaucoma, I have no idea. We were interested in looking at hypoxia and the possible role of excitotoxicity (as we heard to be an important process in ischemic damage) and the role of certain stress proteins and, if we could possibly take advantage of any differential susceptibility P cells, that may provide the key to unlocking some secrets that we have not been able to explore yet. If we can take advantage of differential susceptibility between different classes of ganglion cells, and see what their differences are, then we may learn more about the process.

We used retinal ganglion cells from rats that are seven to 11 days old. On the left is a Müller cell culture that we used as a substrate for our retinal ganglion cells. Here we have a retinal ganglion cell which has been stained with the monoclonal antibody Thy-1, donated to us by Dr. Colin Barsible, of our Department, and this is one way to identify retinal ganglion cells in this dissociated culture. You have to remember in these cultures there are all sorts of retinal cells. We do not see any photoreceptors but there are certainly retinal ganglion cells, bipolar cells, laminar cells, horizontal cells, and Müller cells. Another way to positively identify the retinal ganglion cells is by retrograde labeling. Here you see a retrogradely labeled cell with granular blue. The problem with granular blue is that it fades fairly rapidly and it complicates our analysis of survival.

*Optic Nerve in Glaucoma, pp. 233–242*
*edited by S.M. Drance*

**Hoffman**: Do you say these are retrogradely labeled cells?

**Dr. Caprioli**: Yes, these were injected into both superior colliculi, two days before harvesting the eyes and in this case with granular blue. But more recently we have gone to the use of Di-I, which seems to be a more stable label and is around quite a lot longer.

Therefore, most of what I am going to tell you about retinal ganglion cells in our culture are from these labeled, retrogradely labeled cells with Di-I. This is the survivorship that we see on various substrates. We have used laminin-coated dishes, cortical astrocytes, and retinal glial cells (Müller cells) as substrates. Not too surprisingly, the retinal ganglion cells seemed to do best on a Müller cell substrate. Here we have a little less than 50% survivorship at the end of seven days. We can see cells that survive for a month or more, though these are relatively few, I think we are really below the 5% level. There may be something very special about those cells that last so long. But certainly you do not see that kind of survival on laminin-coated dishes.

We notice spontaneous synaptic activity, this is from a patch clamp recording of a labeled retinal ganglion cell. So there is some evidence that these cells do have some functional activity.

**Dr. Quigley**: Joe, you said synaptic activity. Is one cell being stimulated to spike, or was it one cell being recorded when another cell was being stimualted?

**Dr. Caprioli**: That was one cell being recorded, and that cell had synaptic connections to other cells around it. So it was not stimulated by any current that we were passing through, that was spontaneous spiking behavior.

**Dr. Quigley**: Spontaneous spiking, not synaptic connections.

**Dr. Caprioli**: Spontaneous spiking behavior. However you do not see that spiking behavior unless you develop synaptic connections or you pass a current through the cell and depolarize it. These are solitary retinal ganglion cells that have been depolarized with currents. And we have seen a couple of different types, and I do not want to make too much of this because I am not an electrophysiologist, but we did see phasically and tonically firing types of cells when depolarized with a current.

This follows the work that has been done in the central nervous system by Dr. Choi and others. These are the responses of solitary retinal ganglion cells which have been patch-clamped to glutamate, kainate, aspartate, NMDA, acetylcholine, and glycine. This is what happens to a cell that has some synaptic interaction with other cells and is spontaneously spiking, in which we locally apply with a micropipette 100 μM glutamate in the region of the cell, and it again depolarizes and spikes at a high frequency (Fig. 1). So we were happy to see this kind of electrical activity in our cells in culture.

We looked at the survivorship of these cells as a function of concentration of the excitatory amino acids, kainate, glutamate, and NMDA (Fig. 2). This is after exposure of six hours, so we are not likely to see any differential effects between the AMPA and NMDA receptors here. In these graphs, we can see the concentration-related effect on survivorship. And we see, in the presence of 200 μM glutamate, a survivorship as a function of time. We are counting only the retinal ganglion cells that have been labeled.

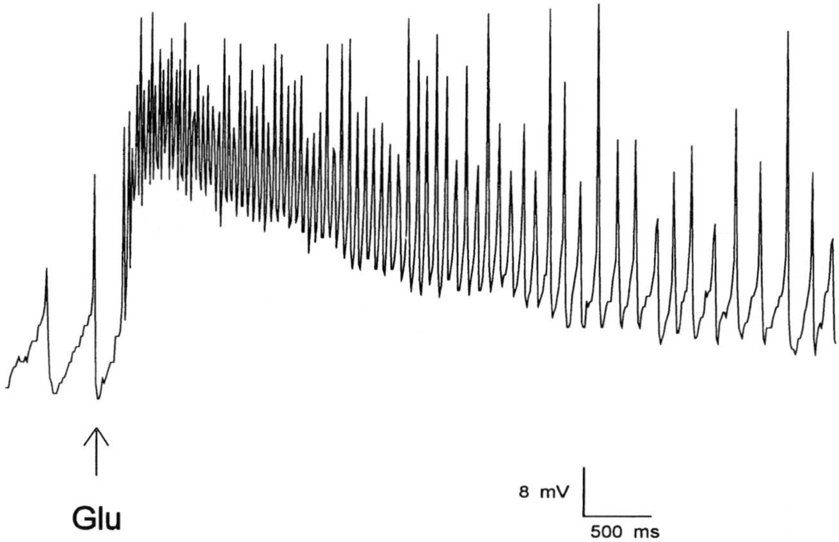


*Fig. 1.* A spontaneously spiking retinal ganglion cell in culture on a glial monolayer is depolarized by glutamate. Simultaneously, spiking frequency is increased.

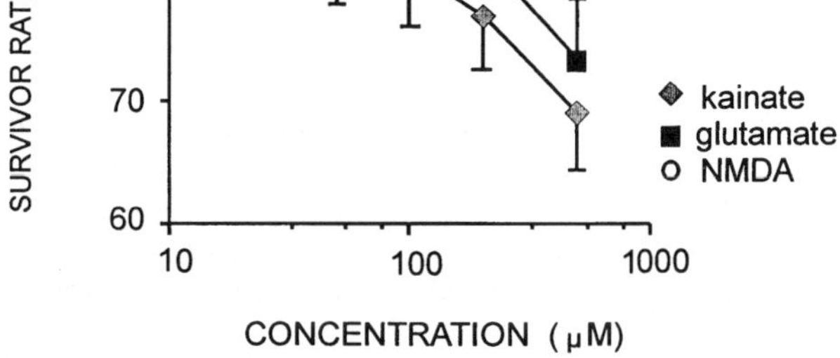


*Fig. 2.* The survivorship of retinal ganglion cells in culture (percentage of control) as a function of the concentration of the excitatory amino acids kainate, glutamate, and NMDA. Survival after six-hour exposure to the excitatory amino acids compared to control are given.

MK-801 prevents this excitotoxic death completely. This is a concentration of MK-801 and this is a cytotoxic death induced by 200 μM of glutamate (Fig. 3). This appears to be dose-related.

Here we have survival rate (as percent of control) as a function of $O_2$ concentration, and, in general, when I say hypoxia I am talking about 9–10% $O_2$ concentration, and when I say anoxia, I make the mistake of saying anoxia, but it really is not completely anoxic; it is hard to get the cell culture medium to be completely anoxic,

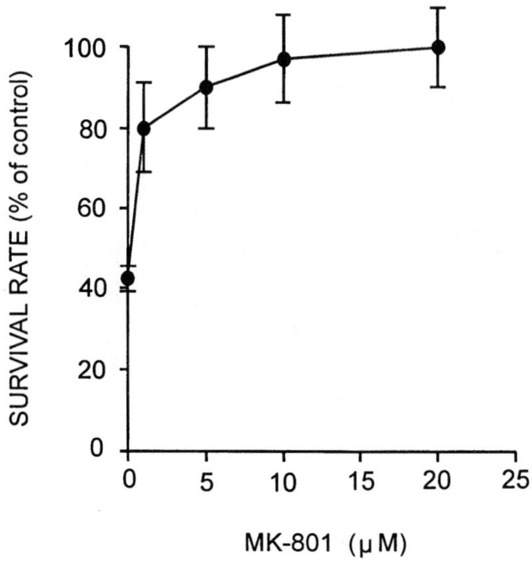


*Fig. 3.* The NMDA antagonist MK-801 blocks the excitotoxic effects of 200 μM glutamate in a dose-related fashion. Survival refers to the survival rate as a percentage of control, after six hours of exposure to 200 μM glutamate and progressive concentrations of MK-801.

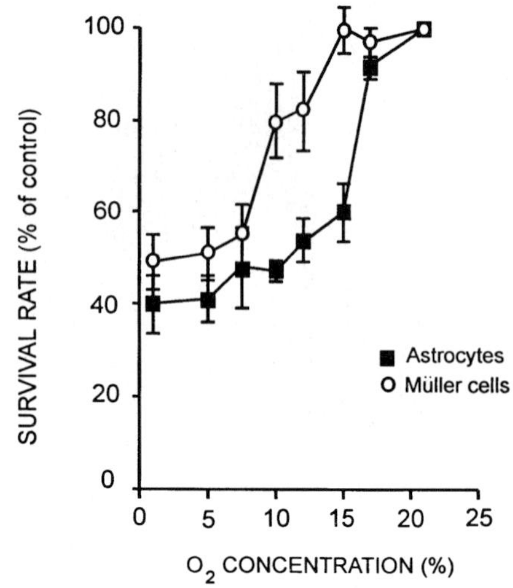


*Fig. 4.* Survival rate of cultured retinal ganglion cells as a function of ambient oxygen concentration. Data are given separately for a substrate of cortical astrocyte and for a substrate of retinal Müller cells.

we are really talking about 2–3% $O_2$ concentration (Fig. 4). We see this dose-response relationship. Retinal ganglion cells seem to do somewhat better in the presence of Müller cells than they do with cortical astrocytes under hypoxic conditions.

Here is a relationship with time and this is the effect of hypoxia, that is, about a 9% oxygen concentration, and at the end of 24 hours, in the presence of Müller cells, you still see that about 75%, as a percent of control, again, of the retinal ganglion cells are still surviving.

**Dr. Siesjö**: I am a bit intrigued by what you say that the minimal oxygen concentrations you come down to are 2–3%. That would imply that your oxygen tensions would exceed 10 mmHg, and your diffusion distances can not be very large, particularly not if you have a monolayer of cells. So I can not see that you could come to critical oxygen tensions if you do not reduce the oxygen tension down to zero.

**Dr. Caprioli**: We really do not have a monolayer of retinal ganglion cells. We have a monolayer of glia, and the retinal ganglion cells are scattered fairly sparsely on top of that glia...

**Dr. Siesjö**: But they are supplied from above, are they not?

**Dr. Caprioli**: They are supplied from the atmosphere.

**Dr. Siesjö**: Yes. So if the diffusion distances are really very small and the critical mitochondrial oxygen tension is a fraction of 1 mmHg, I can not see how that could reduce the viability of the cells if there are no other factors involved.

**Dr. Caprioli:** Well, there may be other factors involved. I can not really answer your question, I can just show you the results we have. And these oxygen concentrations are measured with an electrode in the media, so I think these are fairly accurate concentrations in the media itself.

**Dr. Quigley:** Why can not you make it airtight, Joe, and give it 100% nitrogen?

**Dr. Caprioli:** Well, we have done that, and even if you wait for several hours after you have done that, you really still can not get rid of all the oxygen, at least that we can measure.

**Dr. Quigley:** I also want to know what you mean by percent of control. Do you mean that at 25 hours a culture which did not get exposed to oxygen had a certain number, and this is the number that did in the oxygen, or is this the percent of the original number that were present in a similar dish.

**Dr. Caprioli:** These are parallel controls. So that this is the percent that is present compared to a control that has not been exposed to a decreased oxygen concentration.

**Dr. Quigley:** So at 25 hours you had how many percent, I am sorry I have forgotten the original control graph, the original control graph at 25 hours had 25% of the original numbers, so this is now really something like 10% of the original number.

**Dr. Caprioli:** Yes, that is right.

In the presence of MK-801, at least in these cells under these conditions, we can completely block the effect of hypoxia on the survival of these cells. We made some recordings, and it is hard to make recordings in sick cells, but we have made some recordings, and showed that in the presence of hypoxia, and again, hypoxia (9% oxygen) there is a significant reduction in the resting membrane potential of the retinal ganglion cells as measured with patch clamping.

**Dr. Quigley:** Joe, this comes back to where is the oxygen coming from. You say it is dissolved in the medium, well, why do you not drive it out with something else.

**Dr. Caprioli:** It is in equilibrium with the atmosphere, and if we perfuse our hypoxic chamber with 100% nitrogen it takes a long time to get all of the oxygen out of the media.

**Dr. Quigley:** I would take it out first. I mean, you know, if you took your medium, and the problem is, what would it do to the pH and other things in the medium.

**Dr. Caprioli:** The cells are initially in oxygen-containing media; they need to be before we expose them to an anoxic conditions. We can change the media but there are small amounts of oxygen present. This is not a problem that is unique to our laboratory; actually, this is a problem that exists in this work in general, even in the CNS.

This may be more interesting to you. We poison glycolysis with iodoacetate and we see also a dose–response relationship with respect to survival. There is a time relationship, and we have about a 40% survival after 24 hours, compared to our control cultures.

Now we see preliminary data with respect to the possible differential effects on cells of different sizes. We divided the cells into small, medium, and large: less than 12 μm average diameter, between 12 and 18, and greater than 18 μm. In cell culture, one does not of course have the dendritic elaborations that may make morphologic distinctions of the cells possible as it is in intact retina, so we made these rather arbitrary decisions about cell size. This is the percent of control with respect to each population of size that we have divided these cells into. And this is after six hours of hypoxia, and we saw a significant difference between the survival rate of the small cells and of the large ones. Now, one possible problem here might be that the large cells were not always large, but they started out small, and these cells were destined to die and they have already swollen and become large. I do not think that is happening because we have observed cells over time, the same cell over some time in culture, but we are investigating that a little bit more thoroughly right now. This is a preliminary finding,

These are similar data with respect to time under hypoxic conditions, again as percent of control. This is survival of large cells and this is the survival of the small and medium-sized cells, and there appears to be a significant difference.

That was, by way of some introduction, to give you an idea about our cell culture system and how it is behaving, even if it behaves as you might not expect. A few words about heat shock proteins. Heat shock protein was first uncovered in Italy by Ritossa in the 1960's. He observed puffs in the polytene chromosome in the salivary glands of Drossophila. These polythene chromosomes are unique in that there are thousands of copies of identical DNA lined up all together, and it was quite fashionable in those days to observe the development of the organism in terms of where the puffs of chromosomes were located, which were the areas of active replication. This is a normal chromosome, and this is a heat shock chromosome that displayed these typical puffs, indicating that there is active DNA replication. Heat shock protein is remarkably highly conserved genetically. It is present in bacteria, yeast, plants, and animals, the homology between the proteins in yeast compared to humans, for instance, is about 50% or greater. There are constitutive and inducible forms of heat shock protein. The stress proteins, as they are called more generally, have been divided into heat shock and glucose regulated proteins. The glucose regulated proteins have been observed in glucose starved cells, simply another type of stress. There are families of these proteins. Heat shock protein A is otherwise known as ubiquitin, which as its name suggests, is present in all living cells. The heat shock protein of the 72-kDa family is the major inducible one in the central nervous system. The 73-kDa protein seems to be constitutively expressed.

Hightower, at the University of Connecticut, first proposed that these heat shock proteins, or the synthesis of these proteins, are induced by protein denaturization. Subsequently, in an important piece of work, it was discovered that injection of denatured proteins into individual cells can induce the synthesis of heat shock proteins. Subsequently, hyperthermia was found to be protective against light damage in the rat retina. Heat shock proteins probably have something to do with the maturation of proteins and their folding, and have been called molecular chaperones for this reason.

Figure 5 is a small cartoon that shows the proposed function of these proteins. This is a newly synthesized protein that has not yet folded. This protein, on the basis of its thermodynamic properties may fold in the correct way, but it may not; it may wind up as a non-functional protein if it folds in the wrong way. It was previ-

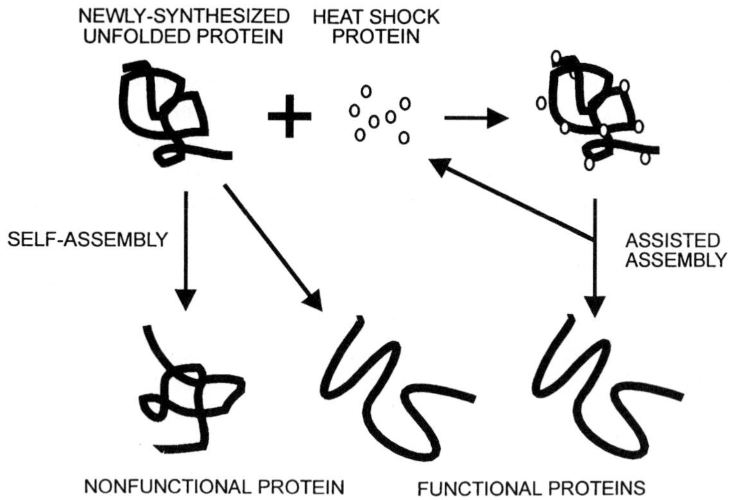


*Fig. 5.* A cartoon which depicts the proposed mechanism of heat shock proteins in the assembly of functional proteins.

ously thought that these proteins would simply fold naturally into the correct conformation, but many times they do not, and heat shock proteins appear to assist these proteins to fold in the correct way to produce functional proteins. There are other proposed functions for the heat shock proteins as well. It seems, though, that the synthesis of heat shock proteins is induced whenever there is an increased demand for protein synthesis or protein secretion. Whenever there is an accumulation of abnormally folded or denatured proteins (such as with heat), heat shock protein synthesis is turned on and the heat shock proteins assist the proteins fold back into their original and functional conformation.

Heat shock proteins have been used simply as a marker of stress and cell injury. They have also been used to mark the stress response in immunology. There are certain heat shock proteins that bind to immunoglobulins and help them form in the right conformation so that they can function properly. Stress proteins have been recognized to perhaps be useful in toxicology, as a marker of toxicity. And finally, and this has not yet been realized, perhaps stress proteins can be induced as a form of rescue therapy.

What do we find in retinal ganglion cells. This is an intact retina, actually, and this is a phase contrast photograph. Here are Di-I labeled retinal ganglion cells, and this is a control. Here is the same set of photographs from a rat who has been given a warm bath at 42°C for one hour. There is some induction, you can see here, of heat shock protein; we are staining for the 72-kDa heat shock protein.

With exposure to glutamate, again this is the Di-I labeled retinal ganglion cell, exposure to glutamate also turns on the synthesis of heat shock protein, you can see this cell, for instance.

This is the result after hypoxic injury. Again, this is hypoxia after six hours, this is the control, and this is the hypoxic culture, here is the retinal ganglion cell, and this is the retinal ganglion cell which is staining positive for HSP72.

**Dr. Quigley:** Could the glia also stain?

**Dr. Caprioli:** Yes. This is a relationship, actually, Harry, between retinal ganglion cells and the glia. The glia seem to express heat shock protein at a later time. The black boxes of Figure 6 show the time course of expression of heat shock protein by retinal ganglion cells and the open circles represent the Müller cells. We believe that all types of retinal cells in this culture dish are expressing heat shock proteins. This figure shows heat shock protein expression as a function of time under hypoxic conditions and after exposure to iodoacetate, which is a glycolysis inhibitor, and kainate. Under all three conditions we were able to see retinal ganglion cells synthesize heat shock protein. This is an immunoblot, a Western blot. The control lane is number 1, in which we do not see expression of heat shock protein, and here are various degrees of hyperthermia and exposure to excitotoxicity, and the last two are hypoxia; hypoxia, actually, and anoxia, at least as we defined it.

It is very interesting (and this is consistent with previous work in the central nervous system) that the pre-induction of the heat shock protein response seems to protect against further injury. These are two groups of cells: the first group has not been preheated before exposure to kainate (200 μM), and this is their survivorship. When you take a similar group of cells, heat them for an hour, let them recover for several hours, and then expose them to the same concentration of kainate, survival is enhanced.

The same result is found for exposure to hypoxia. Anyway in which we can induce the synthesis of heat shock protein, either by heating cells, by exposing them to a prelethal dose of hypoxia and then coming along with a lethal dose, by exposing them to lower concentrations of kainate, any of these things seem then to be protective against further, more lethal insults.

What does all that mean? It is not surprising that the retinal ganglion cells behave much as central neurons do with respect to hypoxia and excitotoxicity and with respect to their synthesis of heat shock proteins. It is interesting that the pre-induction

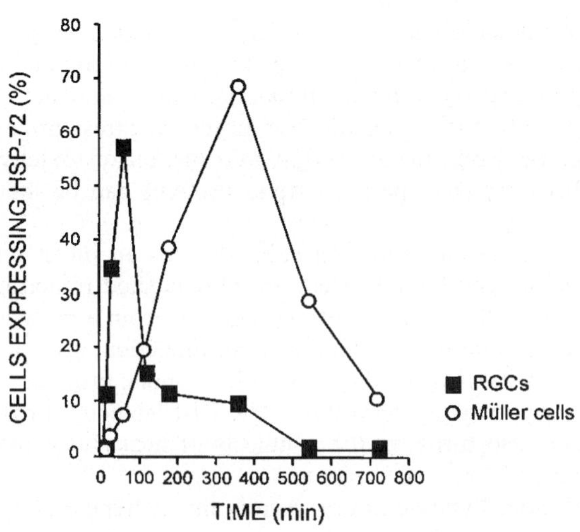


*Fig. 6.* The time course of expression of heat shock protein (72-kDa) in labeled retinal ganglion cells in culture and in Müller cells in culture.

of heat shock protein seems to be protective against further insults. Whether or not any of this has something to do with glaucoma, I think that is our challenge, that is the bridge that we need to build. I think the reason we hear is that the clinicians among us are frustrated, because patients who have progressive damage at relatively low pressures often continue to get worse and lose field despite all efforts to lower IOP. We need to explore other possible avenues for the treatment of such patients, and only by the elucidation of basic mechanisms will we be able to start to figure out what avenues we should approach.

**Dr. Choi:** Those were pretty studies. Have you tried to block the protective effect of heat pretreatment with protein synthesis inhibitors or antisense oligonucleotides or something like that?

**Dr. Caprioli:** That is a very good question. Much of the work was done in our laboratory by Dr. Shigehiko Kitano, originally from the University of Tokyo. He has since gone back to the University of Tokyo, and I came to Venice the long way around, actually stopped in Tokyo to visit him on my way here, and he tells me that he has done that, he has blocked the heat shock protein with quercetin, and this inhibits the protective effect.

**Dr. Anderson:** How do you tie this to our glaucoma problem?

**Dr. Caprioli:** Well, I have been trying to do that for the last two days. If ischemia is a problem, I like to think of ischemic damage to the nerve as a glaucomatous process only if it is occurring in very discrete areas, is a recurring insult affecting small bundles at a time, but the damage is relatively acute for those individual cells, then I think it is rather apparent how this may fit into that sort of scheme.

**Dr. Anderson:** Is the protein manufactured at the cell body or at the axon in the optic nerve, and does it have its protective effect at the axon or at the cell body?

**Dr. Caprioli:** This is exclusively cell body work, and of course the proteins are manufactured in the cell body. Whether they have any protective effect against an insult that is going on downstream on the axon, I have no idea.

**Dr. Hoffman:** When you cultured your retinal ganglion cells, how long were they in culture and what sorts of things did you throw in the culture to keep them going, did you put in any growth factors, for instance?

**Dr. Caprioli:** No growth factors were used, it was just garden variety Eagle's media; we had no growth factors in the culture.

**Dr. Hoffman:** How many hours or days did you keep them? Or did you keep them?

**Dr. Caprioli:** Typically, we kept the cells around for three to five days, and most of these experiments were done after they had been harvested and they had been on glia for three to five days. But as I mentioned, some of them can survive for four to six weeks. But if we had waited much longer than a few days, we might be getting into some selected population from which I would be afraid to draw any conclusions.

**Dr. Hoffman:** Do you think that the heat shock proteins may be a good marker to look at in glaucoma patients to see whether or not you can identify retinal ganglion cells that had been in some way injured, even though they are still alive?

**Dr. Caprioli:** Yes, I think that is a great idea. I think it would be difficult to get the eyes to do that, but that would be great if we could show that.

**Dr. Ransom:** Joe, I had a short list of questions. Were these experiments done at 37°?

**Dr. Caprioli:** Yes.

**Dr. Ransom:** Good. I think that that is important for us to know about.

**Dr. Caprioli:** The hyperthemia to induce heat shock, was at 42° for one hour.

**Dr. Ransom:** The hypoxia business that was briefly discussed, it may turn out actually that working at more than zero oxygen tension might be more relevant, because it could well be that if one does try to relate these things back to graded kinds of injury, as opposed to the all or none sort of injury that occurs in the context of stroke, that hypoxia, rather than anoxia, really might be valuable. But having said that, there is always the possibility that you may have a fairly steep gradient, so that, although the average amount of oxygen in the solution overlying your culture is above zero, what it actually is at the tissue level may be considerably less than that. A couple of people have been interested in this sort of problem. There is a man in Switzerland by the name of Sykopolis who has done very nice studies with oxygen electrodes, and he finds that in certain culture models there can be extraordinarily steep gradients, and oxygen can vary considerably. The final point is the observation about differential sensitivity between large and small cells. Dennis spoke this morning about NADPH, or actually what we now recognize as nitric oxide synthase containing neurons are relatively resistant to certain kinds of injury. I wonder if it would be useful or reasonable to consider staining your neurons for nitric oxide synthase?

**Dr. Caprioli:** We have not done that, but it is a useful idea. The other thing that we are pursuing is to look at the glutamate and NMDA receptors in subpopulations of different size retinal ganglion cells. We do not have the results yet.

**Dr. Zeimer:** This is an answer to Bruce Ransom's question. Certainly in *in vivo* sections of retina or flat mounts of retina, we have been unable to demonstrate the presence of any NADPH positive neurons. This may be different in culture.

# 16. OPTIC NERVE CIRCULATION

JOSEF FLAMMER, M.D.

Let me introduce this session more from a clinician's point of view. After having done a fellowship with Stephen Drance in '81/'82, he convinced me that some type of vascular insufficiency might be involved in the pathogenesis of glaucomatous damage, at least in some glaucoma patients. Then, in 1983, a patient with normal-tension glaucoma came to see me for a second opinion. This lady was in excellent general condition and was working as a university professor. She explained to me that all ophthalmologists she had consulted had come to the same conclusion: that she had progressive glaucomatous damage although her intraocular pressure was always within the normal range. When greeting this patient, I noticed that her hands were very, very cold. She told me that she had had cold hands since her youth. She emphasized that she had had many check-ups by internists and that everything had been found to be normal. I referred her once more to an angiologist and asked how he would explain her cold hands. He did a nailfold capillaroscopy and wrote me that this patient had a vasospastic syndrome that responded well to nitroglycerin. At that point I said to myself that this patient had two diseases, namely a vasospastic syndrome and normal-tension glaucoma, and nobody in the world could tell me whether these two entities are really independent. The first entity we can treat, at least partially. The second we do not know how to treat, at least at that time.

The patient was so highly motivated to try anything that she agreed without hesitation to take nifedipine for a period of time. Two days later, she called me to tell me that she had the subjective feeling that her vision might have improved. As of that time I was writing my thesis on fluctuations of visual fields, I asked the patient if she would allow me to repeat perimetry, and there was no doubt that the visual fields were better, repeatedly better. After this first observation, we examined a large number of patients with the help of nailfold capillaroscopy, and we found a relationship between acral blood flow and visual fields, and we postulated vasospasm to occur somewhere in the ocular circulation. We described the so-called ocular vasospastic syndrome, which is a combination of a general tendency towards vasospasm, for example in the fingers, together with visual field defects.

Such visual field defects can sometimes be provoked by cold or by emotional stress. The optic discs of these patients are mostly normal or slightly pale. The visual field defects are reversible, either spontaneously or by antivasospastic treatment, such as a calcium-channel blocker. In patients with excavated optic nerve discs, that is, in patients that we would call glaucomas, the reversibility is much less or totally absent. I would like to emphasize this because this might explain the controversy in the literature. The reversibility under treatment with a calcium-channel blocker depends on three factors. One is age: the younger the patient, the more often and the larger the reversibility. Second is the status of the optic nerve head. Obviously, if you have lost all the fibers, you can no longer expect any reversibility. The third and very important factor is the presence or absence of vasospasm. In patients in whom we found vasospasm in the finger, we rarely or never saw any reversibility of the visual fields. Thus, I think this explains the different findings of the different studies.

After this clinical digression, let me come to our question of this session. What is the role of vascular pathology in the pathogenesis of glaucoma. There is enough evi-

*Optic Nerve in Glaucoma, pp. 243–245*
*edited by S.M. Drance*

dence – and you have heard it many times during this session - both from an experimental standpoint as well as from clinical observations, that increased ocular pressure alters structural and neural elements of the optic nerve head; the clinical consequence of this is pressure-reducing therapy. This, however, does not imply an identical pathomechanism in all chronic open-angle glaucomas. Many clinical and laboratory parameters have been described to be on the average different in chronic glaucoma patients compared to normals. The main factors are hemodynamic variables. Besides a few reports on rheological factors, most investigations have dealt with vascular factors, such as decreased blood pressure, decreased ciliary perfusion pressure, decreased blood cell velocity in the fingers, decreased blood cell velocity in the ophthalmic arteries, increased prevalence of silent cardiac ischemia, and others. Hemodynamic alterations, therefore, might independently or in concert with IOP be involved in the pathogenesis of glaucomatous damage.

Before discussing the potential role of vascular insufficiencies in the pathogenesis of glaucoma, let us first summarize a few anatomical and physiological aspects of the optic nerve head blood supply. In humans, the ocular vessels are derived from the ophthalmic artery. The ophthalmic artery is the first major branch of the internal carotid entering the orbit through the optic canal. The ophthalmic artery crosses the optic nerve and branches in a variable pattern. Two separate vascular systems are involved in the nutrition of the eye: the retinal vessels and the uveal or ciliary vessels. It is important to realize that they are two totally separate systems.

The central retinal artery enters the optic nerve about 10 mm behind the eyeball and appears at the optic disc, where it branches into four major vessels, forming the vascular network of the inner layers of the retina. Two, less commonly three, posterior ciliary arteries originate from the ophthalmic artery. Each posterior ciliary artery divides into 10 to 20 branches which penetrate the sclera at the posterior pole to form the choroidal capillaries, a dense, one-layer network.

The most superficial layer of the optic nerve head is to some extent supplied by the retinal circulation. The prelaminar portion of the optic disc is primarily supplied by branches of the short posterior ciliary arteries and partially by the peripapillary choroidal arteries. Neither the peripapillary choroidal capillaries nor the central retinal artery contributes to this prelaminar portion. The lamina cribrosa portion of the optic nerve receives blood mainly from branches of the short posterior ciliary arteries and recurrent branches of the peripapillary choroidal arteries. The retrolaminar part of the optic nerve receives blood to some extent from the central retinal artery but mostly from pial vessels. The vessels of the retina have tight junctions and are not fenestrated like the vessels in the brain. The choroidal capillaries, however, are fenestrated and leak low molecular substances. The optic nerve head, although mainly supplied by the ciliary circulation, also has tight junctions and non-fenestrated capillaries. There is, however, no diffusion barrier between the choroid and the optic nerve head.

**Dr. Quigley**: Your diagram, a typical picture of the choroid and the sclera next to the optic nerve head, does not take into account the fact that in the human the choroid is actually largely blocked from direct contact with the optic nerve head substance by a flange of sclera which comes up, and it is present much more in humans than it is actually in monkeys. So while the choroid does have a diffusional possibility into the optic nerve head, the extent of that in vertical height is in the order of 50 to 100 μm, maximum, surrounding the disc.

**Dr. Flammer:** Thank you. Another peculiar aspect is the venous outflow. Although the optic nerve head is mainly supplied by the ciliary arteries, the veins are drained by the central retinal veins.

Now, what about the regulation of blood flow? Based on present knowledge, the circulation of the optic nerve head seems to be autoregulated. In this respect, the optic nerve head behaves like the retina and differently from the choroid. Autoregulation means that the blood flow in a defined range is independent of the perfusion pressure, in this context independent of intraocular pressure and blood pressure. The mechanism of this autoregulation is not yet fully understood, and the deficiency of this autoregulation in some instances is conceivable.

There is a rich nervous supply of the ciliary and uveal vessels. This may also influence perfusion under normal and pathological conditions. The endothelial cell layer plays a crucial role in local regulation of blood flow and most probably also a crucial role in autoregulation.

# 17. MICROCIRCULATION

ANDREAS ZEIHER, M.D.

Speaking about the microcirculation in general is going to be a very difficult and broad field, because, as you will see, there are some specific differences with respect to different microcirculatory fields within the body. I will try to summarize the current knowledge, how the microcirculation works, what it is actually doing, and at the end I will hopefully have set the stage for Tom Lüscher to go directly to the ophthalmic blood supply regulation, especially with respect to some endothelial functions, which have become very important and have actually revolutionized the research in blood flow, not only in the heart or in the peripheral circulation, but also in the brain.

In terms of microcirculation, the traditional concepts of physiologists have been that we can divide the circulation into two parts or two compartments. The large conductance vessels and the resistance vessels or the microvessels or microcirculation. This is not entirely correct because conductance vessels do actually contribute to resistance to blood flow, and they contribute in different amounts in different regions. If you look for example at the brain circulation, up to a diameter of 7.8 mm in vessel diameter, there is already a drop in aortic pressure by more than 20 or 25%. The carotid artery, for example, contributes about 20 to 25% to the vascular resistance of the central circulation.

There is quite a similarity between the cerebral circulation and the coronary circulation, such that these curves are actually almost parallel, although the heart circulation has shifted a little bit to the right, indicating that conductance vessels in the heart contribute a little bit less to overall drop in resistance. In sharp contrast, in the skeletal muscle circulation and the mesenteric artery circulation, most of the vascular resistance is regulated by a very narrow size class of vessels. Now, let us look, to begin with, at the heart. As I said, there are some similarities to the brain, though the heart has been extensively studied.

We have a number of different components affecting vascular resistance. One is metabolic control. The other, Dr. Flammer already mentioned, is autoregulation. There are some extravascular compressive forces, of course, which will act upon the vessels directly. There are a number of humoral factors, which I will discuss in detail later, and there is, even in the heart, a neural control that importantly participates in the regulation of the microcirculatory tone, and therefore in the regulation of vascular resistance and blood flow. All this has to be finely tuned to give the right supply according to the demand.

Which size classes of vessels actually participate in the different mechanisms of blood flow regulation: if you reduce perfusion pressure to 16 mmHg, then autoregulation takes place. Autoregulatory vasodilation actually takes place only in the very small vessels, smaller than 100 µm in diameter, and the dilatory response of these vessels actually is in parallel with the smaller size. The larger size vessels do not at all respond, or even constrict, in response to a reduction in perfusion pressure. In contrast, the metabolic regulation of blood flow in the coronary circulation, and I assume it is the same in the cerebral circulation, occurs when all size classes of vessels, from 0–400 µm, dilate in response to increased demand. Thus there is a clear-cut difference in the size class contributing to autoregulation and to metabolic regulation of blood flow.

*Optic Nerve in Glaucoma, pp. 247–258*
*edited by S.M. Drance*

If you go further and look at what happens to some neural stimulation, induced via sympathetic stimulation or by intracoronary norepinephrine infusion, there is a very heterogeneous response. The larger microvessels, up to 400 μm constrict, whereas the very small vessels dilate and therefore increase blood flow in response to sympathetic stimulation and in response to norepinephrine infusion.

**Dr. Quigley:** Dr. Zeiher, what are the smallest blood vessels on this graph? It looks to me as if they are about 50 μm in diameter...

**Dr. Zeiher:** Fifty μm.

**Dr. Quigley:** We will find that interesting, since when we get to talking about the optic nerve, the smallest vessels in your graph are about three times the size of the largest vessels that are in the optic nerve. I presume they might behave the same, though.

**Dr. Zeiher:** Yes. It is obviously a problem of measuring, because these measurements are performed by stroboscopic illumination, and the heart is beating too, so you will have some motion blur in the image, so you cannot actually go to smaller size vessels of the heart for measuring.

And we now come to some humoral substances which are very common, in the coronary circulation, probably less in the cerebral circulation. We focus first on serotonin. Again, there is a very heterogeneous response. We have dilation in the very small vessels, but vasoconstriction in the larger vessels. This altogether will result in no change in blood flow at all because this vasoconstriction will actually offset the vasodilation in the small vessels.

**Dr. Zeimer**: Excuse me. Do these vessels have sphincters?

**Dr. Zeiher:** Whether they have sphincters or not, they have a smooth muscle layer, which actually does the vasoconstriction. They have an endothelial cell layer and beneath that a smooth muscle cell layer, and this is actually the active vasoconstricting part of the vessels. And the difference between large vessels and small vessels is that the ratio between the endothelial cell layer and the smooth muscle cell layer is much more optimized in the very small vessels than in the large vessels. I will discuss this later on.

In contrast, if you look at vasopressin, it has a less heterogeneous response. In general most of the vessels actually do vasoconstrict, especially the smaller vessels.

In recent years it has become very apparent, and Dr. Flammer already pointed it out, we do have an endothelium in the vessels, and this endothelium very importantly modifies the response to all of the stimuli I just showed you. The overall blood flow response in a given regional vascular bed depends not only on what happens by the direct effect of these substances on the smooth muscle layer of these individual vessels, but also on how the endothelial cell layer functions and coordinates and integrates all the responses throughout the entire circulation.

The endothelial cells are oriented in the direction of blood flow. It is a monolayer tapestry of the vessel. There are a number of substances which we encounter, and which every blood vessel encounters every minute, which importantly modulates its tone.

First of all, acetylcholine has been very useful to us as a pharmacological tool to study endothelial function. We all agree that acetylcholine does not appear in the circulating blood because it is rapidly inactivated by the cholinesterases, but as a pharmacological tool it is very helpful to assess the functional integrity of this cell layer. Platelet products are, however, very common in the blood stream. First of all, ADP and ATP and 5-HT or serotonin are very common humoral substances circulating with the blood. Platelet activating factor, thrombin, and histamine also exert a dilatory response through the endothelium if the endothelium is functionally intact. If we have no endothelial cell layer, all these substances will induce direct vasoconstriction, because, for example, serotonin has direct receptors on the vascular smooth muscle cell causing vasoconstriction. In contrast, if it comes in contact first with the endothelium, there are two serotonin receptors which will release a so-called endothelium derived relaxing factor, which then dilates the vascular smooth muscle cells instead of constricting it.

The same is true for neuropeptides. For example, substance P dilates through the endothelium. Bradykinin has receptors on the endothelium which will release endothelium derived relaxing factor. The calcitonin gene-related peptide also does this.

I showed you previously the effect of norepinephrine. Norepinephrine acts via the two receptors on the endothelial cells to release endothelium derived relaxing factor and thereby counteracts the obvious direct constricting effect on the smooth muscle cells, which is exerted by norepinephrine.

And then probably the most important stimuli for the basal release of these endothelium derived relaxing factors are these physicochemical stimuli like shear stress, pulsatility, and the partial oxygen pressure. I would like to focus on the shear stress mediated release of EDRF.

**Dr. Anderson**: May I interrupt to ask you a question before you go on. What you have just explained makes it very important to know for each vascular bed, in every experimental condition, whether or not the stimulus was presented to the luminal side of the vessel or to the abluminal side of the vessel. In understanding the response of the coronary arteries, for instance, when you said there was a certain stimulus, and one portion of the vascular bed dilated while the other constricted it may reflect an intrinsic difference in their reaction, but a difference in how that size vessel had the agonist presented. With something like sympathetic stimulation, you would have to know where the nerve fibers end. Do they go to these very small vessels, or are the small vessels only exposed to the simultaneous release of *circulating* catecholamines that would occur during sympathetic stimulation. One must also know whether or not there are fenestrated vessels or tightly closed vessels (as in the central nervous system) to interpret these responses. This means all vascular beds are very different from each other, and you need to know the exact microanatomy to known bio-exposure to agonists in addition to knowing receptor locations.

**Dr. Zeiher**: That is a very important point, as I showed in the beginning, I had sympathetic stimulation and then at the same time, the norepinephrine infusion which goes directly from the luminal side of the vessel to the endothelium. You are absolutely correct, there are regional differences in the responses to various stimuli, and probably differences in the various mechanisms.

When the so-called endothelium derived relaxing factor (EDRF) was detected, they had an artery that was perfused, and then the perfusate was dripped onto an arterial strip from which the endothelium had been removed. This so-called EDRF has now been identified as nitric oxide and is nothing else than the endogenous nitrovasodilator. If you give nitroglycerin, as a source of nitric oxide, you get the relaxing response. If you just perfuse the artery and let the pure perfusate drip on these arterial strips you get some relaxation. If you use acetylcholine to induce a stimulated release of EDRF, you get a relaxation which is comparable to what you get with nitroglycerin. And then if you use authentic nitric oxide, you get the same response. This is all inhibited by some scavengers. So this was actually to show that this EDRF is actually nitric oxide and is endogenous nitroglycerin.

In the meantime, the whole process has been very nicely elucidated. To form nitric oxide, there are receptors, probably mediated through G inhibitor proteins. Then there is calcium increase, and this calcium increase, together with carmodulin, activates the nitric oxide synthase, the enzyme, and this enzyme does nothing else than convert the amino acid L-arginine to L-citroline, and as a product we will have nitric oxide. This nitric oxide then diffuses into the vascular smooth muscle cell layer, there activates guanyl cyclase, and induces relaxation of the vascular smooth muscle cell. There is some calcium influx which is necessary for the guanyl synthase to be activated.

One of the most important and basally active mechanisms of release of EDRF or nitric oxide is the flow and the shear stress exerted by the flow on the endothelial cell layer. Thus we can actually view endothelial cells as so-called mechano-transfusers, transfusing flow into nitric oxide formation, and through this nitric oxide formation, into a vasodilatory response of the vessel wall.

**Dr. Zeimer**: Could you tell us, so while we hear the presentation we can think about what kind of vessel has the same mechanism, which of the vessels in the optic nerve head have vascular smooth muscles. What size of vessels and what size of capillaries.

**Dr. Alm:** Well, I asked Harry that question before, and one of the reasons why this is attractive for me is that we never could explain why you have autoregulation in the optic nerve head. And the reason was that, as far as I understand, you do not have a continuous layer of smooth muscles in the optic nerve head, which means that, at that time there was no real way to explain how it could transmit a signal to the more proximal part of the vascular bed. But with the endothelial cells they may act independently of contact with other smooth muscles. Is that reasonable?

**Dr. Zeiher**: Yes, it definitely is, because flow is translated into a signal by the endothelial cells and into a substance, namely nitric oxide. There has been a long debate, there are some circulations in which there is ascending dilatation about the mechanism but, as it is called, so that the pulse jumps from one endothelial cell to another in an ascending way. But the easiest way to transduce flow changes into caliber changes is just by using the endothelial cells as a mechanotransducer, as it happens.

**Dr. Flammer**: Is that also true for the venous part?

**Dr. Zeiher**: Yes, for the venous part too. Although the amount of nitric oxide released in veins is a lot less compared to arteries.

**Dr. Flammer**: The reason I am asking is that in the so-called venous thrombosis we have very much dilated veins and we have little flow, so, this would not explain that, but anyway, it is interesting.

**Dr. Zeiher**: But shear stress levels are a lot lower, of course, in the veins.

**Dr. Alm**: You showed many substances that will release nitric oxide, but some of them, as I understand it, have a very brief effect because there is a rapid tachyphylaxis. What I was thinking about was, you have no epinephrine. Is epinephrine also releasing nitric oxide, and is that sustained effect?

**Dr. Zeiher**: Norepinephrine activates endothelial alpha-2 receptors, which do release nitric oxide. It is a transient effect.

**Dr. Alm**: And epinephrine, would that also?

**Dr. Zeiher**: It is the same with epinephrine and norepinephrine, yes.

**Dr. Alm**: So in everyday life you probably would not have much effect from a constant level of circulating epinephrine, because of tachyphylaxic or transient nature of the effect.

**Dr. Zeiher**: Yes. What this schematic shows too is that the amount of nitric oxide is directly proportional to the blood flow and inversely proportional to the diameter of the vessel. This is a very important aspect, and again, comes to some kind of vasoconstrictor stimuli, how actually the endothelium interacts with all vasoconstrictor stimuli even if they do not act via the endothelium. If you keep blood flow rate constant, and you have a relaxed vessel, you will have this amount of cyclic GMP production, indicative of or equivalent to the amount of nitric oxide production. If you then go ahead and constrict a vessel with any agent you use, and you keep the volume of blood flow constant, the nitric oxide production will massively increase because of the reduction in diameter. The vessel will come back to a more relaxed state, and therefore counteracts any constrictor effect of any substance acting on the smooth muscle cell layer. Thus the endothelium is very important as a feedback mechanism.

If we talk about endothelial nitric oxide formation for a moment, I should remind you that there are a number of different nitric oxide synthases. One was mentioned just before, that is the brain nitric oxide synthase, which has nothing to do with the endothelium, and there is nitric oxide formation in macrophages. With respect to the endothelial nitric oxide formation, we have a basal constitutive nitric oxide production. We can stimulate this nitric oxide formation, as I mentioned, by receptor dependent stimulation, but also by receptor independent stimulation. Nitric oxide synthesia is calcium dependent, so if you increase calcium concentration in the endothelial cells by calcium ionophore, we get an increase in nitric oxide formation. And also receptor independent, we can do it by physical stimuli.

Now, let me come to this point. Does a constitutive basal release of nitric oxide mean anything for the circulation. This is just a study we did a couple of months ago. If you look at the messenger RNA level of the nitric oxide synthesis in aortic cells, you can also use microvascular cells, and you look at the message of native and freshly harvested cells, and then you culture the cells for 48 hours, you can see a dramatic decrease in the message for nitric oxide synthesis, indicating that as long as the endothelial cells are exposed to blood flow, there is a high production of nitric oxide. Once you take them out of the blood vessel and you culture them, your message decreases dramatically. As it should be, because blood flow is an important stimulus for the release of nitric oxide.

So what does it mean for the regional blood flow in different circulatory beds. In an experiment done by Gardner and co-workers, they plot the nitric oxide formation just by infusing an analog of L-arginine. This analog LMMA is a stereospecific inhibitor of the nitric oxide synthesis and prevents formation of basal nitric oxide. After infusion of the inhibitor, aortic pressure dramatically increases by almost 40% in these rats, and at the same time regional blood flow in various circulatory beds in the hindquarter, in the renal bed, and in the mesenteric vascular bed, dramatically decreases. Thus, indeed there is a tremendous amount of basal nitric oxide release which obviously keeps the vasculature in a dilated state. The same is true for the human forearm circulation, the microcirculation of the forearm (as shown by Vallens *et al.*) They infused these inhibitors of nitric oxide formation into the forearm circulation, and what you can find is a reduction in blood flow by more than 60%. Once you stop the infusion, it comes back again. Thus, indeed in the human circulation the basal production of nitric oxide is very important for keeping regional blood flow.

The same happens in the cerebral circulation. The basilar artery will contribute to the reduction in pressure by at least 20 or 25%, and if you use the same analog to block basal nitric oxide formation, you get a decrease in basilar artery diameter of about 30%.

**Dr. Flammer**: There was a paper last week in the German Society meeting, they blocked nitric oxide formation in dogs and compared the reduction of blood flow in the different organs, and the organ in which the drop was most pronounced was the eye, especially in the choroid. They measured with labeled particles, microsphere technique.

**Dr. Quigley**: Is that a good measure for the choroid?

**Dr. Alm**: I cannot judge that.

**Dr. Zeiher**: So the very obvious conclusion from these experiments is that basal formation of nitric oxide keeps the vasculature in a dilated state. What we call hypertension is not hypertension, but is actually hypovasodilation, which means a chronic state of reduced nitric oxide production. And indeed, the first human studies looking at this phenomenon using acetylcholine and assessing the stimulated release of nitric oxide revealed that if you do this in normotensive and hypertensive patients, the hypertensive patients respond a lot less to acetylcholine infusion, indicative of a reduced capacity of the endothelial cells in the forearm to release nitric oxide. Tom Lüscher's group has obtained the same data, and this I think is very established. There have now been studies using LLNMA, in which you actually can see that this analog has less effects in hypertensive patients, indicating that there is a clear-cut defect in the nitric oxide synthesis in at least the peripheral circulation of these patients.

Does this also happen in the brain or in the cerebral circulation? These are paired arterioles of normal and spontaneously hypertensive stroke-prone rats. And what you can see is that in response to bradykinin, which is an endothelium dependent dilator, the response in the hypertensive rat is dramatically reduced compared to the Wistar-Kyoto rats despite the fact that if you give authentic nitric oxide there is the same response, indicating that the effector cells, the smooth muscle cells, are acting correctly onto nitric oxide. Thus there is indeed a reduced production of nitric oxide by bradykinin. This experiment using the calcium ionophore, A23187, shows that it is not only confined to a disturbance in receptor-mediated nitric oxide production, but to receptor independent mechanisms because this substance, again in the spontaneously hypertensive rat, produced less vasodilation compared to Wistar-Kyoto rats.

Now comes the drawback. These authors, Mayhan and co-workers, looked, what kind of mechanisms might be responsible for the phenonemon. They used indomethacin to block some cyclooxygenase product, and were able to reverse this abnormal vasoconstrictor response in the spontaneously hypertensive rat, to produce a dilator response. Although the result was not exactly similar to the control rats, at least in part cyclooxygenase product might be responsible for this effect in the paired arterioles, so it is not all nitric oxide.

In humans, in the forearm, indomethacin and aspirin had no effect, indicating that there are not only differences in various vascular beds, but there are also differences between different species. I think Tom Lüscher will go into detail with this afterwards, because he did a lot of studies using cyclooxygenase products.

If you look at different patient groups, one with normal coronary arteries and no risk factors for coronary artery disease, another with coronary artery disease but normotensive blood pressure values and no hypercholesterolemia, at hypertensive patients, and patients who have elevated cholesterol, and we look at the acetylcholine blood flow response in these patients, we see that especially patients with elevated cholesterol levels have a significantly impaired vasodilatory response to acetylcholine. Obviously they have a defective EDRF production in response to acetylcholine, whereas hypertensive patients are not different from patients with coronary artery disease but normal blood pressures. Thus, we conclude from these experiments that, in the coronary circulation, hypertension *per se* is not associated with a reduced production of nitric oxide. This is in sharp contrast to the peripheral circulation, but there are, as you know, obvious differences between these two circulations.

**Dr. Alm**: Is it not true that you have muscarinic receptors also in the smooth muscles in the coronary ..... So what you can see in the last group that maybe a combination of vasodilation and vasoconstriction .....

**Dr. Zeiher**: Anytime you use acetylcholine, the measured blood flow is a combined effect of vasoconstriction and vasodilation, vasoconstriction due to the muscarinic receptors on the smooth muscle cells, and vasodilation due to receptors on the endothelial cells. So you actually get the balance between vasodilation and vasoconstriction. This makes acetylecholine a nice pharmacological tool to assess the functional intactness of the endothelial cell, but it does not tell you, obviously, how much your defect in nitric oxide production is, and so on, because you have this additional vasoconstrictor effects.

In terms of the microcirculation, you will always get increases in blood flow with acetylcholine, unless you have a significant vasoconstriction of the large conductance vessels. The large conductance vessels will finally determine when your blood flow decreases, but not the microcirculation. This is simply because the relationship between the endothelial cell layer and the smooth muscle layer is a lot better for this dilating effect in the microcirculation compared to the large conductance vessels, where you have only a monolayer of endothelial cells, but a number of layers of smooth muscle cells.

These altered responses are not related to any kind of structural alterations in these vessels of hypercholesterolemic patients, because if you give them endothelium independent vasodilators, for example papaverine, which we use as a very potent vasodilator, you see that normals and hypercholesterolemic patients do not differ in their relaxatory response, but still they differ in their response to acetylcholine.

**Dr. Flammer**: Does it depend how long you have hypercholesterolemia? Because this may end up as some type of atherosclerosis, changing the endothelial cell layer, or is it just the acute level of cholesterol?

**Dr. Zeiher**: It would obviously be a very good study to do if we would know when the patient first had elevated cholesterol levels. But we do not know in patients. In animals you can actually induce hypercholesterolemia and you will get impaired vasodilator response after one week. The beauty of using the microcirculation and using coronary vascular resistance changes is that you will never get atherosclerotic lesions in the microcirculation. The microcirculation differs from the large conductance vessels such that atherosclerotic lesions develop in the large conductance vessels but never in the microcirculation. So these effects cannot be attributed to atherosclerosis.

**Dr. Zeimer**: Could you define what you call microcirculation. Because in the eye we may call microcirculation something else.

**Dr. Zeiher**: Yes. As you see here, these are studies in patients. So what do we actually measure is blood flow which is determined by the microcirculation, and we have no way to define which size class of vessels was actually giving this response. All we can do is exclude vasoconstriction of the large conductance vessels which we can see by angiography. So these are vessels, let us say, between 1 mm and 10 μm. But this is the sum of the overall result of the acetylcholine infusion. In clinical studies it is not possible to exactly define which vessel did dilate.

**Dr. Zeimer**: The only comment I want to make is that what you call in the heart microcirculation are central retinal arteries in the eye, so I would like to qualify what you meant. A 1 mm vessel is something we never see in the eye, and so we typically, and I think people would agree, that the microcirculation size is well below 100 μm, and one of the big differences between what you talk about and what we see in the eye in a lot of areas is that we do not have smooth muscles in very small vessels.

**Dr. Zeiher**: I am not sure, I actually do not know up to what size class in the eye there are no smooth muscle layers at all, but as I know from the heart, there is a smooth muscle layer to the very very small size class of 10–20 μm vessels. So I do believe that it might be the same in the eye.

**Dr. Zeimer**: Doug, you correct me if I am wrong, I understand in the retina, I do not know in the optic nerve head, there are no visible smooth muscle sphincters throughout the whole retina.

**Dr. Lüscher:** May I just make a comment as well. I mean, basically, if you talk about vasomotion there must be smooth muscle cells or something else, just to lead me to confusion here. If you do not have smooth muscle cells, you cannot measure changes in blood flow. These vessels will not determine your blood flow, will they?

**Dr. Zeimer**: I disagree.

**Dr. Lüscher**: Then you consider pericytes or some other structure...

**Dr. Zeimer**: Exactly.

**Dr. Lüscher**: Yes, but then this is a matter of semantics. I think what he measures here is flow, and flow is determined by very small vessels, and of course, the contribution to changes in flow becomes bigger as blood vessels become smaller. But there is a limit, if you have capillaries with no smooth muscle cells or any contractile structure, there is no contribution to changes in flow. There can be contributions to the basal level, but the changes he measured, they have to relate to some contractile or dilating structure, which is smooth muscle cells or pericytes.

**Dr. Zeimer**: The point I want to make...Well, two points. One is that, in areas without smooth muscle, like in the eye, you may not see these effects and you may not see the response to nitric oxide that you see here.

**Dr. Lüscher**: Well, we can talk about that later...

**Dr. Anderson**: But to clarify the anatomic situation, which is what Ran Zeimer is asking, the arteries, as they become smaller, have three, and then two, and then one layer of smooth muscle, and they finally get to the point where they merge into the capillary layer. But throughout there is an endothelial layer and externally there is another layer. It transforms from being a single layer of smooth muscles into a layer of pericytes as the transition is made from arteriole to capillary. It is more or less a continuous coat in the particular vascular bed that we are interested in. Precapillary sphincters, which exist in other vascular beds, would be at the branching point, where a capillary branches from the smallest arteriole. The sphincter is a collection of circularly arranged contractile cells that may close off this capillary loop for a time and then open again, so that there is intermittent perfusion of different capillaries in rotation. So, if you look at the mesentery, one capillary will be perfused for a moment and then another and then another and then another. Such sphincters do not seem to occur in the retina, so that there is continuous perfusion of all vascular beds.

**Dr. Zeiher**: Not in the retina, but Michael van Buskirk showed that constrictions exist in between the choroid and optic nerve head after stimulating with alpha-adrenergic drugs.

**Dr. Anderson**: I do not think that the anatomical structure of a sphincter has actually been observed, that is to say, a collection of muscular cells. The physiologic constriction at that branch point might have other explanations due to elastic structures and so on, besides smooth muscle cells. It is a difficult thing to sort out in the optic nerve head.

**Dr. Zeiher**: But besides this probably important heterogeneity in different capillaries being perfused, I would like to reiterate that what we actually do measure is blood flow, the integral sum of all the effects of acetylcholine and all the integrated effects of released nitric oxide.

Let me just go over what we do have now for evidence in humans. We do not know the exact site and the class of vessels that are impaired in their regulation. With respect to impaired endothelium-mediated regional blood flow, we are very sure that it happens. It is a very specific feature of hypertension, if not even the cause. It happens in hypercholesterolemia and is associated with atherosclerosis but whether it is secondary or primary remains to be defined. It clearly has been shown in diabetes mellitus in the corpus cavernosum and also in the cerebral circulation. We have severely impaired endothelium-mediated blood flow regulation in chronic obstructive pulmonary disease, which actually correlates very closely with the extent of chronic obstructive pulmonary disease. With respect to the coronary circulation, there is one disease which is called idiopathic dilated cardiomyopathy which has been shown to be associated with hypercholesterolemia, atherosclerosis. Advanced age, and this is I think a very important aspect, is associated with an impaired endothelium-dependent vasodilatory capacity of the coronary microcirculation.

With respect to the brain and the cerebral circulation, I mentioned that diabetes has been shown in the corpus cavernosum to be associated with a reduced dilatory response. As shown before for the spontaneous hypertensive rats, this diabetic impairment, or the impairment in endothelium-dependent relaxation in diabetic rats, appears to be related to some kind of a cyclooxygenase product, because giving indomethacin almost normalizes the dilator response to acetylcholine. This has not been the case for the corpus cavernosum, and this is also not the case for reduced blood flow response in the forearm in diabetic patients. Thus again there is heterogeneity in different vascular beds and probably species.

What does it mean if you do have, and I think this is an important point we have to make, what does it mean if we do have impaired endothelium-dependent dilatory capacity of any kind of vascular bed? If you just look at postischemic forearm blood flow in normal patients and in hypercholesterolemic patients, they have a significantly impaired and reduced post-ischemic forearm blood flow increase, which can be almost normalized after treatment for two years. In addition, if we just look at what happens to the shear stress in a vessel which is not able to dilate, in contrast to those who are able to dilate, the shear stress, with an increase in flow, is dramatically increased in these vessels. And if you take shear stress as not only a mechanism to release nitric oxide but also as a mechanism by which platelets are activated and blood-borne particles are in contact with the vessel wall and might be damaged, this might be an important aspect. As we have seen, even if your flow changes by 90%, your shear stress does not change at all because of the dilatory response of the vessel.

Finally, and I think this is the most important aspect of it, we studied what happens to coronary vascular resistance during sympathetic activation. We used cold-pressor testing, a mechanism that induces an increase in blood pressure, increases the heart rate, is associated with increased circulating norepinephrine and epinephrine levels, and it is associated with an increased myocardial oxygen consumption.

In normal patients, the coronary vascular resistance decreases during this intervention. In coronary artery disease patients with normal endothelial function, the same happens. In the group with impaired endothelial function there is actually an increase in coronary vascular resistance despite the fact that myocardial oxygen consumption increases. You can interpret this as endothelial dysfunction. That induces ischemia in these patients because the metabolic demands are not met due to the failure of the endothelium to produce dilation.

There is, in addition, increasing evidence that endothelial dysfunction might account for ischemia in patients with normal coronary arteries. At least in the coronary circulation, a defective endothelium-dependent dilatory response of the microcirculation importantly not only fails to modulate the blood flow, but might very well contribute to the development of ischemia in the first place.

And let me come to the last part of my talk. Do we have any chance to affect this system by some kind of treatment that affects this arginine-nitric oxide pathway. As I mentioned in the beginning, we have the nitric oxide synthesis, which activity might simply be decreased, in hypertension. We can have an increase in deactivation of nitric oxide, we can have an impaired signal transduction mechanism, and, since nitric oxide is formed from L-arginine, we can have a reduced intracellular availability of L-arginine which may interfere, then, with the production of nitric oxide. And at least in hypercholesterolemia, this reduced intracellular availability of L-arginine appears to be at least one mechanism for the reduced nitric oxide production and for the reduced vasodilatory response. Because if you give hypercholesterolemic patients acute L-arginine and supplement their L-arginine levels, their vasodilatory response to increasing dosages of acetylcholine again is normalized, whereas before it was severely reduced, compared to normal cholesterolemic patients.

The same is not only true for the coronaries, but you can get the same effect in the peripheral circulation in hypercholesterolemic patients, so that we indeed do have a way of interfering with this system. L-arginine has no effect in hypertensive patients, neither in normal cholesterolemic nor in hypocholesterolemic patients, indicating that the defects are different between hypercholesterolemia and hypertension. Also, and this is also important, what we call the age-related decrease in acetylcholine-induced blood flow responses, which means that with increasing age the ability to dilate the blood vessels via releasing nitric oxide is reduced, is also not affected by the infusion and supplementation of L-arginine.

If we now summarize these thoughts with respect to the effects on cerebral blood flow, we have what we term autoregulation: an increase in aortic pressure will induce an increase in arteriolar pressure, and this will result in a constant blood flow over the so-called autoregulatory range. When the blood pressure is very much increased, this autoregulation does not function anymore. The same is true with neuronal activity or some kind of metabolic demand. We have a decrease in arterial pressure, which calls for a dilatory response of the resistance vessels, and this will increase blood flow. Sympathetic nerve activity will decrease arteriolar pressure and therefore keep cerebral blood flow constant. The hormonal effect depends on which hormone, but also whether the endothelium is functional or not. If you have an impaired endothelial dilatory function, your homeostasis is severely disturbed with respect to autoregulatory modulation of blood flow, definitely in sympathetic nerve activity regulation, and definitely also in the hormone effect. And finally, since the microcirculation is the final part of the circulation, connected to large arteries, we should not dismiss that atherosclerotic lesions in large conductance vessels, while far away from the microcirculation, may none-the-less affect the microcirculation just by release of vasoactive factors in these atherosclerotically altered vessels. Substances, like, for example, serotonin or thromboxane, then diffuse into the distal part and reach the microcirculation, and there, depending on the functional integrity of the endothelium, will have either a dilatory or a constrictor effect. Tom Lüscher will answer some more questions because he has done some studies specifically with the ophthalmic circulation.

# 18. ENDOTHELIAL MEDIATORS AS REGULATORS OF THE OPHTHALMIC CIRCULATION*

THOMAS F. LÜSCHER M.D., PETER MEYER M.D., IVAN O. HAEFLIGER M.D., JOSEF FLAMMER M.D.

## Abstract

The eye is one of the best perfused organs of the body. Blood flow to the eye is regulated by neuronal factors as well as circulatory and local mediators. The endothelium modulates vascular tone by the release of relaxing factors such as nitric oxide, prostacyclin and a putative hyperpolarizing factor. In isolated ophthalmic arteries and perfused eyes, all endothelial factors participate in the regulation of local vascular tone. While in larger ophthalmic vessels this is due to their effects on vascular smooth muscle cells, in capillaries, pericytes can be influenced as well. In addition, contracting factors are formed, *i.e.* the peptide endothelin-1 and cyclooxygenase products such as thromboxane $A_2$ and prostaglandin $H_2$.

In the peripheral circulation endothelial dysfunction occurs in several cardiovascular diseases. An imbalance of endothelium-derived relaxing and contracting factors could be important for the development of vascular ophthalmic complications, for instance in hypertension, diabetes, arteriosclerosis and retinal ischemia. Endothelial dysfunction may also contribute to vasospastic events in retinal migraine and low-tension glaucoma associated with Raynaud phenomenon and migraine. Drugs modulating the effects of these local mediators may be promising therapeutic tools in these disorders of the ophthalmic circulation.

## 1. Introduction

The eye is a highly perfused organ[1]. In humans and in many experimental animals, the eye has two separate types of blood vessels, which differ anatomically and physiologically: the retinal vessels, which supply part of the retina, and the uveal or ciliary blood vessels, which supply the rest of the eye. Alterations in ophthalmic blood flow are involved in many diseases of the eye. Hence, the characterization of the mechanisms involved in the regulation of ophthalmic blood flow are of great clinical relevance. There is autonomic innervation of the extraocular vessels as well as of choroidal vessels, while vessels of the retina and optic nerve head are not innervated. Hence, local factors may be particularly important in these vessels[1].

Local blood flow is determined by three major factors: (1) perfusion pressure of the arterial circulation; (2) tone of resistance arteries; and (3) physical properties of the blood (*i.e.* viscosity). This chapter will exclusively focus on the influence of endothelial mediators on the contractile state of smooth muscle cells and pericytes. It is obvious that other factors such as neurotransmitters, circulating hormones as well as myogenic and metabolic factors also contribute (see ref. 2).

## 2. The endothelium as a regulator of local vascular tone

Endothelial cells are a source of numerous substances; some of them do regulate vascular tone, in particular nitric oxide, cyclooxygenase products and endothelin-1.

*L-arginine/nitric oxide pathway:* Nitric oxide, a powerful vasodilator and inhibitor

* Supported by grants of the Swiss National Science Research Foundation (No. 32-36571.92) and a grant-in-aid by the Karl Mayer Foundation, Triesen, Fürstentum Liechtenstein

*Optic Nerve in Glaucoma, pp. 259–281*
*edited by S.M. Drance*

of platelet function[3-5], is formed from L-arginine by the constitutive form of nitric oxide synthase[6,7] (Fig. 1). Nitric oxide synthase is also found in nerves and platelets and an inducible form (by endotoxin, tumor necrosis factor and interleukin-1) in macrophages, neutrophils and smooth muscle cells[8].

In endothelial cells, nitric oxide is released in response to products released from platelets[9,10], hormones and autacoids[see 2] (Table 1; see ref. 2). Shear stress (*i.e.* the viscous drag exerted by the circulating blood) activates potassium current across the endothelial cell membrane[11-14]; this in turn causes hyperpolarization which triggers the release of nitric oxide and prostacyclin and mediates flow-dependent vasodilation. Nitric oxide has a short biological half-life and is inactivated by hemoglobin[4] and oxygen-derived free radicals[15].

In vascular smooth muscle and platelets, nitric oxide activates soluble guanylyl cyclase which leads to the formation of cyclic 3',5'-guanosine monophosphate (cGMP) and in turn to relaxation and anti-aggregation respectively via a decrease in intracellular $Ca^{2+}$ and dephosphorylation of myosine light chains[16-18] (Fig. 1). Nitric oxide production can be inhibited by analogs of L-arginine (*i.e.* L-$N^G$-monomethylarginine; L-NMMA; nitro-L-arginine methyl esther: L-NAME)[19,20]. Circulating methyl- and dimethylarginines in plasma act as endogenous inhibitors of nitric oxide[21]

*Other endothelial vasodilators:* Endothelial cells (and to a lesser degree also smooth muscle) form prostacyclin from arachidonic acid after activation of phospholipase $A_2$ and cyclooxygenase[22]. Prostacyclin acts as a vasodilator and inhibitor of platelet function, but through stimulation of cyclic AMP rather than cyclic GMP. Nitric oxide and prostacyclin potentiate each other's effects as vasodilators and platelet inhibitors.

In addition, an endothelium-derived hyperpolarizing factor (EDHF)[23] has been proposed based on the fact that endothelial cells are able to increase the membrane potential of vascular smooth muscle via activation of ATP-dependent potassium channels[24]. Its chemical nature remains elusive. EDHF contributes to endothelium-dependent relaxation particularly with certain agonists such as bradykinin[25].

*Endothelin:* Endothelial cells produce the 21 amino acid peptide endothelin[26] (Fig. 2; for review see 27) of which three isoforms exist: endothelin-1, endothelin-2 and endothelin-3. Endothelin-1 is the only isoform produced by the endothelium; it is generated from precursor molecules stimulation by several factors (Table 1) Endothelin production is inhibited by nitric oxide, prostacyclin and a putative inhibitory factor produced by vascular smooth muscle cells[28,29].

In vascular smooth muscle, endothelin binds to $ET_A$-, but also $ET_B$ receptors, linked to phospholipase C[30-32]; the formation of inositol triphosphate and diacylglycerol increases intracellular $Ca^{2+}$ and evokes long-lasting contractions (Fig. 2; see ref. 27). In certain vessels, endothelin activates voltage-operated $Ca^{2+}$ channels via its receptor and a $G_i$ protein[33]. At concentrations at which endothelin-1 exerts no direct contractile effect, it potentiates contractions to norepinephrine and serotonin[34]. In vivo, endothelin causes a transient vasodilation which precedes its pressor effect[26]. The dilatator response to endothelin involves activation of endothelial $ET_B$ receptors linked to nitric oxide and prostacyclin release[35-36].

Under normal conditions the circulating endothelin levels are very low[37] suggesting that it primarily acts as a local regulatory factor; indeed, two thirds of the endothelin formed by endothelial cells is released abluminally towards vascular smooth muscle[38].

*Cyclooxygenase-derived contracting factors:* The endothelial cyclooxygenase pathway produces several contracting factors like thromboxane $A_2$, prostaglandin $H_2$ or superoxide anions particularly in the cerebral circulation and in veins (see ref. 27).

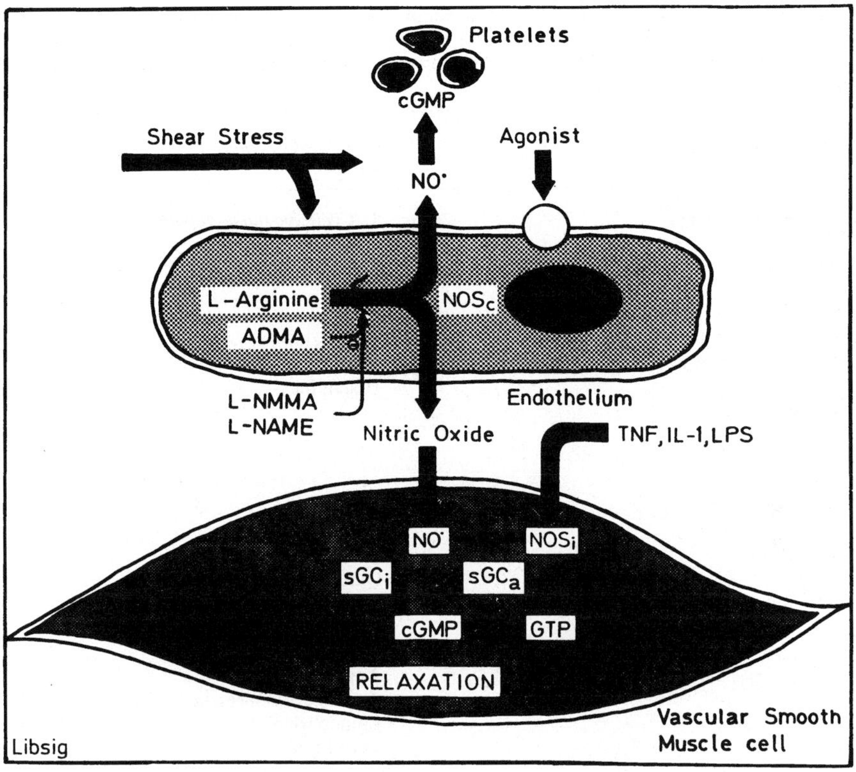


*Fig. 1.* Schematic representation of the L-arginine nitric oxide pathway: cGMP=cyclic 3'-5'guanosine monophosphate; GTP=guanosine triphosphate, NO=nitric oxide; $NOS_i$=inducible nitric oxide synthase; $NOS_c$=constitutive nitric oxide synthase.

Prostaglandin and thromboxane $A_2$ cause contraction and activate platelets. Oxygen-derived free radicals cause direct contraction and chemically inactivate nitric oxide.

## 3. Endothelial mediators in the ophthalmic circulation

Although endothelial regulatory systems are present in the entire cardiovascular system, a great heterogeneity exists from one vascular bed to another, both in the arterial and venous circulation. Endothelial responses are more pronounced in arteries than in veins and with decreasing vascular diameter in the same vascular bed (see ref. 2).

*Basal release of nitric oxide:* In isolated porcine and human ophthalmic and ciliary arteries, inhibitors of nitric oxide formation induce endothelium-dependent contractions[38-40]. In the perfused porcine eye, L-NAME reduces ophthalmic flow by 40%[41] (Fig. 3). Hence, the ophthalmic circulation is in a constant state of vasodilation due to the basal release of nitric oxide. The basal release of nitric oxide assures local blood flow, protects against vasoconstrictor stimuli and prevents activation of platelets and other blood cells.

*Stimulated release of nitric oxide:* In the human as well as porcine and bovine ophthalmic artery, acetylcholine, bradykinin and histamine evoke endothelium-dependent

*Table 1.* Agonists which evoke endothelium-dependent relaxations or endothelial-dependent contractions in certain blood vessels. Not all these agonist have already been tested in the ophthalmic circulation. Those who are known to evoke endothelium-dependent responses in the ophthalmic arteries are marked with an asterisk

| *Endothelium-dependent relaxations* | *Endothelium-dependent contractions* |
|---|---|
| *Autacoids and hormones* | 1. *Cycloxygenase-dependent contractions* |
| Acetylcholine* | Arachidonic acid |
| Bradykinin* | |
| Histamine* | |
| Substance P | |
| Adenosine triphosphate, | Acetylcholine |
| Adenosine diphosphate | |
| Serotonin | Histamine |
| Arginine vasopressin | |
| (cerebral vessels) | |
| Thrombin | |
| Calcium ionophore A23187 | |
| *Mechanical forces* | |
| Shear stress | Quick stretch* |
| Transmural pressure | |
| | *Endothelin-1* |
| | Angiotensin II |
| | Arginine vasopressin |
| | Epinephrine |
| | (thrombin) |
| | Interleukin-1 |
| | A23187 |
| | Phorbol ester |
| | Oxidized low density lipoproteins |

relaxations which are mediated by nitric oxide[38-44] (Fig. 4). In the extraocular porcine circulation, the sensitivity to bradykinin increases in vessels with a smaller diameter[40].

In the perfused porcine eye, bradykinin increases flow and reverses decreases in flow induced by a thromboxane analog[41] (Fig. 4). The response to bradykinin is prevented by L-NAME suggesting that nitric oxide is the only mediator. In contrast, in the porcine ophthalmic artery L-NMMA reduces the response to bradykinin, but a considerable relaxation persists[38]. This indicates that in extraocular arteries, bradykinin releases both nitric oxide and another endothelium-derived relaxing factor, most likely EDHF.

*Endothelin:* In isolated ophthalmic and retinal arteries, endothelin-1 evokes potent contractions[38-40,45] (Figs. 2 and 5). The sensitivity to endothelin increases with decreasing vascular diameter[40].

In the perfused porcine eye, endothelin-1 increases ophthalmic flow at very low dosages and reduces it at higher doses for prolonged periods of time[41]. Endothelin-3 evokes similar increases in flow, but it is less potent as a vasoconstrictor. This dual action of endothelins is due to the activation of endothelial $ET_B$ receptors releasing prostacyclin (mediating the transient vasodilation) and by the activation of $ET_A$ receptors on vascular smooth muscle at higher concentrations of endothelin (Fig. 2).

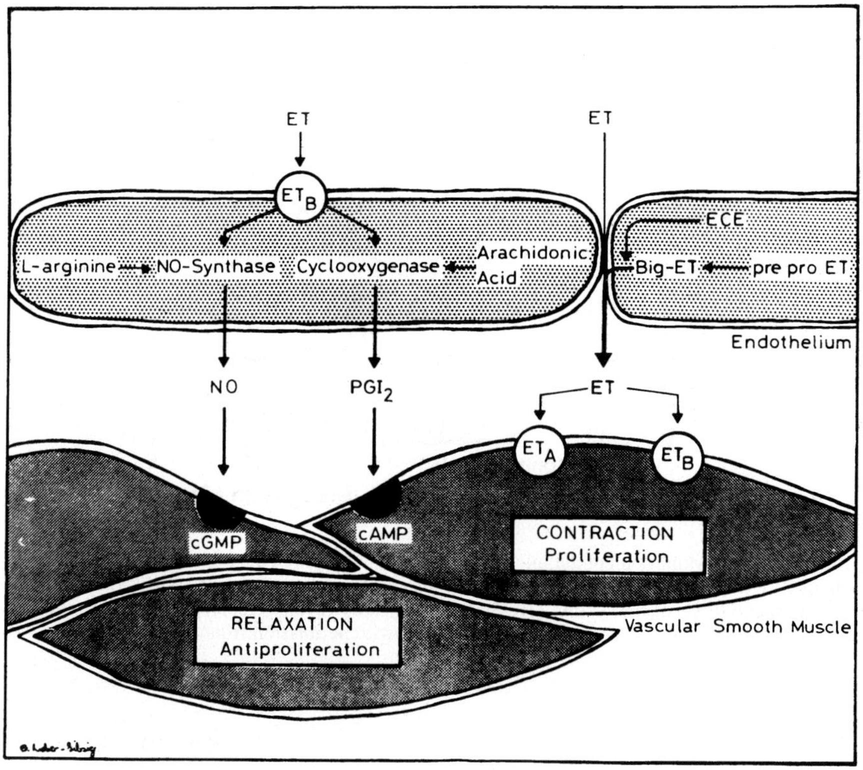


*Fig. 2.* Production and action of endothelin in the blood vessel wall: cAMP=cyclic 3'-5'adenosine monophosphate, cGMP=cyclic 3'-5'guanosine monophosphate; circles=receptors; ET=endothelin; NO= nitric oxide; $PGI_2$=prostacyclin.

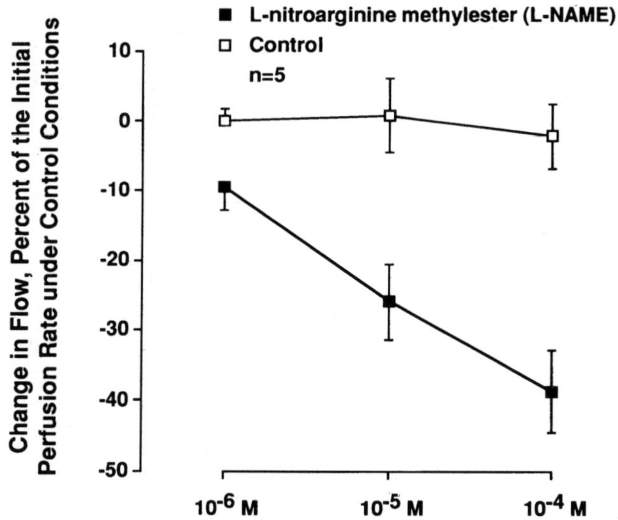


*Fig. 3.* In the isolated perfused porcine eye, L-NAME causes marked decreases in flow (■; measured by the outflow of perfusion solution through the ophthalmic veins), while the time control remains constant (□). (Reproduced with permission from Meyer *et al.*[41].)

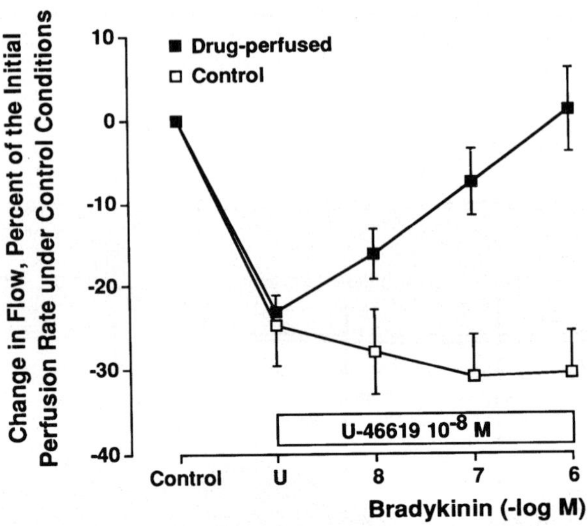


*Fig. 4.* Effects of bradykinin on ophthalmic flow in the perfused porcine eye: the thromboxane analogue U-46619 markedly decreases ophthalmic flow over a long period of time ( □ ). Co-infusion of U-46619 plus increasing concentrations of bradykinin (10/-8 - 10/-6 M) fully reverses the decrease in an ophthalmic flow induced by the thromboxane analogue (■). (Reproduced with permission from Meyer *et al.*[41].)

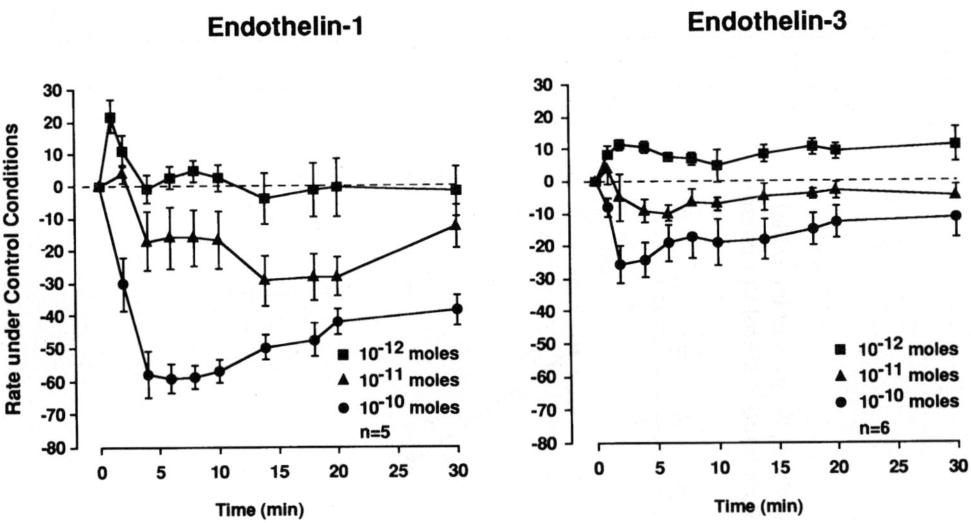


*Fig. 5.* Effects of endothelins in the perfused porcine eye: Intraluminal infusion of endothelin-1 (left) and endothelin-3 (right) both cause mild increases in ophthalmic flow at a low dose (■) and marked decreases in ophthalmic flow at high doses (▲ ; ●). The vasodilation is equally potent with both isoforms indicating that an $ET_B$ receptor is involved (on the endothelium), while ET-1 is the more potent vasoconstrictor suggesting a predominant $ET_A$ receptor mediated response. (Reproduced with permission from Meyer *et al.*[41].)

*Cyclooxygenase products:* In porcine ophthalmic arteries with endothelium, quick stretch induces a transient increase in tension, which is prevented by inhibitors of cyclooxygenase (*i.e.* indomethacin)[38]. Hence, the contracting factor most likely represents thromboxane $A_2$ or prostaglandin $H_2$. Stretch-activated ion channels in endothelial cells[14] may initiate the response.

*Endothelium-derived factors and pericytes:* Pericytes are contractile cells adjacent to the endothelial lining of capillaries. Pericytes are likely to modulate blood flow in very small ophthalmic arteries and capilaries. Cultured pericytes relax to sodium nitroprusside which releases nitric oxide from its molecule and in turn increases cGMP[46]. In addition, pericytes respond to endothelin-1 and prostacyclin[47-49].

## 4. Endothelial dysfunction

Endothelial dysfunction occurs in various disease states such as hypercholesteremia and atherosclerosis, hypertension, diabetes, vasospastic syndromes as well as in ischemia and reperfusion (see ref. 2). Most of these conditions are associated with impaired endothelium-dependent vasodilator responses and/or increased endothelium-dependent contractions. This suggests that endothelial cells are an important target for mechanical factors, noxious circulating substances and cardiovascular risk factors. Hence, it appears that endothelial cells may represent important vascular mediators of the effects of cardiovascular risk factors. Whether a primary endothelial dysfunction *per se* is able to cause vascular disease in any vascular bed is unknown.

*Potential importance of endothelial dysfunction in ophthalmology:* As in the majority of systemic vascular diseases endothelial function is impaired, similar alterations are likely to occur in the ocular circulation, especially in hypertension, diabetes, atherosclerosis or cerebrovascular ischemia. Endothelial dysfunction may also participate in vasospastic syndromes particularly ocular or retinal migraine and in some forms of low-tension glaucoma associated with Raynaud's phenomenon and migraine[50-53]. Indeed, circulating endothelin levels are higher in low-tension glaucoma than in high-tension glaucoma (unpublished observations).

## 5. Endothelium-dependent effects of cardiovascular drugs

A certain number of drugs used in clinical ophthalmology have the ability to modify endothelium-dependent responses.

*Local anesthetics:* In porcine ciliary arteries, lidocaine, bupivacaine or mepivacaine impair endothelium-dependent relaxations to bradykinin which may explain the reduction in local blood flow during retrobulbar anesthesia[54]. Interestingly, exogenous substitution by L-arginine restores the response even in the presence of the drugs. Hence, local anesthetics may reduce the intracellular availability of the precursor amino acid.

*Angiotensin-converting enzyme (ACE) inhibitors:* ACE is part of the endothelial cell membrane and identical to kinase II which inactivates bradykinin[55,56]. This explains why ACE inhibitors such as enalapril or benazepril increase endothelium-dependent relaxation to bradykinin in isolated ciliary arteries and augment the increase in ophthalmic flow induced by bradykinin in the perfused porcine eye[57].

*Endothelin receptor antagonists:* In the perfused porcine eye, FR139317, a specific $ET_A$ antagonists, markedly reduces the decrease in ophthalmic flow induced by

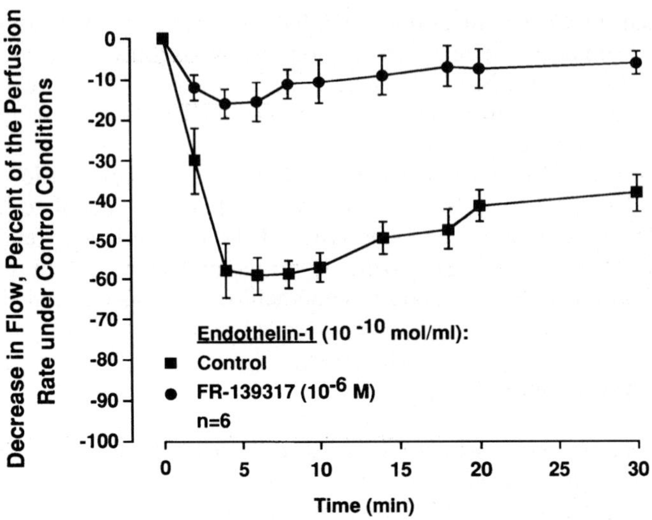


*Fig. 6.* Effects of the endothelin ETA receptor antagonist FR139317 in the perfused porcine eye. Under control conditions, intraluminal injection of endothelin-1 causes a marked and sustained decrease in ophthalmic flow (■ ; as measured by the outflow of perfusion solution through the ophthalmic veins) which is markedly reduced by FR 139317 (●). (Reproduced with permission from Meyer *et al.*[41].)

endothelin-1[41] (Fig. 6). As endothelin is increased in several disease states in which the eye also is involved (*i.e.* certain forms of hypertension, diabetes, Raynaud's syndrome, migraine, etc.), these newly developed drugs may provide important tools to characterize the role of endothelin in these disease states and potentially also may represent a new therapeutic approach in ophthalmology.

## 6. Conclusions

Through the local secretion of vasoactive substances, endothelial cells profoundly modulate local vascular tone in the ophthalmic circulation both under basal conditions and in response to mechanical forces and local hormones and platelet products. In the ophthalmic circulation, nitric oxide and endothelin-1 therefore are important regulators of blood flow. A dysfunction of these local regulatory systems may be involved in diseases of the ophthalmic circulation and may offer new therapeutic approaches.

## References

1. Alm A: Ocular circulation. In: Hart WM (ed): *Adler's Physiology of the Eye (Ninth Edition)*, pp 198-227. St. Louis: Mosby-Year Book, Inc., 1992
2. Lüscher TF, Vanhoutte PM: *The Endothelium: Modulator of Cardiovascular Functions*, pp 1-228. Boca Raton: CRC Press, 1990
3. Furchgott RF, Zawadzaki JV: The obligatory role of endothelial cells in the relaxation or arterial smooth muscle by acetylcholine. *Nature 299:* 373-376, 1980
4. Furchgott RF: Studies on relaxation of rabbit aorta by sodium nitrite: the basis for the proposal that acid-activable inhibitory factor from bovine retractor penis is inorganic nitrite and the endothelium-derived relaxing factor is nitric oxide. In: Vanhoutte PM (ed): *Vasodilatation: Vascular Smooth Muscle, Peptides, Autonomic Nerves and Endothelium*, pp 401-414. New York: Raven Press, 1988

5. Palmer RMJ, Ferrige AG, Moncada S: Nitric oxide release accounts for the biological activity of endothelium-derived relaxing factor. *Nature 327:* 524-526, 1987
6. Palmer RMJ, Ashton DS, Moncada S: Vascular endothelial cells synthesize nitric oxide from L-arginine. *Nature 333:* 664-666, 1988
7. Bredt DS, Snyder SH: Isolation of nitric oxide synthetase, a calmodulin-requiring enzyme. *Proc Natl Acad Sci USA 87:* 682-685, 1990
8. Moncada S, Radomski MW, Palmer RMJ: Endothelium-derived relaxing factor. Identification as nitric oxide and role in the control of vascular tone and platelet function. *Biochem Pharmacol 37:* 2495-2501, 1988
9. Cohen RA, Shepherd JT, Vanhoutte PM: Inhibitory role of the endothelium in the response to isolated coronary arteries to platelets. *Science 221:* 273-274, 1983
10. Yang Z, Stulz P, Von Segesser L, Bauer E, Turina M, Lüscher TF: Different interactions of platelets with arterial and venous coronary bypass vessels. *Lancet 337*, 939-943, 1991
11. Pohl U, Holtz J, Busse R, Bassenge E: Crucial role of endothelium in vasodilator response to increased flow in vivo. *Hypertension 8:* 37-44, 1986
12. Rubanyi GM, Romero JC, Vanhoutte PM: Flow-induced release of endothelium-derived relaxing factor. *Am J Physiol 250:* H1145-H-1149, 1986
13. Olesen S-P, Clapham DE, Davies PF: Haemodynamic shear stress activates a $K^+$ current in vascular endothelial cells. *Nature 331*: 168-170, 1988
14. Lansman JB, Hallam TJ, Rink TJ: Single stretch-activated ion channels in vascular endothelial cells as mechanotransducers? *Nature 325:* 811-813, 1987
15. Rubanyi GM, Lorenz RR, Vanhoutte PM: Bioassay of endothelium-derived relaxing factor(s): inactivation by catecholamines. *Am J Physiol 249:* H95-H101, 1985
16. Rapoport RM, Draznin MB, Murad F: Endothelium-dependent relaxation in rat aorta may be mediated through cyclic GMP-dependent protein phosphorylation. *Nature 306:* 174-176, 1983
17. Radomski MW, Palmer RMJ, Moncada S: The anti-aggregating properties of vascular endothelium: interaction between prostacyclin and nitric oxide. *Br J Pharmacol 92:* 639-646, 1987
18. Radomski MW, Palmer RMJ, Moncada S: Endogenous nitric oxide inhibits human platelet adhesion to vascular endothelium. *Lancet 2:* 1057-1058, 1987
19. Rees DD, Palmer RMJ, Moncada S: The role of endothelium-derived nitric oxide in the regulation of blood pressure. *Proc Natl Acad Sci USA 86:* 3375-3378, 1989
20. Yang Z, Von Segesser L, Bauer E, Stulz P, Tschudi M, Lüscher TF: Different activation of the endothelial L-arginine and cyclooxygenase pathway in the human internal mammary artery and saphenous vein. *Circulat Res 68:* 52-60, 1991
21. Vallance P, Leone A, Calver A, Collier J, Moncada S: Accumulation of an endogenous inhibitor of nitric oxide synthesis in chronic renal failure. *Lancet 339:* 572-575, 1992
22. Moncada S, Vane JR: Pharmacology and endogenous roles of prostaglandins endoperoxides, thromboxane $A_2$ and prostacyclin. *Pharmacol Rev 30:* 293-331, 1979
23. Vanhoutte PM: The end of the quest? *Nature 327:* 459-460, 1987
24. Standen NB, Quayle JM, Davies NW, Brayden JE, Huang Y *et al.*: Hyperpolarising vasodilators activate ATP-sensitive $K^+$ channels in arterial smooth muscle. *Science 245:* 177, 1989
25. Richard V, Tschudi M, Lüscher TF: Different activation of the endothelial L-arginine pathway by bradykinin, serotonin and clonidine in porcine coronary arteries, *Am J Physiol 259:* H1433-H1439, 1990
26. Yanagisawa M, Kurihara H, Kimura S, *et al.*: A novel potent vasoconstrictor peptide produced by vascular endothelial cells. *Nature 332:* 411-415, 1988
27. Lüscher TF, Boulanger C, Dohi Y, Yang Z: Endothelium-derived contracting factors (Brief review). *Hypertension 19,* 117-130, 1992
28. Boulanger C, Lüscher T.F.: Endothelin is released from the porcine aorta: inhibition by endothelium-derived nitric oxide (Rapid publication). *J Clin Invest 85:* 587-590, 1990
29. Steward DJ, Langleben D, Cernacek P, Cianflone K: Endothelin release is inhibited by coculture of endothelial cells with cells of vascular media. *Am J Physiol 259:* H1928-H1932, 1990
30. Sakurai T, Yanasigawa M, Takuwa Z, Miyazaki H, Kimura S, Goto K, Masaki T: Cloning of a cDNA encoding a non-isopeptide-selective subtype of the endothelin receptor. *Nature 348:* 732-735, 1990
31. Arai H, Hori S, Aramori I, Ohkubo H, Nakanishi S: Cloning and expression of a cDNA encoding and endothelin receptor. *Nature 348:* 730-732, 1990
32. Masaki T: The discovery, the present state, and the future prospects of endothelin. *J Cardiovasc Pharmacol 13 (Suppl 5):* 1-4, 1989
33. Goto K, Kasuya Y, Matsuki N, Takuwa Y, Kurihara H, Ishikawa T, Kimura S, Yanagisawa M, Masaki T: Endothelin activates the dihydropyridine-sensitive, voltage-dependent $Ca^{2+}$ channel in vascular smooth muscle. *Proc Natl Acad Sci USA 86:* 3915-3918, 1989
34. Yang Z, Richard V, Von Segesser L, *et al.*: Threshold concentrations of endothelin-1 potentiate contractions to norepinephrine and serotonin in human arteries: a new mechanism of vasospasm? *Circulation 82:* 188-195, 1990

35. Dohi Y, Lüscher TF: Endothelin-1 in perfused hypertensive resistance arteries: different intra- and extraluminal dysfunction. *Hypertension 18,* 543-549, 1991
36. Wright CE, Fozard JR: Regional vasodilation is a prominent feature of the haemodynamic response to endothelin in anesthetized, spontaneously hypertensive rats. *Eur J Pharmacol 155:* 201-203, 1988
37. Suzuki N, Matsumoto H, Kitada C, *et al.*: Immunoreactive endothelin-1 in plasma detected by a sandwich-type enzyme immunoassay. *J Cardiovasc Pharmacol 13 (Suppl 5):* 151-152, 1989
38. Wagner OF, Christ G, Wojta J, Vierhapper H, Parzer S, Nowotny PJ, Schneider B, Waldhäusl W, Binder BR: Polar secretion of endothelin-1 by cultured endothelial cells. *J Biomed Chem 267:* 16066–16068, 1992
38. Yao K, Tschudi M, Flammer J, Lüscher TF: Endothelium-dependent regulation of vascular tone of the porcine ophthalmic artery. *Invest Ophthalmol Vis Sci 32:* 1791-1798, 1991
39. Haefliger IO, Flammer J, Lüscher TL: Nitric oxide and endothelin-1 are important regulators of human ophthalmic artery. *Invest Ophthalmol Vis Sci 33:* 2340-2343, 1992
40. Haefliger IO, Flammer J, Lüscher TL: Heterogeneity of endothelium-dependent regulation in ophthalmic and ciliary arteries. *Invest Ophthalmol Vis Sci 33:* 2340-2343, 1992
41. Meyer P, Flammer J, Lüscher TF: Nitric oxide and endothelin-1 in the revelation of the ophthalmic microcirculation. *Invest. Ophthalmol Vis Sci 34:* 3614-3621, 1993
42. Benedito S, Prieto D, Nielsen PJ, Nyborg NCB: Role of the endothelium in acetylcholine-induced relaxation and spontaneous tone of bovine isolated retinal small arteries. *Exp Eye Res 52:* 575-579, 1991
43. Benedito S, Prieto D, Nielsen PJ, Nyborg NCB: Histamine induces endothelium-dependent relaxation of bovine retinal arteries. *Invest Ophthalmol Vis Sci 32:* 32-38, 1991
44. Nyborg NCB, Nielsen J: The level of spontaneous myogenic tone in isolated human posterior ciliary arteries decreases with age. *Exp Eye Res 51:* 711-715, 1990
45. Nyborg NCB, Prieto D, Benedito S, Nielsen PJ: Endothelin-1-induced contraction of bovine retinal small arteries is reversible and abolished by nitrendipine. *Invest Ophthalmol Vis Sci 32:* 27-31, 1991
46. Haefliger IO, Tschauer, A, Anderson DR: Relaxation of retinal pericyte contractile tone through the nitric oxide-cyclic GMP pathway. *Invest Ophthalmol Vis Sci 35:* 991-997, 1994
47. Chakravarthy U, Gardiner TA, Anderson P, Archer DB, Trimble ER: The effect of endothelin-1 on the retinal microvascular pericyte. *Microvasc Res 43:* 241-254, 1992
48. Kelley C, D'Amore P, Hechtman HB, Shepro D: Vasoactive hormones and cAMP affect pericyte contraction and stress fibres in vitro. *J Musc Res Cell Mot 9:* 184-194, 1989
49. Dodge AB, Heechtman HB, Shepro D: Microvascular endothelial-derived autacoids regulate pericyte contractility. *Cell Mot Cytoskelet 118:*180-188, 1991
50. Gasser P, Flammer J: Blood-cell velocity in the nailfold capillaries of patients with normal-tension and high-tension glaucoma. *Am J Ophthalmol 111:* 585-588, 1991
51. Kline LB, Kelly CL: Ocular migraine in a patient with cluster headaches. *Headache 20:* 253-257, 1980
52. Phelps CD, Corbett JJ: Migraine and low-tension glaucoma. A case control study. *Invest Ophthalmol Vis Sci 26:* 1105-1108, 1985
53. Wolter JR, Burchfield WJ: Ocular migraine in a young man resulting in unilateral transient blindness and retinal edema. *J Pediatr Ophthalmol 8:* 173-176, 1971
54. Meyer P, Flammer J, Lüscher TF: Local anesthetic drugs reduce endothelium-dependent relaxations of porcine ciliary arteries, *Invest Ophthalmol Vis Sci 34:* S 2730-2736, 1993
55. Vanhoutte PM: Why are converting enzyme inhibitors vasodilators? *Br J Clin Pharmacol 28:* 1S-10S, 1989
56. Vidal M, Vanhoutte PM: Endothelium-dependent effects of the converting enzyme inhibitor trandolapril. *FASEB J 2:* 2410, 1988
57. Meyer P, Flammer J, Lüscher TF: Local vascular action of the angiotensin system in the porcine ophthalmic major circulation. *Invest Ophthalmol Vis Sci* 1995 (in press)

## Discussion

**Dr. Drance:** Dr. Lüscher, can you tell us something about the responses of the circulation to cold. You have worked extensively with this. What happens, let us say, in ocular circulation, the cerebral circulation, the coronary circulation? Is it all on a sympathetic basis, or how does it occur?

**Dr. Lüscher:** That is a very good question. We have not cooled down our eyes, yet, but maybe we should do it, because it would enable to us to delineate between reflex effects and direct effects. Clearly, as you know, cold immersion produces pallor in whatever part of the body is cooled, but there is also a marked general activation of the sympathetic nervous system, there is no question about it. An interesting aspect in the context of the endothelium is that the endothelium modulates responses to norepinephrine. In fact Andreas Zeiher and Helmuth Drexler have shown that if you immerse the hand in a cold environment you see nothing or small vasodilation in the normal coronary circulation, while in patients with disease you have marked vasoconstriction. It has also been shown that cold immersion of one hand increases endothelin production in the other hand. So clearly, cold has a lot of effects on the circulation which relate to the sympathetic nervous system as well as to the endothelium. I think the endothelium is primarily a modulator, I should say, probably primarily by inhibiting the vasoconstriction that occurs under these conditions. The teleologic function is that normally if you run and the sympathetic nervous system is activated, you do not want coronary vasoconstriction. You want to avoid that, and I think the role of the endothelium is to buffer these responses. If you get sick, this may importantly contribute to the level of angina you develop in the coronary circulation. What it all means in the eye we do not know yet, so we really should look at that.

**Dr. Langer:** You mentioned several antagonists of the endothelin receptors. Are they peptidic or not peptidic, and do they possess any degree of intrinsic activity as agonists or as partial agonists? And the second question is, are there compounds that would inhibit the endothelin converting enzyme and thus prevent the formation of endothelin, which would be one way to act directly on both receptors, since this seems to be the strategy.

**Dr. Lüscher:** The endothelin converting enzyme, to my knowledge, has not been cloned yet (it has now: *Editor*), but there are methylproteases which are known to inhibit this enzyme but may inhibit a lot of other enzymes as well. One rather useful tool which we have used is phosphoramidone. One can demonstrate that if you give big endothelin, that phosphoramidone would prevent conversion to a considerable extent, Yanagisawa works heavily with this enzyme, and certainly this is one approach to try to block the endothelin system. There is a disadvantage, however, because big endothelin may have some effects also by itself, without conversion, which, perhaps, as previously with thromboxane synthase inhibitors, may be a slight problem.

Now, with regard to the endothelin antagonists, not all the structures are known, because the companies are quite secretive about it. Not all of them have been patented, and some of them are peptide-like, but most are not. Most of them except two, the structure of which I do not know because it has just been patented but should be published soon, are orally available, but not to a great extent.

**Dr. Siesjö:** Just a comment to Dr. Drance's question. I think that the general consensus, when it comes to the cerebral circulation and cold, is that when you reduce temperature of the brain you reduce the oxygen and glucose consumption by about 5% per degree of lowering of brain temperature. And the circulation follows, if you adjust the pH according to the shift in temperature, there is a parallel decrease in cerebral blood flow and metabolism.

**Dr. Drance:** Thank you very much, I appreciate that comment, but my question was not directed so much as to what happens to the brain when it is cooled, but rather when a limb is cooled. Now, what happens to the circulation of the brain, the eye, and the coronary circulation. If cold produces some visual changes in the eye, which has been reported by many people now, the question is how does it do it and which vessels are responsible. Our measurements of the ophthalmic artery velocity show very quickly changes in the velocity to a half cigarette. In contrast we have not been able to measure a change in the ophthalmic artery after cooling one hand even though we can measure a change very easily, in the other hand. If you cool one hand and blood flow changes in the other hand, I wonder if you had information about the mechanisms.

**Dr. Flammer:** It could be again that, Michael van Buskirk, you may have an answer to that, because you showed a nice picture in which endothelin depressed the circulation quite specifically in the optic nerve head.

**Dr. Lüscher:** I am sure that within a year's time we will be able to do crucial experiments with specific antagonists.

**Dr. Flammer**: I think you mentioned the paper of Moriya *et al.* in which they found, and we are looking for the same, you know, the endothelin blood level in patients with normotension glaucoma was increased, although the blood pressure was low, because if I understand it correctly, normally it correlates somehow with the blood pressure.

**Dr. Lüscher**: Not necessarily. Depending on the degree of vascular disease and renal failure it correlates rather nicely. But the literature on hypertension is very controversial. Most of the papers we reviewed had normal values, while there are two or three papers reporting increased values.

**Dr. Flammer**: I do not mean the people with systemic hypertension. In the same individual, if he increases his blood pressure by activity, does the physiologic response include an increase in endothelin?

**Dr. Lüscher**: Yes, during exercise on a bicycle there is some increase.

**Dr. Seisjö**: I am sorry, Dr. Drance, I think I misunderstood you. I do not know of any data about the cerebral circulation when the subject is cold, but predictably it would not be changed unless your change the $CO_2$ tension or the oxygen tension to low levels or you changed metabolic rate in the brain. But for the eye, I mean, I have no idea; it can be completely different.

**Dr. Lüscher**: Sure. I mean, obviously there are different mechanisms. Cold to the body may produce a reflex, or humoral mediated responses. The eye is obviously also exposed directly to temperature, in contrast to the brain, so it could also respond directly. Certainly we know from experiments that you can put your hand in cold water and you can have changes in the eye, so reflex or humoral mechanisms certainly are involved.

**Dr. Alm**: Well, I have really one question and one comment. The question is about what you just talked about, the effect of cold on the ocular circulation. If we can imagine for instance that you have an increased sympathetic tone, you should remember that there are no sympathetic nerves to the retina. But what I would like to ask, what happens in the other hand with regard to sympathetic tone and blood flow if you have an increased sympathetic tone by dipping one hand into cold water?

**Dr. Flammer**: Yes, it decreases blood flow in the other hand, this has been published many times.

**Dr. Lüscher**: And endothelin goes up in the other arm as well, that is Freequist's paper in BBRC three years ago.

**Dr. Alm**: But I am a little bit confused about endothelin, the idea that that should be involved in for instance, low-tension glaucoma. First of all, you showed that there is a rapid tachyphlaxis...

**Dr. Lüscher**: It is not rapid, but there is tachyphlaxis, yes.

**Dr. Quigley**: Would you give us an idea of the time course that you mean by rapid or not rapid?

**Dr. Lüscher**: Well, what we do is a concentration response curve, which takes maybe half an hour, 45 minutes, and then you wash out, and it is very difficult to get rid of endothelin. You have to wait for quite some time, and then the next concentration response curve *in vitro* is tachyphylactic. But for instance, if you infuse endothelin in the forearm of human subjects with relatively low concentrations, you maintain a continuous decrease in flow, so there is no loss of vasoconstrictor activity.

**Dr. Quigley**: Over what time course was that experiment done?

**Dr. Lüscher**: Hours. I mean, basically, you can drop down flow locally with endothelin, and if you do not do anything else, it is quite dangerous. It is an important point. I do not think we should hold the tachyphylaxis data against it, because *in vivo*, and also in isolated vessels, if it remains close to the vessel wall, there is a tremendous continuation of responses, which I have never seen with any other agonist, and this shows that it binds very tightly to the receptor.

**Dr. Alm**: That is not the only argument. You have also the blood–brain barrier, and in this case, the blood–retinal barrier. You have also shown that if you infuse endothelin intravenously in cats, you will find practically no effect on either choroidal or retinal blood flow. Also, endothelin is surprisingly weak for the retinal vessels if you give it into the vitreous body, which is a way to surpass the blood–retinal barrier. Also it seems to release nitric oxide in both vascular beds and also prostacyclins in the choroid, and probably PGH2 or some vasoconstrictive arachidonic acid metabolite in the retina. So it does not have, at least in acute experiments, very impressive effects on either the choroid or the retina, at least, *in vivo*, in cats.

**Dr. Lüscher**: Yes, of course. I mean, clearly in the porcine it differs, but I do not know whether this is also occurring in the retinal circulation. We have studied the entire ophthalmic circulation. We have also to be careful not to extrapolate too much from infusion experiments, because as you have seen with slow intravascular infusion we have this vasodilator effect. Endogenous endothelin may produce a different effect, and keep in mind that endogenous endothelin release would be primarily abluminal and local.

**Dr. Alm**: Then you would not find, as you say the Japanese did, increased levels in the blood. An abluminal release and increased concentrations in the blood are two different things.

**Dr. Lüscher**: I am not saying that it is not also released luminally, but what I am saying is that most of it is released abluminally. That has been recently demonstrated. A year ago the Vienna group showed that three quarters is released abluminally rather than luminally. But what I am saying is that if the plasma endothelin levels are increased, it means that in some part of the circulation there must be considerable production, but you do not know where, and you do not know how much you will have locally at the site of your interest.

**Dr. Epstein**: In your porcine preparation, what is the effect of catecholamines on endothelin?

**Dr. Lüscher**: We have not infused it in the porcine eye, I must say. We have used serotonin because it is the most reliable and most stable vasoconstrictor in the extraocular arteries, but we have no data in the perfused eye, but we probably should do it, but we have not done it yet.

**Dr. van Buskirk**: I just wanted to address the tachyphylaxis issue as well as the ocular issue. My colleague, Dr. Chalsey, has used an ALZA minipump delivery system to deliver endothelin into the perineural area by using a little tube, and produced profound vasoconstriction in the affected eye but not in the fellow eye. He has delivered it for most of the eyes for a week, and has now delivered it for two weeks and still gets profound vasoconstriction at extremely low doses in a dose-dependent manner.

**Dr. Drance**: In cats?

**Dr. van Buskirk**: Oh, I am sorry, that was in the rabbit. I can not remember whether we have done that also in cats.

**Dr. Lüscher**: Just for the tachyphylaxis comment, of course that is a very important one, and we have data *in vivo* and *in vitro* in the human for bradykinin, substance P, and endothelin. And for instance, if you infuse bradykinin or substance P in the hand veins of patients or normal subjects, you get rapid tachyphylaxis. With bradykinin you can do a concentration response curve with three or four dosages, otherwise it is not reproducible. With substance P it is very difficult to get more than one dose reliably. But with endothelin we never have a problem. To the contrary, a group in Edinburgh has reported that if you continue to infuse low concentrations of endothelin for hours that you get a continuous increase in vasoconstriction, rather than a decrease, as I mentioned earlier.

**Dr. van Buskirk**: The biggest problem was to get the dose small enough to get the response low enough.

**Dr. Quigley**: People have been infusing endothelin into hand veins of humans?

**Dr. Lüscher**: Yes we have.

**Dr. Quigley**: Did they go blind?

**Dr. Lüscher**: No.

**Dr. Quigley**: Did they say they had any effect at all on their vision, or did anybody bother to look?

**Dr. Lüscher**: Well, you see, these are very low concentrations.

**Dr. Quigley**: But this thing works at 10 to the minus 8, 10 to the minus 9, I would be interested, would not you?

**Dr. Lüscher**: The dilution effect is tremendous...

**Dr. Quigley**: Well, you are already telling me you would not *expect* to see an effect. I was just interested in whether somebody bothered to look. No one actually looked, right?

**Dr. Lüscher**: That is right, basically we might have overlooked an effect, I agree. But what I am saying is, we use concentrations that have no effect on blood pressure, we can not say more than that.

**Dr. Zeimer**: I would like to bring the discussion we had outside back here and try to go back to glaucoma. If we take what Joe Caprioli tells us, that the interest in glaucoma would be a very local effect, affecting only a few neurons, therefore it must be an effect at the capillary level. We know that, and correct me if I am wrong, I just read what Doug Anderson circulated among us, that glaucoma is different from shutting down the central artery supply to the optic nerve, therefore glaucoma is not a central, homogenous shut-down of the circulation to the optic nerve. If anything, like Joe says, it is a very local effect. If it is a local effect to a microscopic region, it means on the capillary level. Therefore in order to apply what you say here to glaucoma, we would have to assume that the endothelial cells know to talk to somebody else except smooth muscle. And maybe Doug Anderson can tell us if endothelial cells can talk to pericytes. If this effect exists, then it could be extremely interesting to glaucoma, because then maybe local endothelium, being affected by stretching, could talk to their pericyte and cause a local defect in the regulation. So I think the central question, and Doug, maybe you can help us, is: can endothelial cells talk to pericytes and cause vasoconstriction or vasodilation.

**Dr. Anderson**: As moderator I am trying to stay out of the discussion, because there are so many people with raised hands in line waiting patiently to speak but I think the questions at hand here are very relevant. We do want to talk about the implication of all this toward physiology, what role do these things play in controlling regional versus local blood flow, and that sort of thing. And secondly we need to consider disease states. You made a long list where there was a high endothelin level: is that primary to the process that produced the disease, or is the high endothelin level a reflection of a general compensatory response. What implications might it have if one vascular bed has a disease, brings forth a compensatory response with spillover of endothelin, which now has another effect somewhere else in the body. Is that what vasospasm is? Is vasospasm a disease some place that produces an effect elsewhere? These are the kinds of questions that I would like to learn from you, but I am seeing from your head nodding that I am not going to get those answers because these things are not known yet. But Dr. Zeimer is correct, we might turn our attention to the pathophysiologic implication of Dr. Lüscher's presentation.

**Dr. Lüscher**: Maybe Ivan Haefliger can comment on the pericytes, because that is what he works on.

**Dr. Anderson**: Yes, you evidently read what we had circulated ahead of time, and so far the pericytes seem to show very much the same responses, or the capabilities of response, as smooth muscle cells. That is, they respond to neurotransmitters, they respond to second messengers of various kinds, they respond to paracrines. We are going to get into that tomorrow, when I have the opportunity to give my presentation, provided there is anything left to say by that time.

**Dr. Lüscher**: I would also like to actually ask you a question related to Dr. Zeimer's. And that is, how solid are the data about where vasoconstriction, if any, occurs in glaucoma? Do you actually know in these patients where it occurs? It does not occur in the main ophthalmic artery or in the central retinal artery, but where does it occur? Is it in a branch of the retinal artery, or is it further down the line, where is it?

**Dr. Anderson**: The answer is that we do not know. We are trying to figure that out. We are trying to learn from you the level and type of vessel in which such constriction generally occurs because no one has observed where there is a vasoconstriction in glauocma, and among us we are not even in agreement as to whether vasoconstriction is an important element of the process..

**Dr. Lüscher**: The reason I ask, obviously, if the work on pericytes is very important, I think we have to learn more about that, that is obvious. But the question is, could it also be that this occurs in larger vessels, which still do have vascular smooth muscle cells around.

**Dr. Anderson**: Tomorrow we will talk more about pericytes. And yes, that is exactly the question.

**Dr. Quigley**: In the visual system we have the tremendous advantage that when something happens dysfunctionally we can test it topographically. So I would like to know something about the vasospastic patients. I have not had the good fortune to see them in my practice so I have to ask those who have, where do they lose visual field? And if the topographic loss of visual field is somehow regular and predictable, then that would tell us something about where the regionality of the poor blood supply is. So what do they look like?

**Dr. Anderson**: As moderator I will permit Drs. Flammer and Drance to answer that, and then we will get to Dr. Langer who has been waiting patiently to speak.

**Dr. Flammer**: First of all, in most of the cases both eyes are involved, but the visual field defects are never symmetrical. In young people mostly we observe quite a diffuse change, but about one-third have also very localized changes, and you can not distinguish these changes from the visual field of a glaucoma patient. If you show only the visual field to an ophthalmologist, I would guess in 90% of the cases he would say the patient has glaucoma. You can observe everything, bundle defects, diffuse things, you can really observe everything. But in young, including children, it tends to be quite diffuse.

**Dr. Quigley**: You include children among glaucoma patients in this case. Or the children have vasospasm.

**Dr. Flammer**: No, I am speaking about vasospasm, not about glaucoma.

**Dr. Lüscher**: That would mean that this may be also quite diffuse in the supplying arteries and not necessarily at the very small ones.

**Dr. Drance**: Well, I think we are confusing things. We have been confusing many things for a long time, and we are confusing them again. I think what Dr. Flammer is talking about is what he calls the vasospastic syndrome, and that he has not said it has anything to do with glaucoma necessarily.

**Dr. Quigley**: But what he is talking about is vasospastic syndrome...

**Dr. Drance**: Yes, we are talking about vasospastic syndrome and he has just told you what the field defects look like during vasospasm in the absence of glaucoma. In the glaucoma picture we certainly see lots of patients who are very vasospastic to cold. We have not been able to find that they had different visual field defects from the patients who had low-tension glaucoma, open-angle glaucoma, and who were not vasospastic. We have been looking to try and identify clinically whether they behave differently and have not been able to do so. I do not see the non-glaucomatous patients with vasospastic syndrome, because I do not work in that area, but I see lots of glaucoma with vasospasm, and I cannot differentiate it clinically by any parameter that I have tried to find yet. So that I can look at somebody and say from his discs or visual field, you are vasospastic, but I can diagnose vasospasm as a concomitant to the glaucoma by many examinations, questions, and all other sorts of things.

**Dr. Anderson**: Please excuse us, Dr. Langer, for having completed this discussion before going on to the topic that you will bring up.

**Dr. Langer**: It is stimulating enough. My question concerns the circulating levels of endothelin, but I think you can answer those questions. The first one is, how specific is the method to determine the levels, whether it can discriminate between endothelin-1, -2, and -3, and thirdly, how robust are the changes that were recorded? Do we get twice baseline, 10 times, what is the nature of the difference?

**Dr. Lüscher**: Well, as usual, when a new peptide comes up, the literature is pretty messy, because everybody is impatient to measure it and some are not capable to do so yet but they still publish it. We have spent a year on establishing a reliable assay, and we now feel very confident that we can measure it reliably. The extraction is a problem. And the assay is good or bad if the extraction is bad or good. If you look at the values in the literature, and we have reviewed that extensively, the normal values are different by a ratio of 1 to 20, which is unacceptable. I think that the lower values, in the picogram per milliliter range, are probably the right ones. Now, how specific is it. Obviously you can measure endothelin-1, -2, and -3, and you can also measure big endothelin and other peptides. The cross-reactivity of the antibodies available, and a lot of them are available commercially now, differs. Some cross-react with big endothelin 80%, some are very specific for endothelin-1, so it really depends also on the question you raise. If you want just to measure endothelin overall you can have an assay which cross-reacts with endothelin-3, it does not matter, but it is not very useful to have too much cross-reactivity to big endothelin, because this gives you background noise to see changes. But on the other hand, most of the changes which have been looked at by people able to distinguish big endothelin and the final product have shown that this goes parallel. So, the third aspect, how robust are these changes, I think that most of the changes are at most a doubling of endothelin levels, sometimes threefold, but not much more than that.

**Dr. Langer**: May I follow this by another question. What are the changes in angiotensin II levels in plasma in hypertensive patients with regard to normotensive patients?

**Dr. Lüscher**: For endothelin or angiotensin?

**Dr. Langer**: No, angiotensin.

**Dr. Lüscher**: Well, I am not the person to address this question, because that is not our primary interest. But I can only say that the same problem with measuring, or even the bigger problem applies to angiotensin too. I think the only person in the world who can measure angiotensin II is Jürg Nussberger in Lausanne, and he would be the one to answer the question.

**Dr. Langer**: The point was not perhaps to get the answer, but to say that the changes in circulating levels of a mediator like endothelin may not necessarily predict the involvement in a disease state. It may be locally produced and never get into significant changes in circulating plasma, and yet have physiopathological importance.

The point I wanted to make is that angiotensin II receptor antagonists are antihypertensive agents, and angiotensin converting enzyme inhibitors are antihypertensive agents. And the question of circulating levels, you know, may still be open, perhaps, for angiotensin.

**Dr. Lüscher**: I could not agree more with you. I am very glad for your comment. Indeed, I am consulting with different companies on the indications for endothelin antagonists. In first studies, they tend to be fixed on these elevated levels. I remember when we tested captopril in 1979, I had a patient who almost went into shock. We measured the angiotensin levels, we did even an angiography for renal artery stenosis, she had nothing. She had normal levels of renin, everything. And the same applies for endothelin, indeed. It is possible that with endothelin antagonists you lower blood pressure and the hypertensive rat has absolutely normal or low levels of endothelin in plasma. So one has to be careful, I agree.

**Dr. Anderson**: The effect could be by removing the physiologic effect that is present even if there is no pathological level of angiotensin.

**Dr. Lüscher**: I think normally you have so much dilution that you would not see anything. You may have increased levels in the fingers or other local sites of disease, but because of dilution you do not see anything if you measure it in the general circulation.

**Dr. Anderson**: No, my point about your patient who went into shock is that an elevated angiotensin production may not have been important in producing that patient's hypertension, it may have been a physiologic level, but by removing the physiologic basement, you can go into hypotension no matter whether it had anything to do with the pathologic state of hypertension or not.

**Dr. Lüscher**: Sure, or bradykinins may be involved, we do not know.

**Dr. Flammer**: I have a question as a clinician to Dr. Zeiher and Dr. Lüscher. I am well aware that we have more questions than answers in what is going on in glaucoma, but if you have a patient with very low blood pressure and is spastic at the same time, what would you treat first? Well, first of all, would you treat? And if yes, should we first try to bring the pressure up, because this may also reduce the spastic syndrome, or should we first treat the spasm? Let us say it is a 40-year-old lady or something like this. What would you recommend to do first?

**Dr. Zeiher**: That is really a very difficult question. I think it depends what the lady feels worse about, if she actually suffers from having low blood pressure, and she is symptomatic about it.

**Dr. Flammer**: She suffers because she has a normal-tension glaucoma, let us assume that, and we have many of those cases. You do not need to treat because the patient is suffering traditional symptoms, but let us assume that there are some statistical indications that there is at least some relationship between low perfusion pressure and normal-tension glaucoma, whether this is causal or not I do not know. If at least there is a statistical relationship, so the patient is losing function and we would like to do something. What shall we do?

**Dr. Lüscher**: A trial, a randomized trial.

**Dr. Anderson**: If I translate the question? The question is, if we make the assumption that there is normal-tension glaucomas on the basis of poor perfusion, and this patient has both a low blood pressure and vasospasm, each of which contribute to low perfusion, which one would you treat first because treating one may have an aggravating effect on the other. That is the question.

**Dr. Lüscher**: But how solid is that. This is only a correlation, a statistical correlation. We do not know whether in fact if we increase blood pressure, whether this decreases the episodes, do we know that?

**Dr. Flammer**: We know that many patients with a spastic syndrome are much less spastic if you increase the blood pressure by systemic mineralocorticoids, for example. If you treat with adrenalin or similar drugs, then we do the opposite. We increase the spasm. But what would you do, what would you recommend?

**Dr. Quigley**: What is the outcome parameter of this experiment going to be, what is it you are going to be monitoring?

**Dr. Drance**: We are measuring visual field, for example.

**Dr. Quigley**: Well we do not know any treatment besides intraocular pressure lowering that I know conclusively affects glaucoma. I think you are asking the doctor a very unfair question. It is a wonderful hypothetical question, which blood flow parameter might you change, but if I were the committee for evaluating this experiment, I would have trouble understanding what the sample size was and other things about it.

**Dr. Flammer**: The sample size of what?

**Dr. Quigley**: How many subjects are required if you are going to treat some patients and not treat other patients; and if you are going to watch their visual field, are you looking for improvement on their field or non-progression, what are we looking at?

**Dr. Flammer**: No, I did not ask for a study, I ask as a clinician. In other words, you would say you would not treat this patient.

**Dr. Quigley**: Naturally not. There is no evidence whatever that treating the blood pressure........

**Dr. Flammer**: There is no evidence that we should reduce the intraocular pressure in these cases.

**Dr. Quigley**: There is only minimal evidence that lowering intraocular pressure helps, you are absolutely right. But there is more evidence of that than there is of changing blood pressure.

**Dr. Anderson**: And the problem for a clinician is always this: that you run out of information that is solid as to how you should treat the patient. Then you must make a *judgment* as to which way is best. So here we have a patient in whom lowering the pressure seemingly is not going to be of much benefit, because you have it as low as you can get, and yet they are losing vision. You are asking for a judgment from these very knowledgeable people about vascular events. If you have to make a judgment, which one would you choose? That is the clinician's dilemma, they have to make a judgment without facts.

**Dr. Lüscher**: Exactly.

**Dr. Anderson**: So we need a randomized trial.

**Dr. Lüscher**: No, no, you have an individual patient who is facing you today.

**Dr. Quigley**: No, I would love to have a randomized trial, but I would not want you treating the vascular system of an individual patient outside the context of a study. Let us hear about the randomized trial, I am not interested in case by case discussions.

**Dr. Flammer**: I have not yet any results. We treat half the patients with fluocortisone and the others we do not treat.

**Dr. Quigley**: And what does that do. I am not trying to be an iconoclast, I want to hear about your study.

**Dr. Flammer**: It just increases the blood pressure, and we would like to know whether this is of any benefit to the patient, we do not yet know the answer. But as a clinician treating an individual patient, I do not have an answer, and I would like to know from the internist what he would recommend, what makes the most sense.

**Dr. Kaufman**: You are increasing the blood pressure in these?

**Dr. Flammer**: Yes. We have many normal-tension glaucomas, you have observed and many others have done so too, and many publications are under way, that a low blood pressure is a risk factor for glaucoma.

**Dr. Kaufman**: Right, you might need many thousands of patients to do this, but are you saying at the same time the increased risk of heart attack and stroke is acceptable, because there is evidence from the internal medicine literature, that even within the normal blood pressure range the risk of these things goes up with the blood pressure. So it may be like the beta blockers and heart attacks, you do not know what other parameters you are changing when you try to treat glaucoma.

**Dr. Drance**: Semantics! What Joseph does not mean is elevating the blood pressure to 150/90. What he is presenting is a patient who has had a maximal intraocular pressure reduction, is now running a pressure of 9 or 10, is 48 years young, he is a dentist, and he says, I am continuing to lose my vision in that eye and your fields confirm this. And he has a blood pressure of 70/50 and he is strongly vasospastic. And having said to him, I may kill you with unproven drugs, he says, I am going blind. One therefore wonders what one can possibly do for this individual. Joseph is asking the question, under these circumstances, which of the two might you do first, elevate the blood pressure or use a calcium channel blocker, and the calcium channel blocker may reduce the blood pressure further. But it might improve perfusion by virtue of vasodilation, I think that is what Joseph is asking. Not the study; the person says, I would love to join your study, but I am going to blind now.

**Dr. Flammer**: I just would like to add this copy from the internal medicine literature showing that if the blood pressure is going very low, the risk of getting some heart attack or whatever is increasing again. But we are observing, and many others are observing the same, that many of our normal tensions, and also the open-angle glaucoma patients, are here, in this range.

**Dr. Lüscher**: And that is the J curve discussion, yes?

**Dr. Flammer**: This is not in ophthalmology, it might be different in ophthalmology, but just saying that low blood pressure may not always mean this person is very healthy. In the past we always said, low blood pressure can only be of benefit, you are a lucky person you have very low blood pressure, and I do not think this is true. At least statistically there is a very clear relationship. We need a study which would show very clearly that the progression of glaucomatous damage in high-tension and in normal-tension glaucoma was statistically very high, and very significantly related to the level of the blood pressure. And the patients who had very low blood pressure had a much higher risk of losing field.

**Dr. Quigley**: Well, I have not read the doctor's study, and he has not as yet read the Baltimore Eye Surgery data because it is being submitted for publication at the present time. Dr. Jim Tielsch has looked at a population of 5,500 people in Baltimore, Maryland, that were population based. They had a diagnosis of glaucoma. Their eye pressure was low or high, glaucoma was not diagnosed by level of eye pressure. Each of these people had their blood pressures measured and medical histories taken as well. And we can talk about the relationship between hypertension and glaucoma in that population at some length, but there was no association between low blood pressure, and no general association between high blood pressure, and glaucoma in that population. Likewise in a longitudinal study in which we followed 800 persons with ocular hypertension, and now this, Joseph, may be the selection factor that of course ruins the correlation for the non-population based sample, but in a recruited group of ocular hypertensive persons followed for a period of 12 years, those who developed new field loss, first field loss, incident field loss, had no relationship between the level of their blood pressure measured at onset of the study and whether or not they later developed visual field defects. Now perhaps that second study is selected against the kind of person that you are thinking of, because they were ocular hypertensions. But the persons in the population based study were not selected for any reason at all except they existed in the U.S. Now we can talk about details of it. The duration of their hypertension was related. What we estimate to be the duration of their high blood pressure was a risk factor, but having high blood pressure in general was not, and in particular having lower blood pressures was not. There may be different populations perhaps.

**Dr. Flammer**: But they measured just once the blood pressure? We monitor over 24 hours and we saw that if you would take just one blood pressure we would have missed all the relationships.

**Dr. Quigley**: I guess we could take it thousands of times, but if you take it in a group of 5,000 people, you have given each person an equal chance to show you their random low blood pressure that is going to happen. So statistically what you just said is not necessarily a criticism of what I just presented.

**Dr. Epstein**: The hour may be late so I am not thinking so clearly, but it seems to me we are arguing about the wrong thing. We just had several lectures on mechanisms of vascular relaxation and contraction, and I thought that was the context of the question. They were very specific about mechanisms. If you assume that there is a vascular component to some form of glaucoma, and you have a patient with low blood pressure, the question is, I would say, if you raise the blood pressure, and the nerve head vasculature autoregulates, then it should not make a difference unless there is a defective autoregulation in glaucoma. And if you think there is a vascular spasm, then if you had something that would relieve the spasm, I guess the question is, would you increase blood flow even if systemic blood pressure were lower. I guess you do not have the answer to the questions, but based on these studies and mechanisms, what should we be thinking about studying, forgetting about whether it is one patient, a controlled study. What is the mechanism that might prove most fruitful to treating or understanding a vascular component that may or may not exist with this disease.

**Dr. Anderson**: You are actually creating the transition from today's discussion and the major impact of our discussion tomorrow. That is, where is the relationship between blood pressure and flow? Where should we measure the blood pressure, in the brachial artery or in the last arteriole that enters the disc, for example.

# 19. REGULATION OF CEREBRAL BLOOD FLOW

GARY L. BAUMBACH, M.D.

As a neuropathologist, and at one time an ophthalmologist, I found the proceedings to be very stimulating, and I suspect that if I had not ended up in cerebral circulation looking at vascular mechanics and structure of cerebral blood vessels, that it would have been fun to have gotten into glaucoma, looking at effects of glaucoma on structure and function of the various parts of the eye.

I want to take just a minute to introduce my topic. Prior to my arrival in Venice I spent a fair bit of time thinking about how I was going to relate regulation of cerebral blood flow to the topic of glaucoma. During the course of the meeting, however, it became apparent that I really did not need to work at it very hard. As an extension of the central nervous system, the optic nerve and retina have several characteristics in common with other parts of the brain, including mechanisms that regulate blood flow. For example, it is likely that blood flow in retina and optic nerve is tightly autoregulated in much the same way as cerebral blood flow. So in my talk today I am going to use the concept of autoregulation as a springboard to discuss structural factors that may impair autoregulation of cerebral blood flow. The rationale for this approach is the consideration that dysfunction of autoregulation of blood flow in the optic disc may, at some level, contribute to damage from glaucoma.

In attempting to illustrate the concept of autoregulation (Fig. 1), I want to emphasize three points. First, within the range of autoregulation, cerebral blood vessels react or respond to changes in perfusion pressure by actively adjusting their diameters, thus vessels dilate in response to reductions in perfusion pressure and constrict in response to increases in pressure. Second, once outside the autoregulatory range, the vessels are no longer able to compensate, flow becomes pressure-dependent, and not infrequently tissue damage occurs. For example, reductions in perfusion pressure below the autoregulatory range may result in anoxic, hypoxic, or ischemic damage. Finally, critical reductions in perfusion pressure may come about either as a result of reductions in arterial pressure, but more importantly for the topic of this meeting, through increases in intracranial pressure. To my way of thinking, one might consider increases in intracranial pressure to be a counterpart to increased intraocular pressure.

Reductions in cerebral perfusion pressure become even more critical when the autoregulatory curve is shifted to the right (Fig. 2). An implication of this rightward shift is that cerebral vasodilatation is impaired. Another implication is that damage related to vascular insufficiency may occur with even smaller reductions in perfusion pressure. So let us now consider some of the changes in vascular structure that might contribute to impaired dilatation. These would include hypertrophy, reduced distensibility, and remodeling of the vessel wall (Fig. 3).

Hypertrophy of the vessel wall will result in impaired dilatation when the increased wall mass is forced inward and encroaches on the vascular lumen. Reductions in distensibility will produce impaired dilatation because of limitations that are imposed on the ability of the vessel wall to stretch in response to a given level of intravascular pressure. Remodeling is a relatively new concept that we have proposed as yet another mechanism of impaired cerebral vasodilatation. By remodeling we are referring to a reduction in external diameter. Reductions in external diameter would be expected to

*Optic Nerve in Glaucoma, pp. 283–299*
*edited by S.M. Drance*

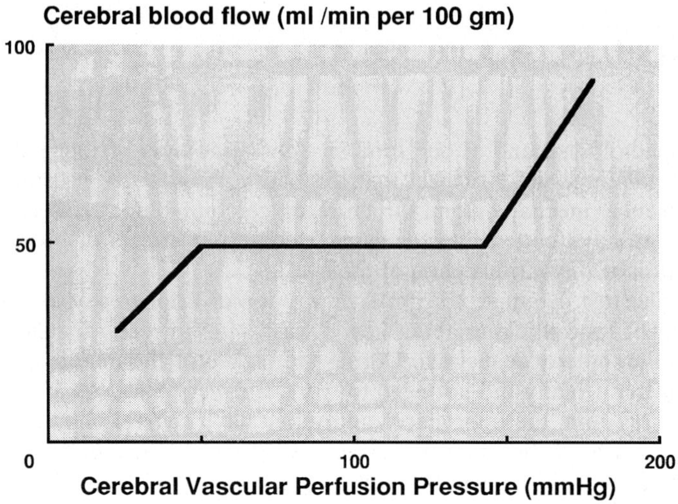


*Fig. 1.* Concept of cerebral blood flow autoregulation. Under usual conditions cerebral blood flow remains constant over a wide range of intravascular pressure and becomes pressure-dependent only at the extreme lower and upper ends of the pressure–flow relationship.

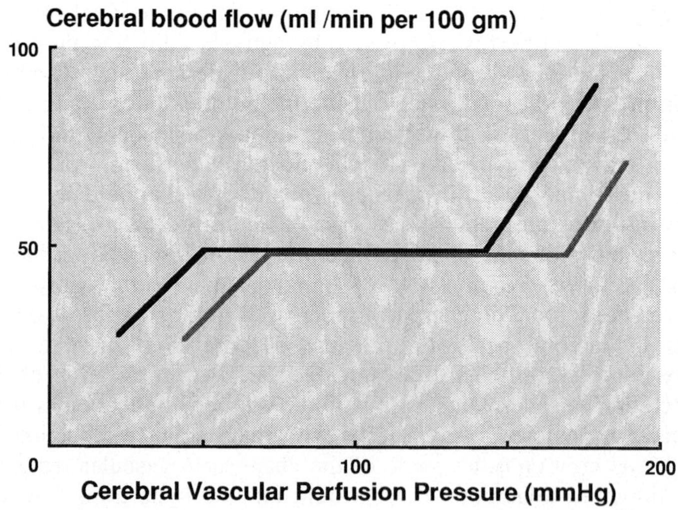


*Fig. 2.* Concept of rightward shift in cerebral blood flow autoregulation that often accompanies chronic hypertension.

result in impaired dilatation in much the same way as hypertrophy, *i.e.*, by forcing wall mass inward and producing encroachment on the vascular lumen.

I would now like to illustrate these changes more fully by showing you some of the findings from our studies of aging and chronic hypertension. The reason for considering these conditions together is the commonly held perception that the effects of chronic hypertension and vascular structure merely represent an acceleration of the ag-

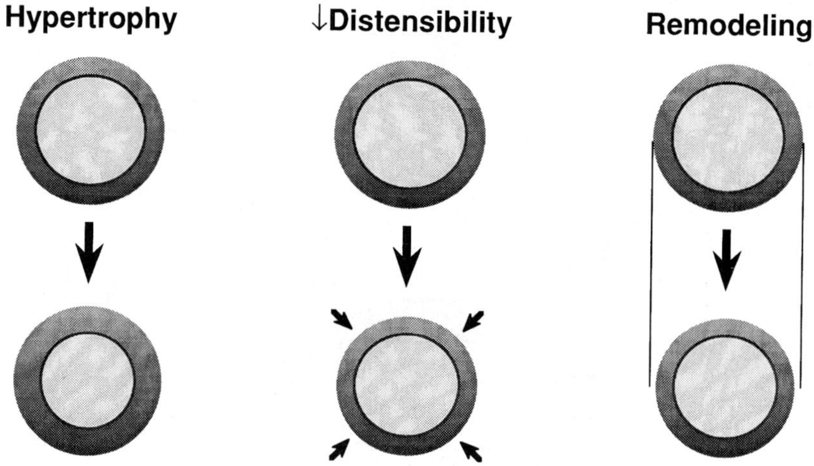


*Fig. 3.* Schematic representation of some of the factors that may contribute to impaired dilatation of cerebral blood vessels during chronic hypertension.

ing process. In our studies of aging we have used adult and aged Fisher rats, adult rats being nine to 12 months of age, and aged rats being 24 to 27 months old. In the studies of hypertension that I am going to present today we have used normotensive Wistar-Kyoto rats and stroke-prone spontaneously hypertensive rats.

The purpose of both of these studies was to examine vascular mechanics in pial arterioles. Measurements in pial arterioles include pressure, diameter, and cross-sectional area of the vessel wall. Because we are interested in wall structure as opposed to the effects of active changes in smooth muscle on the vessel wall, we do most of our measurements with the vessels during maximal dilatation with EDTA. In other words, we use the EDTA to remove smooth muscle tone.

Figure 4 shows the method that we use to measure pial arteriolar pressure. The brain is exposed through a craniotomy and artificial cerebrospinal fluid is continuously suffused over the brain to maintain physiological conditions. By using a micropipette attached to a servo-null pressure measuring system, we are able to measure pressure within exposed pial arterioles. This system has a couple of advantages. First, we are able to measure pressure in quite small blood vessels, down in the range of 20 to 30 μm. Secondly, this system is capable of giving us good measurements of pulse pressure in addition to mean pressure. We also measure diameter through this window using a videomicroscopy system.

To measure cross-sectional area of the vessel wall we use a histological preparation. The arteriole was fixed by suffusing gluteraldehyde over the cranial window, with the animal still alive, so that we were able to use the animal's blood pressure to keep the vessel distended during fixation. This is evidenced by the presence of blood cells and plasma within the lumen of the vessel. The vessel is nicely distended. To get cross-sectional area of the vessel wall we use a computer-assisted image analyzing system to trace the inner and outer edges of the wall.

These slides show these measurements of systemic arterial pressure and pial arteriolar pressure and diameter in adult and aged rats and normotensive and hyperten-

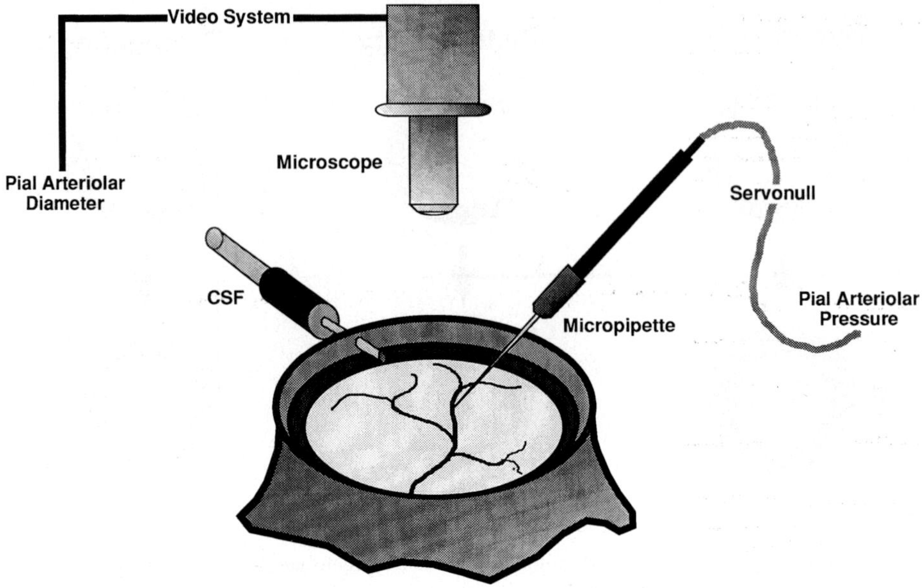


*Fig. 4.* Method used to measure pressure and diameter in pial arterioles. Pial arteriolar pressure was measured through a micropipette attached to a servo-null pressure measuring device.

sive rats. One of the points that I wanted to emphasize here is that, in contrast to the expected increases in both systemic and pial arteriolar pressures that we have in hypertensive rats, pressure in the aged rats was not increased, and if anything was maybe a little bit lower than in the adult group. And secondly, I want to point out the range of vessel diameters. These measurements were made before we removed vascular tone, so these vessels are in a baseline state, so to speak. In both our studies the vessels ranged between about 40 to 50 μm in diameter, so we are not really quite down to the 20-μm diameter that it sounds like we might expect to find in the eye, but we are getting there.

Now, what about the effects of aging and hypertension on wall mass? Figures 5 and 6 show measurements of cross-sectional area of the vessel wall in adult and aged rats (Fig. 5) and the normotensive and hypertensive rats (Fig. 6). We used cross-sectional area of the vessel wall as an indicator of wall mass. We found that hypertensive rats have a greater cross-sectional area than their normotensive counterparts. In contrast, with aging we found a reduction in cross-sectional area of the vessel wall. This was somewhat surprising to us, because we had anticipated that, if anything, aging would result in hypertrophy similar to chronic hypertension. If anything, we found the opposite result, so that whereas we have cerebral vascular hypertrophy in hypertension, we have atrophy with aging.

The following figures show measurements of pial arteriolar diameter taken at several different levels of pial arteriolar pressure in adult and aged (Fig. 7) and normotensive and hypertensive rats (Fig. 8). These measurements were made after the vessels were deactivated with EDTA, so we are now looking at the vessels in their maximally dilated state. I would also point out that pial arteriolar pressure is typically about half of systemic pressure, so that at 70 mmHg pial pressure, systemic pressure would be about 130 to 140 mmHg.

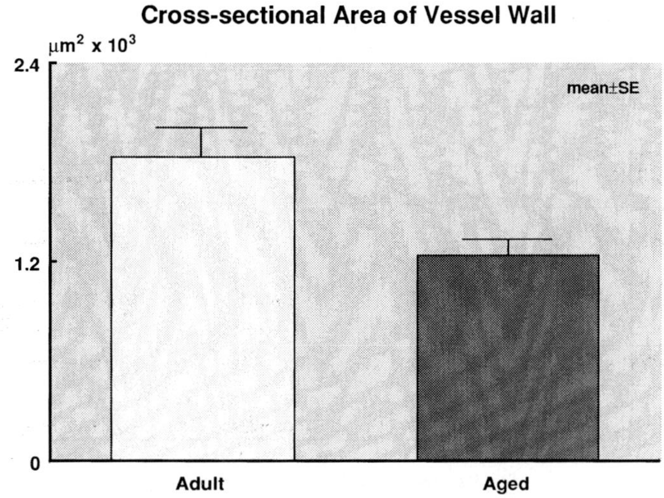


*Fig. 5.* Measurements of cross-sectional area of the vessel wall in pial arterioles in adult and aged Fischer rats.

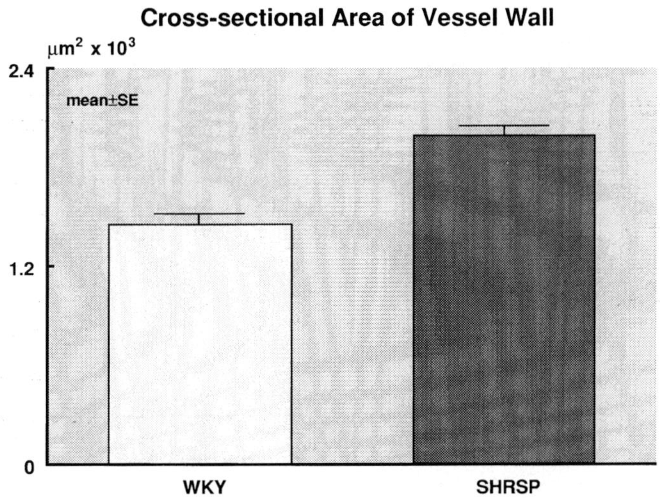


*Fig. 6.* Measurements of cross-sectional area of the vessel wall in pial arterioles in normotensive Wistar-Kyoto (WKY) and stroke-prone spontaneously hypertensive (SHRSP) rats.

The first thing we note here is that with reductions in pressure, the vessels react passively, that is diameter is dependent on pressure. In the aged group, at the higher levels of pressure, diameter was significantly less than in the adult group, whereas at lower pressure it looks as though the pressure diameter in the two groups converge. In hypertensive rats we also found a substantial reduction in diameter at the upper levels of the curve. In contrast to aged rats, however, we found that this difference in diameter be-

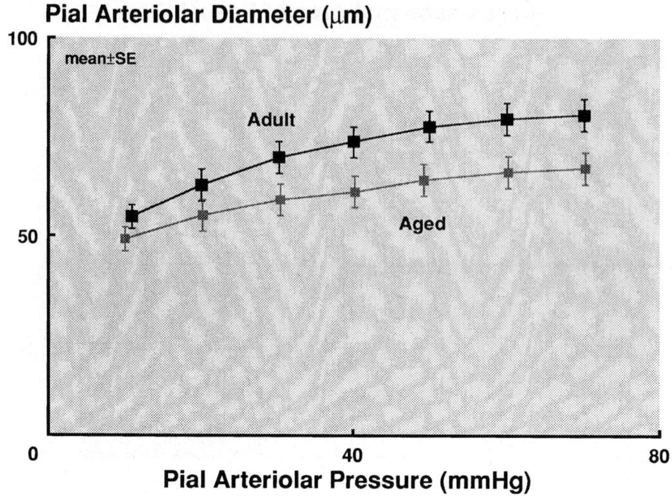


*Fig. 7.* Pressure–diameter relationships in pial arterioles in pial arterioles in adult and aged Fischer rats. Vascular smooth muscle was deactivated with EDTA.

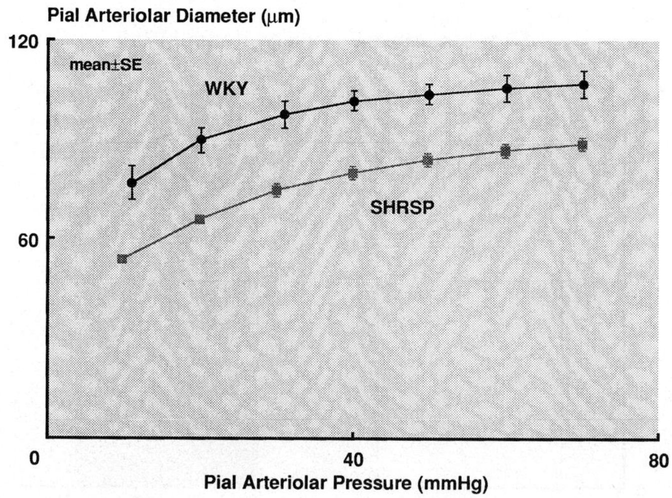


*Fig. 8.* Pressure–diameter relationships in pial arterioles in pial arterioles in normotensive Wistar-Kyoto (WKY) rats and stroke-prone spontaneously hypertensive (SHRSP) rats. Vascular smooth muscle was deactivated with EDTA.

tween the two groups is essentially maintained throughout, so that the pressure diameter curves in this case tend to parallel each other.

These are the stress–strain relationships in pial arterioles of aged and adult rats and normotensive and hypertensive rats. The stress–strain relationship is an indicator of vascular distensibility. The further the curve is shifted to the right, the more distensible the vessel. In aged rats, the stress–strain curve was shifted to the left of the curve in adult rats, which indicates that distensibility was reduced in the aged group. That is what we expected based on the previous findings in large arteries such as in basilar artery.

We expected that chronic hypertension would result in essentially the same shift as aging, but surprisingly we found that the stress–strain curve was actually shifted to the right in the hypertensive group relative to the normotensive group. Our initial response to this finding was skepticism, since at the time we did not have very much experience with the *in vivo* method we were using to examine vascular mechanics. In subsequent studies we not only demonstrated this same finding time and again in SHRSP, we have confirmed it using an *in vitro* method. But that still leaves us with an apparent paradox, that is an increase in arteriole distensibility despite hypertrophy of the vessel wall. This then brings me to the morphometric data that we generated in an effort to explain the paradox.

**Dr. Anderson**: Before you go on, I am not quite clear here. Were these vessels relaxed with EDTA, so you are looking at the residual elasticity of the wall without smooth muscle participation? And you manipulated the intravascular pressure after the animal was killed or something, you perfused it, or how did you do it?

**Dr. Baumbach**: That is correct. The pial arterioles were relaxed with EDTA. We also manipulated arteriole pressure while the animals were in their living state. This was accomplished using controlled hemorrhage in graded steps.

**Dr. Anderson**: And then perhaps you could answer for me whether EDTA enters the cell so that it actually changes intracellular calcium and binds it as well as extracellular, thereby aborting any kind of reactivity that the smooth muscles might have in the process.

**Dr. Baumbach**: I do not know that I can answer that directly. My perception, or my guess, would be that it must be doing something like that, because we went through great pains to demonstrate that these vessels had no vascular tone and were unable to respond to any constrictor stimuli.

**Dr. Zeimer**: One of the procedures that one needs to use when one wants to measure this stress–strain relationship, from what I understand, is preconditioning. In other words, you do not measure the first cycle of pressure, you first run a few cycles and then measure. Is that the procedure that was used in your experiment?

**Dr. Baumbach**: No, we did not. Examining vascular mechanics *in vitro* requires establishing a reproducible baseline since the vessel has been completely separated from its normal environment. Preconditioning the vessel by cycling intravascular pressure up and down accomplishes this goal. With an *in vivo* preparation, on the other hand, the vessel is supported in a normal way by the surrounding structure, making it easier to establish baseline conditions. For this reason, and because the rats do not easily tolerate large, rapid fluctuations in arteriole pressure, we did not attempt to precondition pial arterioles for *in vivo* studies.

At this point, I would like to share with you some of the morphometric data that we have used as a possible explanation for these shifts in distensibility. I am going to show you just the data from the aged study. To obtain a quantitative method of the composition of the vessel wall, we examined the wall ultrastructurally and used point-counting stereology to quantitate smooth muscle, elastin, collagen, basement membrane. These are measurements of cross-sectional area of these various components. The first thing you will notice is that pial arterioles in both adult and aged rats are composed primarily of smooth muscle on the order of 60 to 70% of the vessel wall is smooth muscle. The wall also contains small but significant amounts of elastin and basement membrane. What seems to be missing here is collagen. We did find collagen but in very small amounts, on the order of about 1%. This is a little different than for arterioles in other vascular beds say, in the mesentery, which were examined by Kurt Wiederhelm back in, I believe, the late '60s using a similar approach. Dr. Wiederhelm found as much as 20%, type III collagen in mesenteric arterioles. We incorporated basement membrane into our measurements of collagen because of our concern that it likely contributes to wall stiffness because it contains a fair amount of type IV collagen.

With aging we found that the cross-sectional area of smooth muscle was substantially reduced, and there was also a reduction in the amount of elastin. You can not see collagen down here, but it really did not change much. Basement membrane stayed about the same or maybe tended to increase very slightly. Now, this still does not tell us very much about the possible relationship between composition of the vessel wall and distensibility. The way I have put that together is to look at the ratio of non-distensible components to distensible components in the vessel wall. We have calculated this ratio several different ways (Fig. 9).

To begin with the traditional approach in large arteries has been to calculate the ratio using just collagen and elastin, with the assumption that smooth muscle probably does not contribute much to distensibility when it is completely relaxed. Looking at the ratio of collagen to elastin, we find that it was increased in the aged rats (Fig. 9). However, as I indicated earlier there really is not very much collagen in pial arterioles. Looking at other components in the wall that might be added to collagen, we chose basement membrane because it does contain a lot of type IV collagen. With the addition of basement membrane, the ratio of non-distensible to distensible components is still increased (Fig. 9). Finally, it really did not seem reasonable to leave out smooth muscle, since it composes so much of the wall. Because smooth muscle has elastic modulus similar to elastin, we added it to the bottom of our equation. Again, the ratio of non-distensible to distensible components was still increased in the aged group (Fig. 9). So regardless of how it was calculated we found a relative increase in non-distensible components in pial arterioles of aged rats. Although while that may not necessarily be the cause of the reduction in distensibility, at least the ratio is going in the right direction to account for that.

**Dr. Zeimer**: You showed that in aged rats there is an increased ratio of collagen to elastin. Now, where is the change, look at Figure 9 on the left, it looks like you have a drastic change in the elastin. So what you are saying is, the amount of elastin was half, or dramatically reduced, and the collagen did not change.

**Dr. Baumbach**: Right, but it is questionable whether collagen changes very much, because there was so little begin with.

**Dr. Zeimer**: Well, but then, you have a ratio, so you are not dividing by zero.

**Dr. Baumbach**: No, we are not, so maybe I am overemphasizing the small amount of collagen. Actually the elastic modulus of collagen is at least tenfold that of elastin,

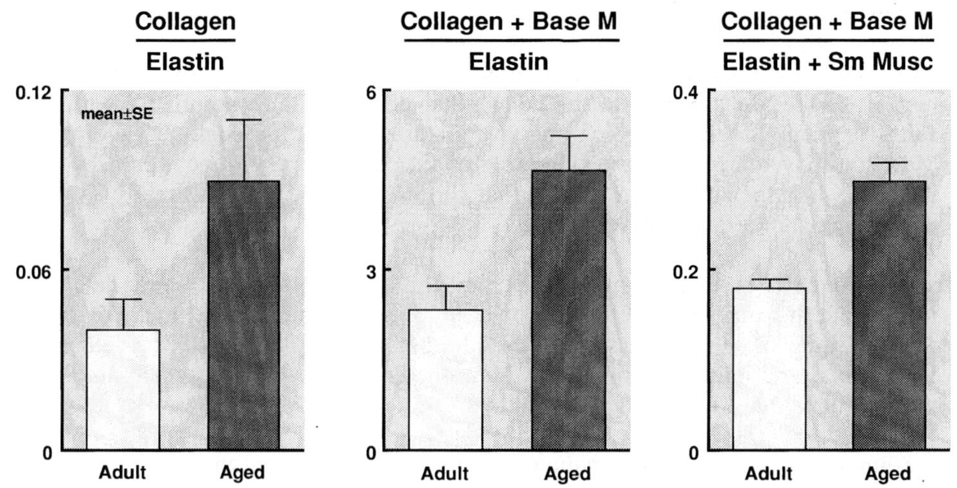


*Fig. 9.* Ratio of non-distensible to distensible components in pial arterioles in adult and aged Fischer rats. To calculate the ratio, collagen and basement membrane (Base M) were considered to be relatively non-distensible and elastin and smooth muscle (Sm Musc) were considered to be distensible.

so it would only take about a tenth as much collagen to counteract the changes of elastin.

At this point, I want to mention our related findings in hypertensive rats. With chronic hypertension we found essentially the opposite, that hypertrophy in the vessel wall was produced primarily by an increase in smooth muscle. We also found a small increase in the amount of elastin, whereas basement membrane stayed about the same. Thus, the ratio of non-distensible to distensible components in pial arterioles was reduced in SHRSP, so it also was going in the right direction to account for the increase in arteriole distensibility that we found.

**Dr. Zeimer**: Can I interrupt you again? You said that in hypertension you found an increase in elastin. Is there any evidence anywhere else where you have creation of elastin in an adult rat, or was the hypertension at an age where elastin was still being formed?

**Dr. Baumbach**: That is a good question. We do not have data to support or refute that possibility.

**Dr. Quigley**: You are looking at elastin amounts by stereology. Can you tell us how you stained the elastin and by EM were you looking at only alpha-elastin or were you looking at the microfibrillar component as well?

**Dr. Baumbach**: We did not try and separate out the microfibrillar component. We did stain the sections with phosphotungstic acid to bring out the elastin component.

**Dr. Quigley**: So this is light microscopy...

**Dr. Baumbach**: No, no, this is electron microscopy.

**Dr. Quigley**: I ask because tannic acid by EM is a way of seeing the alpha-elastin a little better. But in an aging study we did, in the connective tissue, not arteries, in the optic nerve, the younger animal has about the same amount of microfibrillar component. It is the alpha-elastin in the center that becomes more prominent with time. But if I were to guess I think the overall area in our measurements, and John Morrison may remember better, the area of the microfibrillar zone would be about the same. It is the stuff in the middle that sort of changed, so it was really a qualitative change, not a quantitative change.

**Dr. Baumbach**: Yes, that is a good point, and it might be worth at a future date trying to separate this out. We had thought of trying to apply biochemical methods to start making some of those assessments, but the amount of tissue that we are working with in pial arterioles is so small that I am uncomfortable with not being able to see the structures that I am trying to quantitate.

**Dr. Zeimer**: I do not want to be redundant, but if we believe that the viscoelastic property of connective tissue is important in glaucoma, it would be crucial if you could show if there is an example somewhere in the body that you could have an induced change in elastin. That would be very important, because I fail to see that in literature. So, what do you know about that? Do you have any examples? Is that something that could be expected, that you have production of elastin in the adult animal?

**Dr. Baumbach**: I have done some literature searches looking at that question, at least in a peripheral way, and I was never really able to come up with any satisfactory evidence of that, at least in the models of hypertension that we were looking at.

So, to summarize the findings so far, we found with aging that pial arterioles underwent atrophy, became less distensible, whereas with chronic hypertension, at least in SHRSP rats, the vessel wall developed hypertrophy and became more distensible. One might think that chronic hypertension could be considered an antidote to aging, and that it might be a good thing to be a little hypertensive as one gets older, at least as far as the cerebral arterioles are concerned because cerebral vascular changes during aging and chronic hypertension might cancel each other out. However, I do not think that would necessarily be the case, and to explain my reasoning for that I need to go back and consider one more time the pressure diameter relationships in the hypertensive and normotensive rats.

Again, we found that during maximal dilation diameter of pial arterioles in SHRSP rats was reduced at levels of arteriorlar pressure. When we initially considered this finding we assumed that the explanation involved both hypertrophy and reduced distensibility of the vessel wall. When we realized, however, that distensibiity of cerebral arterioles is increased in SHRSP rats, we wondered wether hypertrophy alone was enough to account for this much reduction in diameter. By thinking about it this way, we had a hypothesis to test, that is if the reduction in internal diameter is due only to hypertrophy of the vessel wall, then external diameter of these vessels should be the same in WKY and SHRSP rats (Fig. 10).

There are two ways of visualizing this hypothesis. To test the hypothesis we went back to the drawing board and obtained measurements of external diameter as well as internal diameter during maximal dilatation. Here we have internal diameter and external diameter, in WKY and SHRSP rats. These vessels were maximally dilated and the measurements were performed at 70 mmHg of pial arteriolar pressure. As we found previously, internal diameter was significantly reduced. In addition exter-

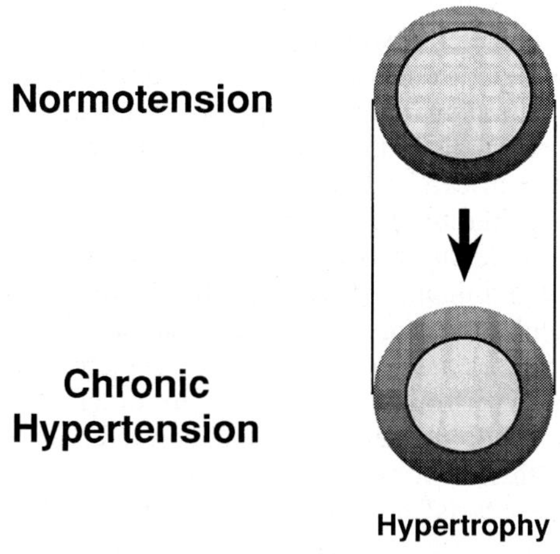


*Fig. 10.* Concept of reduced internal diameter of cerebral arterioles by hypertrophy only.

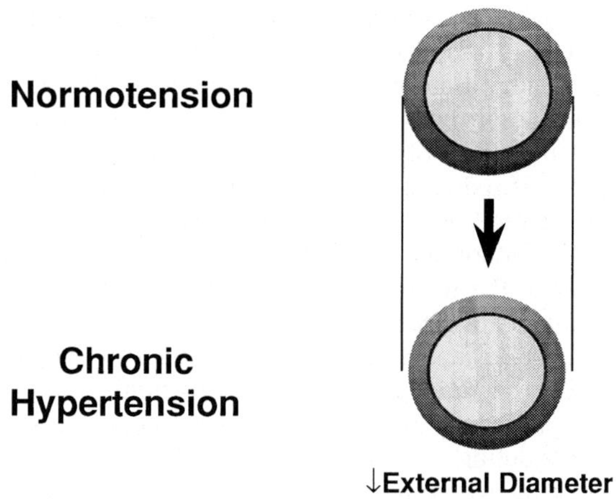


*Fig. 11.* Concept of cerebral vascular remodeling in chronic hypertension.

nal diameter also was reduced. Thus, hypertrophy is not the only factor producing reductions in internal diameter; internal diameter is also decreased by reductions in external diameter. We refer to the reduction in external diameter as remodeling (Fig. 11). By remodeling we mean that the components in the vessel wall have rearranged themselves in such a way as to literally shrink the vessels to a smaller fundamental diameter. In other words, it would not be necessary to have a change in the quantity of the components in the vessel wall. They may simply rearrange themselves to make the vessel smaller.

Just to summarize then, we have not only hypertrophy in pial arterioles during chronic hypertension, but also remodeling. We thought that it was important to separate the contributions of these two processes to the overall reduction in internal diameter that occurred in these arterioles. By using our measurements from normotensive and hypertensive rats, and by making some basic assumptions, we were able to calculate internal diameter assuming only hypertrophy versus internal diameter assuming only remodeling. It turns out that hypertrophy accounts for only about 30% of the total reduction in internal diameter, whereas remodeling accounts for about 70%. Thus, remodeling is the predominant process that contributes to reduction in internal diameter of cerebral arterioles in SHRSP rats.

At this point I would like to change the focus somewhat to consider determinants of hypertrophy and remodeling. Most of our effort in this area, at least until recently, has been focused on determinants of hypertrophy. Possible determinants of hypertrophy include intravascular pressure, neurohumoral factors, and genetic factors. Of these, neurohumoral factors and in particular sympathetic nerves, are known to play an important role in hypertrophy of cerebral arterioles. The role of intravascular pressure, on the other hand, has been more difficult to ascertain. I believe that one of the reasons for this is that most of the studies in the past have used pharmacological methods to manipulate arterial pressure. One of the problems with pharmacological methods is that they affect factors other than pressure, including neurohumoral factors. Thus, it is difficult to interpret the findings of those studies.

We used two different approaches to address this question. The first approach was to place a clip on one carotid artery in WKY and SHRSP rats to completely occlude the lumen. To eliminate neural effects we cut both sympathetic nerves. This procedure was performed when the animals were four weeks of age. We then studied the animals at about 10 to 12 months of age, so that the clip had been in place for about nine to 10 months. At that time we measured pressure, diameter, and cross-sectional area in pial arterioles from both sides of the brain using bilateral craniotomies. So that we have, in effect, a control situation within each animal.

We anticipated that if reductions in pressure contributed to hypertrophy or remodeling, those changes would be reduced on the side with the clip, whereas if pressure were not particularly important, then the changes might be the same on the two sides. So let us look at the results. This is the change in cross-sectional area of the vessel wall and change in external diameter in pial arterioles from the sham and clipped sides of the brain in SHRSP rats. Focusing first on just the sham operated side, the cross-sectional area of pial arterioles was significantly increased, and external diameter was significantly reduced, so that we simply reconfirmed that there is hypertrophy and remodeling.

With carotid clipping we were able to prevent the increase in wall mass, so we prevented hypertrophy. Clipping did not, however, prevent the reduction in external diameter. This then suggests that pressure may play a role in hypertrophy of the vessel wall, but not in remodeling. Another interesting aspect of this study was that the correlation between individual measurements of cross-sectional area of the vessel wall and pulse pressure was very good, in contrast to mean pressure in which there was essentially no correlation. This finding suggests that pulse pressure may be playing a more important role than mean pressure in the development of hypertrophy.

This then raised another question, that is would it be possible to produce hypertrophy of pial arterioles with an increase in mean pressure alone? To answer this question we created an AV fistula in Sprague-Dawley rats by creating a fistula between the descending aorta and the inferior vena cava. The rats also underwent unilateral carotid clipping so that we could compare arterioles from the two sides. We then studied the rats at six months of age. The rationale for the AV fistula was that we anticipated it would result in an increase in systolic pressure and at the same time a decrease in diastolic pressure. Because pulse pressure is equal to the difference between systolic and diastolic pressure and mean pressure is equal to diastolic pressure plus one-third of pulse pressure, it seemed likely that the AV fistula would result in an increase in pulse pressure without having much effect on mean pressure. So now let's look at the effects of AV fistula.

To begin with the AV fistula had essentially no effect whatsoever on systemic mean pressure. Furthermore, the AV fistula had essentially no effect on mean pressure in arterioles from the sham operated side. In contrast, pulse pressure was significantly greater in sham arterioles in the AV fistula rats than in the control rats. Thus, the AV fistula essentially accomplished our goal of increasing pulse pressure without increasing mean pressure. The reason for the carotid clip now becomes apparent. Clipping had a small, but minimal, effect on mean pressure, but normalized pulse pressure in AV fistula rats. Now, what effect did AV fistula have on cross-sectional area?

Beginning again with sham arterioles, the AV fistula resulted in an increase in cross-sectional area of the vessel wall, so it produced hypertrophy. Carotid clipping effectively prevented the development of hypertrophy. To summarize these data we found that AV fistula produced hypertrophy of pial arterioles in association with an increase in pial arteriolar pulse pressure but not mean pressure.

Carotid clipping substantially reduced the degree of hypertrophy, produced by AV fisula and effectively normalized pial pulse pressure. We believe that these findings provide substantial evidence for the concept that pulse pressure may, indeed, be an important determinant of cerebrovascular hypertrophy in chronic hypertension. Also, if we go back and think about the effects of carotid clipping in SHRSP rats, the fact that we were able to prevent hypertrophy with a clip in a genetic model of chronic hypertension would suggest that, at least in that model, genetic factors are not an important determinant of hypertrophy of pial arterioles.

So, in closing, I want to re-emphasize two points. First, remodeling of the vessel wall is a change in vascular structure that in addition to hypertrophy may contribute to impaired autoregulation of cerebral blood flow in chronic hypertension. I am emphasizing this point because we believe that the determinants of remodeling and hypertrophy are not the same.

The second point is that we now have good evidence that pulse pressure may be an important determinant of cerebrovascular hypertrophy. This idea is particularly appealing to us because pulse pressure is a dynamic component of arterial pressure, in contrast to mean pressure which is a static component. Thus the relationship between arterial pressure and vascular hypertrophy may depend to a greater extent on the dynamic components of pressure than on the static components.

**Dr. Siesjö**: I have lost touch with this area, so I hope you can enlighten me on two aspects of your lecture. The first one is, how representative of the surface vessels are the intraparenchymal vessels?

**Dr. Baumbach**: That is a question that comes up all the time. Usually in reviews of our manuscripts, so I should have a pretty good answer for you. We think that there is good evidence that the pial arterioles are representative of what is going on intraparenchymally. When we look at changes in diameter through a closed window as well as through an open window, in response to various stimuli that alter cerebral blood flow, we see comparable changes in diameter going in the appropriate direction.

**Dr. Siesjö**: My second question is, what is the relationship between the reactivity you see of the vessels in terms of distensibility and dilatation to the changes in nutritional blood flow that you have. That is to say, if you have an aged animal or if you have a hypertensive animal, how would the cells react to a given stimulus like a 5-mm change in $pCO_2$. What would be their maximal capacity when you raise the $CO_2$ tension, say, to 80, 90, etc.

**Dr. Baumbach**: With a 5% change in $CO_2$ we see small but significant increases in cerebral blood flow, and also increases in vessel diameter of the pial arterioles. We have never done the calculations to try and determine whether the change in diameter is representative of the change in flow, but I believe Herman Kontos has. He found that the changes in diameter and blood flow are comparable when corrected for certain factors. In terms of very high levels of $CO_2$ which are thought to produce maximal dilatation, there are large increases in blood flow, on the order of two- to three-fold.

**Dr. Siesjö**: Perhaps I did not express myself ideally. What I am really asking is that at the time when I knew something about cerebral blood flow, Murray Harper's series resistance hypothesis was discussed a lot. And what that says is that if you have a constriction upstream in the arterial tree by hypertrophy or by sympathetic innervation, then you can get a dilatation downstream compensating for this, so that the blood flow is unchanged. So what I am asking about is, how would the vascular system in an aged animal, or in a hypertensive animal, be able to respond in terms of blood flow changes, to a given stimulus like an increase in metabolism or an increase in $CO_2$.

**Dr. Baumbach**: It is a little easier for me to answer in terms of chronic hypertension, because there are more data available. The ability of cerebral vessels to respond to dilator stimuli in chronic hypertension is impaired, so that with challenges to $CO_2$ or hypoxia, the hypertensive animal is unable to respond as fully as normotensive animals. Effect of aging, on the other hand, has been a little more difficult to sort out. I think there are some data in the literature that would suggest that maximal dilatation is somewhat impaired with aging, but there is also a body of literature that does not support that. And it is not all that easy to compare our results from aging and chronic hypertension, even though I tried to do it in this presentation, except to say that the only factor in aged rate that was contributing to impaired dilatation of pial arterioles was a reduction in distensibility. We did not find remodeling or hypertrophy with aging. So, it may not be that surprising that with aging cerebral vessel responses are not as impaired as with chronic hypertension.

**Dr. Anderson**: I think that it may be relevant here to point out that when we talk about impaired autoregulation, we have to think in terms of two different things. The thing that you have been studying is the maximum dilatation that can be achieved when you give an extreme stimulus. "Impaired autoregulation" is truncating the curve of autoregulation, seeing where it must stop, because it has reached the maximum dilatation it can. That is different from impairment as a reduced amount of response per amount of challenge, which might be that with a certain degree with which carbon dioxide changes, there may be a certain question of response. I point this out now because later in the morning I know we are going to be talking about this distinction in autoregulation.

Secondly, when you say that hypertensive animals have a lowered autoregulatory response, I guess you mean that with prolonged hypertension, sclerosis develops, and this prevents dilation when the smooth muscle relaxes. But early on in hypertension it might be different. It might be a fact that the vessel is in a contracted state by virtue of either producing the hypertension, or in response to hypertension as an autoregulatory response, and that when some other challenge comes along that calls for dilation, there may be a greater dynamic range for dilation, and in one sense there is an augmented autoregulatory response. In any event, the sense in which we talk about impaired or augmented autoregulatory response is important in the discussion, and I wanted to bring that out at this point.

**Dr. Zeimer**: Before the hypertrophy, we know the wall of the vessel is viscoelastic, and it means that the tissue can elongate but it also can assume a smaller diameter under a reverse stress. Now, if the smooth muscle was constantly constricted, that could induce a reduction in the diameter. In other words, the connective tissue will reorganize to a smaller diameter and also be less elastic.

The one kidney-one clip model of renal hypertension is supposedly a low renin angiotensin model of hypertension, then that might fit with the idea that it is angiotensin that is contributing to remodeling. And we do have studies planned to further explore that possibility. We are not the only ones to find this. Subsequent to our studies Mike Mulvaney's group has been looking at this, actually in human hypertension using their subcutaneous arterial biopsies. They found in hypertensive patients a reduction in diameter but not significant hypertrophy, and at least at this point in time they are attributing that to remodeling. I think that as we go along we may find other evidence to support that this is a more general phenomenon.

**Dr. Kaufman**: You mentioned the importance of pulse pressure in one component of the changes. Though it is sloppy we do have a technique for measuring pulse pressure, at least in the retinal circulation in the human eye, it is called ophthalmodynamometry. And I was just wondering, do we know anything about the pulse pressure in, for instance, normal-tension glaucoma, or hypertensive glaucoma, as compared to, say, age-matched people without that disease? Any of the neuro-ophthalmologist people know anything about that here? Anybody?

**Dr. Baumbach**: You would not get the answers from me.

**Dr. Drance**: There are better ways than ophthalmodynamometry to measure the pulse pressure, namely various oscillographic techniques. I think 20 years ago we showed with ophthalmodynamography that in fact pulse pressures were reduced in patients. Not only was the blood pressure reduced but also the pulse pressures were reduced in patients with normal-tension glaucoma, compared to age-matched normals. Not everybody who had normal-tension glaucoma had this phenomenon.

**Dr. Hoffman**: When you have remodeling does that mean there is hypertrophy, or is there hyperplasia? In other words, do you have more smooth muscle cells or do you have larger ones? And if you have more, what can you say about the response of the vessel to a given level of sympathetic tone? Is the vessel smaller for a given level of sympathetic tone if it is hypertrophic with more cells? Do you have any information?

**Dr. Anderson**: Before you answer, let me ask also if the changes are exclusively cellular, or is there also remodeling of extracellular substance.

**Dr. Baumbach**: First of all, I probably did not make it completely clear, but I would separate the remodeling process from hypertrophy, be it from hypertrophy of individual smooth muscle cells or from hyperplasia and increased numbers of smooth muscle. Now, in thinking about hypertrophy, whether or not you get an increased response to a given constrictor stimulus, such as an increase in sympathetic drive, I think that there is good evidence that you do, but maybe not for the reasons that you would think. I think in the early stages of hypertension research the perception was that the reductions in diameter were probably due to a hypersensitivity or a hyperreactivity of smooth muscle to a given stimulus. Then Dr. Bjorn Folkow came along and proposed the idea that hypertrophy of the vessel wall, being a structural change, could in and of itself account for the smaller diameters, without having to impose the additional constraint that the smooth muscle is more reactive. The rationale for this is that by displacing medial smooth muscle inward toward the lumen, a given amount of shortening of smooth muscle would have a greater effect on diameter than when it was in its normal position. So I think that, depending on how you look at the question, you would say that yes, there is increased reactivity with an increase in smooth muscle mass, but that does not necessarily indicate that there is an increased sensitivity or hyperreactivity of smooth muscle cells *per se*. I would also point out, though, that you can displace the smooth muscle inward with remodeling by just making the vessel smaller, and this could have the same impact as hypertrophy on giving a greater reduction in diameter with a given amount of smooth muscle shortening.

**Dr. Anderson**: If I might, I am curious to know about this distinction you make between remodeling and the hypertrophy. If one is dealing with paralyzed vessels from the point of view of smooth muscle, you are looking at a flaccid wall, which has a certain elastic property. One could, by adjusting the pressure, adjust what the outside diameter of the vessel is. If you adjust the pressure level in both the normal and the hypertensive, you may come upon a pressure level at which the external diameter was the same in both. Then it would look as if it was all hypertrophy, and no sclerosis or restriction. I wonder how artificial this distinction is, because at one pressure level it would look one way, at a different pressure level another.

**Dr. Baumbach**: That is a good point, and we have actually looked at our pressure diameter relationships, not only in terms of internal diameter but external diameter. We find that the decrease in external diameter in chronic hypertension is retained at all levels of intravascular pressures even at very low pressures of 5 to 10 mmHg.

**Dr. Quigley**: I do not know whether it is appropriate now or whether Doug is going to cover this, but it seems to me that if we are going to try to draw some parallel or relevance of what you are talking about to glaucoma, it may be what we need to know is if a change in intracranial pressure affects cerebral blood flow, or arteriolar diameter. One of the things we talk about with glaucoma is the intraocular pressure, and if it is transmitted as a direct tissue effect, then in the retina, at least, it might be comparable to what happens in the cerebral arteries. In the area of the optic nerve where we think some of the damage happens, the vessels are subjected actually to some transmural pressure differences. Has anybody looked at spontaneously cerebrally hypertensive animals, or induced hypertension?

**Dr. Baumbach**: Yes, there actually have been studies looking at effects of acutely changing intracranial pressure on blood flow. And they found that you still have good autoregulation of blood flow during substantial increases in intracranial pressure. In terms of measuring diameters under those conditions, off the top of my head I do not know of any study, but I would be surprised if somebody has not looked at that through a closed window model.

**Dr. Quigley**: Yes, you would have to have a closed window model to have a reservoir high enough, or put it under mercury or something...something really dense.

**Dr. Baumbach**: Yes, very very high. That is true, that is a thought. But the point is well taken, and I was wishing on the plane flight over here that I had done more searching in the neurosurgical literature, looking at effects of raised intracranial pressure, and into overall effects on brain tissue.

**Dr. Siesjö**: Just a very quick comment. From the beginning of my scientific career I remember that when we lowered the arterial mean blood pressure in steps or would increase the CSF intracranial pressure in steps, then you have a breakdown of homeostasis at the same perfusion pressure, which is about 30 mmHg. So you can come up to very high intracranial pressures before you really have a critical lowering of blood flow.

**Dr. Quigley**: If Dr. Alm were prone to smiling he should be smiling, because in the eye it is exactly the same level. A perfusion pressure of about 25 mmHg or 40 $cmH_2O$ is where blood flow nutritionally measured by either antipyrine or deoxyglucose starts to fall off in the retina and in the optic nerve.

**Dr. Alm**: Yes, you have a difference between the brain and the eye, because at least in acute experiments in the brain, if you increase intracranial pressure you have an increase also in blood flow, in blood pressure, which you do not see in the eye.

# 20. ASPECTS OF VASCULAR PHARMACOLOGY RELATED TO OCULAR BLOOD FLOW

S.Z. LANGER, M.D.

First of all, I would like to discuss sympathetic neurotransmission in vascular smooth muscle. Secondly, the molecular biology and the physiological role of alpha and beta adrenoceptor subtypes. Then the pharmacological characteristics of betaxolol, the vasodilating properties of betaxolol, and the probable mechanism for this effect.

A noradrenergic varicosity is the site of release of the neurotransmitter norepinephrine. Two cotransmitters are ATP and neuropeptide Y, but they are not the only ones. In many varicosities that release norepinephrine as a transmitter, one cotransmitter has been established, and it usually contributes partly to postsynaptic responses, like P2 receptors when ATP is the transmitter. The adrenoceptors responsible for vasoconstriction are mainly the alpha-1 adrenoceptor, which is the preferentially innervated adrenoceptor, and sometimes the alpha-2. As you will see from both molecular biology and pharmacology, there are several subtypes of alpha-1 and alpha-2 adrenoceptors. Neuropeptide Y is in some cases also a cotransmitter. The possible role of cotransmitters, and particularly neuropeptides, has been studied in some tissues of several species, and in other ones the question remains open. We know among the cotransmitters, first of all that epinephrine can be coreleased with norepinephrine. Because epinephrine is in the circulation, it can be taken up because it is a substrate for the neuronal uptake mechanism, and it can be released again along with norepinephrine. I mentioned already neuropeptide Y, which has vasoconstrictor properties as a cotransmitter. Galanine is in some noradrenergic nerves, particularly in the dog, and for instance, is well established in the pancreas. ATP is in many vascular beds, and enkephalins, particularly in the adrenal medulla. The possible role of cotransmitters in noradrenergic neurotransmission may come up again in the discussion.

I would like now to move on to receptor subtypes, and there are three main techniques for the identification of receptor subtypes: First of all, and historically the physiological responses in isolated tissues and whole animals. Secondly, ligand binding in membrane preparations. And more recently, molecular biology techniques. As you will see, molecular biology has provided us with the cloning of a number of receptors that exceed the subtypes that we have characterized functionally. One of the challenges of the pharmacologists today is to establish location and function of some of these newly cloned receptor subtypes.

Now, just to review the response that follows the activation of a receptor. Many of those in the adrenergic system are G protein linked. There is an amplifier and a second messenger that will act on a target protein to produce a response at the cellular level. As you well know, all three beta adrenoceptors are linked to cyclic AMP production, and on the other hand, the alpha-1 adrenoceptors are linked to the production of $IP_3$ and diacylglycerol.

Now, let us go back to our noradrenergic nerve terminal and the receptors, and we will concentrate on the alpha and beta adrenoceptor subtypes. The first adrenoceptor to be cloned was the beta-2 adrenoceptor, and that was the work of Lefkovitz. We have seen several examples during the last two days. This was the beginning of a series of cloning of adrenoceptor subtypes, in the alpha-1, alpha-2, and the beta receptor fami-

*Optic Nerve in Glaucoma, pp. 301–310*
*edited by S.M. Drance*

lies. The alpha-1 adrenoceptors, there are at least three that have been cloned: The alpha-1b, the alpha-1c, and the alpha-1d. They all have seven transmembrane domains. It is interesting that the alpha-1a is missing, because it has been described pharmacologically, but it has not been cloned. It is possible that the cloned alpha-1b receptor corresponds to the pharmacology of the alpha-1a. There is in press a paper showing that the alpha-1c receptor is the one present in the human prostate, which has important implications for the therapy of the benign hypertrophy of the prostate. Phenylephrine and other alpha-1 adrenoceptor agonists are used in ophthalmology, but they are not sufficiently selective compounds to separate and characterize the subtypes at the level of the pharmacology. The alpha-2 adrenoceptor subtypes, which were in '74 a single class and defined as the presynaptic release modulating receptors, are now constituted of four subtypes. They are present in different tissues like human platelets for the alpha-2a, neonatal rat lung for the alpha-2b, opossum kidney for the alpha-2c, and the bovine pineal for the alpha-2d. Of course, there is an interest in this area because some of the alpha-2 agonists like clonidine and derivatives of clonidine, decrease intraocular pressure. The human alpha-2 adrenoceptors that are cloned, sequenced, and the chromosomal localization determined, correspond to the alpha-2c10, the alpha-2c4, and the alpha-2c2, which correspond to the a, b, and c subtypes of alpha-2 adrenoceptors.

So we move now to the beta receptor and there are three adrenoceptor subtypes. They all have been cloned. They are all linked to cyclic AMP production. They are all G protein linked, and they possess seven transmembrane domains, and there are selective antagonists that can define the beta-1 and the beta-2 subtypes, but we do not possess yet selective compounds that can define pharmacologically the beta-3 subtype, which so far is called an atypical beta adrenoceptor, and among other places, it is present in adipose tissue. I would like to point out that in a publication in TIPS, which is a sort of a catalog of all the receptor subtypes, betaxolol is included as a reference compound for the selective beta-1 adrenoceptor antagonist.

Now, if we recapitulate, historically the adrenoceptors were first divided in alpha and beta in 1948 by Alquist. The alpha-1 and alpha-2 subclassification came in the early '70s with the discovery of presynaptic receptors. 1977 was the year when beta-1 and beta-2 receptors were defined, and from the contribution of molecular biology and receptor binding, we are now in possession of three subtypes of alpha-1; four subtypes of alpha-2 adrenoceptors; and three subtypes of beta adrenoceptors. So the challenge, as I was saying, is to establish the physiological significance and to produce the pharmacological characterization of these multiple receptor subtypes. In other words, to establish location and function and, in these tasks, the medicinal chemist who has to provide the tools of selective agonists and antagonists, has a very important role. This is why some of these developments are expected to take place in the framework of the pharmaceutical industry research. Of course, one can argue that not all subtypes are targets for drug discovery of agents that will have a therapeutic interest, but many of them.

So, to go to function, and to go back to the noradrenergic varicosity, I would just like to spend a few minutes on the presynaptic receptor sites. First of all, the alpha-2 adrenoreceptors, which are acted upon by norepinephrine released during nerve stimulation. The norepinephrine modulates its own release by acting on alpha-2 adrenoceptors on the nerve terminal of the varicosity to inhibit norepinephrine release. This negative feedback mechanism is not restricted only to norepinephrine, but has been subsequently described for other neurotransmitters. There is for norepinephrine also a positive feedback mechanism, which is mediated by beta-2 adrenoceptors, where epinephrine is more potent than norepinephrine. Activation of these facilitatory presynaptic mechanisms results in an enhancement of the release of the neurotransmitter upon arrival of the depolarization stimulus. There is a sodium-dependent active transport of released norepinephrine from the synaptic cleft back into the varicosity. It represents the main physiological mechanism for inactivation of the released neurotransmitter. It has been cloned recently: it is a protein of 12 transmembrane domains.

Now on to the beta adrenoceptor antagonists. Among the beta-1 selective compounds are betaxolol, atenolol, metoprolol. Among the non-selective compounds, blocking both beta-1 and beta-2 adrenoceptors, are propranolol, timolol, and pindolol.

Betaxolol was synthesized in our laboratories in Paris, and developed for its antihypertensive properties through the oral route. It is now marketed in most countries, including the U.S., for hypertension, and in the late '70s we were fortunate that Alcon Laboratories decided to develop and advance this compound for the treatment of glaucoma because of its properties on intraocular pressure and its other characteristics.

What are the characteristics of betaxolol. First of all, if one looks at it selectivity, as determined by the pA2, which is a measure of receptor antagonism, the higher the pA2, the more potent the compound in blocking the receptor. To compare selectivity we used guinea pig atria, which is a model for beta-1 receptors, and guinea pig tracheal chain, which is a model for beta-2 receptors. Compounds like pindolol or propranolol are equally potent in blocking both subtypes, they are not selective. Compounds like betaxolol have 120-fold selectivity, being more potent in blocking the beta-1 than the beta-2 adrenoceptors. This can be shown also in terms of KD values, comparing the human lung with the guinea pig lung. There is an excellent correlation, which shows the predictability of animal tissues to the human tissue for betaxolol and other beta-blocking agents.

Betaxolol is a competitive antagonist, like other beta blockers, and the pA2 value is 8.9. Another important property of beta adrenoceptor antagonist is the intrinsic activity, namely that some beta adrenoceptor antagonists are able to stimulate the receptor before they produce the blockade. This can be measured by tachycardic effect or an increase in ionotropic properties. Betaxolol has no intrinsic activity while, of course, the agonist isoproterenol, has the full intrinsic activity. Some compounds like pindolol or xamoterol have partial intrinsic activity when compared to the full agonists.

**Dr. Quigley**: Some of the other beta blockers that are of interest to us, could you tell us what their intrinsic activity is, carteolol or timolol, or some of those.

**Dr. Langer**: Carteolol has very little intrinsic activity, it is lower than acetobutalol, which has 20% intrinsic activity. Acetobutalol here is 25%, carteolol would be about 18%, it is very low indeed.

**Dr. Quigley**: And timolol, do you know?

**Dr. Langer**: Timolol has no intrinsic activity, none whatsoever.

One other property which I would like to spend a few minutes on, is the potential to voltage-dependent calcium channels. This is a property of a class of compounds that I call the calcium antagonists, of which dihydroperidines like nifedipine and nitrendipine, are reference compounds. Diltiazem, which is also a calcium antagonist of a different class is, again, a reference compound.

We go back to this possible mechanism of action in describing one property of betaxolol that, in fact, surprised us. And this is the ability to relax vessels contracted by potassium. A vessel contracted by potassium would be dilated mainly by calcium antagonists or directly acting vasodilators. I will show you some experimental results with betaxolol. The vessels are contracted by 80 mM potassium. Papaverine, a classical vasodilating agent, inhibits phosphodiesterase and produces through this mechanism total vasodilation. Papaverine, and betaxolol in micromolar concentration produces a concentration-dependent vasodilatation in these contracted vessels, which is also obtained with bunitrolol, but not with atenolol, a classical beta-1 adrenoceptor antagonist. This on its own was an unexpected observation. Following the lead of the Japanese group that developed the betaxolol, we switched to a more sensitive preparation, which is a blood vessel like the pulmonary artery or the femoral artery of the rabbit, contracted by increasing concentration of calcium chloride. Under these conditions the concentration effect curve to calcium chloride is shifted in a parallel manner to the right. This is a concentration-dependent effect, for 1–10 μM diltiazem, which is a classical calcium antagonist.

Under the same experimental conditions, namely looking at the calcium chloride concentration effect, betaxolol at concentrations 1, 3, 10, and 30 μM produced a parallel shift to the right of the concentration effect curve for the contractile effect induced by calcium. This is qualitatively a behavior that you would expect of a compound possessing calcium antagonist properties. These are concentrations that are higher than those necessary to block beta adrenoceptors. And this is a point that we should not forget, because it is essential when the question comes up as to whether this is a relevant effect under the conditions of its therapeutic use.

**Dr. Lüscher**: Dr. Langer, was this experiment performed in calcium-free solution, and after removal of intracellular calcium, did you add calcium back again?

**Dr. Langer**: Calcium-free solution, and then you add calcium and you get a calcium-dependent contraction.

On the question of the high concentration of betaxolol required to set the calcium antagonist effect of betaxolol, I can immediately say that as far as the oral route of administration, the required concentrations are not present in plasma, they are not that high. But in experiments carried out by Lou DeSantis at Alcon, when tritiated betaxolol was given in the 0.5% concentration usually used locally for the treatment of glaucoma, to pigmented rabbits, under single or multidose administration, a μM concentration is achieved both in the retina and in the choroid, and in the submicromolar range for the albino rabbits. These data, which perhaps might be subsequently commented by Lou DeSantis in more detail, would indicate that in contrast to the systemic oral administration for the antihypertensive indication, local administration of betaxolol may achieve the sort of range of concentration where the second component, namely the calcium antagonist vasodilating effect, can be obtained.

In experiments again carried out at Alcon in which the time course was determined in the choroid, in the aqueous humor, and the retina of the concentrations of tritiated betaxolol in pigmented animals following a single topical ocular dose, you can see that the T½ is rather long, 45, 38, 39 hours, and there is a persistence of betaxolol in still initial micromolar and subsequent submicromolar concentrations after a single dose. Again, it is possible that through this route of administration and with continuous or repeated administrations, quite high concentrations are achieved.

Subsequent experiments were carried out with intra-arterial injection to establish to what extent under *in vivo* conditions these vasodilating effects would be obtained. When measuring femoral flow in anesthetized dogs, papaverine dilates and this is dose-dependent. Betaxolol produces dose-dependent vasodilatation which is less pronounced than papaverine, but in contrast atenolol is entirely devoid of vasodilating properties.

**Dr. Quigley**: Dr. Langer, what kind of dose was relative to the rabbit data or any data you have in humans?

**Dr. Langer**: Compared to doses that would block beta adrenoceptors, they are at least 10 times higher, between 10 and 30 times.

**Dr. Lüscher**: With calcium antagonists, we have done forearm blood flow, and if you give, for instance, verapamil, you can see a measurable forearm blood flow increase. It would be actually quite easy to determine whether this effect occurs *in vivo* in humans; has this been done?

**Dr. Langer**: Not to my knowledge.

**Dr. Lüscher**: Because, I mean, the concentration range alone, it does not tell you much. We have looked at several antagonists, calcium antagonists, and they often are in the micromolar or above range in their concentration range, if they do exert vasodilator effect in isolated blood vessels, and yet if you give it to patients they work at seemingly lower concentrations.

**Dr. Langer**: The purpose of the femoral artery experiment was simply to establish a dose-response curve and to prove that this effect was not blocked by beta adrenoceptor antagonists. In these experiments, the vasodilatation produced by the agonist isoproterenol was blocked by propranolol, while the effect of betaxolol was resistant to blockade by propranolol, and therefore is not an effect associated either with partial beta-2 agonist properties or with any properties linked to beta-1 or beta-2 adrenoceptors. As expected, the effects of papaverine were also not blocked by propranolol. Because one of the working hypotheses is that this compound is devoid of intrinsic activity; however, since intrinsic activity would be manifested in different tissues according to the receptor reserve, and the density of receptors, it is not excluded that in some vascular beds, a weak beta-2 partial agonist action could be manifested, and that, like the effect of isoprenaline, would be entirely sensitive to blockade by propranolol, but that was not the case.

**Dr. Anderson**: You have already pointed out the importance of dose or let us say, concentration, at the tissue level, and how this is higher than is required for beta blockade, and I am thinking back to the information that you presented, where the concentration in the tissues of pigmented rabbits was there. But some of that is bound to the melanin...

**Dr. Langer**: In fact, a lot of it could be bound.

**Dr. Anderson:** ...and that accounts for the long half-life. I presume that the bound form is not active, and what is relevant for the vasodilatory activity is the amount that is unbound and free, and do we know anything about the ratio in the presence of melanin between bound and unbound betaxolol?

**Dr. Langer**: I think Lou DeSantis would be the qualified person to answer that question because he carried out these experiments.

**Dr. DeSantis**: We have no definite data. In looking at that question of how much is free and how much is bound.

**Dr. Langer**: So the answer is, we do not know, but definitely there must be a significant proportion that is bound, although we are globally in the micromolar range, which is the sort of range where this effect can be demonstrated in vitro.

Two more vascular beds when the rat renal artery is perfused, betaxolol shows vasodilatation and atenolol in fact can constrict. In the rat mesenteric artery preparation, betaxolol shows vasodilatation, but there is little or no effect for atenolol. It is dose-dependent, and these are blood vessels that are contracted by potassium. So it is in a variety of preparations, and of species, that this effect can be obtained.

The next question is, does betaxolol have any affinity for the L type calcium channel that can be labeled with nitrendipine. The specific binding of nitrendipine is enhanced by diltiazem, a positive allosteric interaction between diltiazem and the dihydropyridine calcium channel, which is classic by now. Timolol has no affinity, and even at the 100 μM concentration does not inhibit nitrendipine binding. Betaxolol produces a concentration-dependent inhibition of nitrendipine binding in membranes of the rat brain, but we are between 1 and 100 μM. So there is an inhibition of nitrendipine binding by betaxolol which is not obtained by timolol.

So what are the conclusions? First of all, we go back to noradrenergic neurotransmission. Noradrenaline released from sympathetic nerves acts approximately on 10 adrenoceptor subtypes, of course, not in every tissue. I say this because there are either three or four alpha-1's, most likely four alpha-2's, and the discrepancy appears to be due to species differences that for some authors represent additional receptor subtypes. There is a nomenclature committee from the International Union of Pharmacology which has recently decided that species homologs of the same subtype, even if they have minor differences in sequence or in pharmacology, should not be classified as additional different subtypes. So three or four for the alpha-1's and alpha-2's, certainly three for the beta; and these mediate the physiological responses. Several cotransmitters can be released together with norepinephrine during depolarization. It is usually one cotransmitter in a single noradrenergic postganglionic sympathetic neuron. It has not been characterized in many tissues. Only some examples in some species, like neuropeptide Y in the perfused spleen of the pig, like galanine in the pancreas, have been well studied. The rest remains an open question.

Presynaptically, receptors exist on norepinephrine nerve endings and they modulate the release of the neurotransmitter. The autoreceptors that are inhibitory are the alpha-2 adrenoceptors, the autoreceptors that facilitate norepinephrine release are of the beta-2 subtype. Betaxolol is a potent and selective beta-1 adrenoceptor competitive agent. It is an antagonist, and it is devoid of intrinsic activity on either beta-1 or beta-2 adrenoceptors. In several *in vitro* and perfused preparations, betaxolol possesses vasodilating properties that are not shared by other beta adrenoceptor antagonists. However, these vasodilating properties of betaxolol are obtained at doses or concentrations which are 10 to 30 times higher than the pA2 for blockade of beta-1 adrenoceptors. And the relevance of this effect to the rest of the pharmacological properties depends on the concentrations that are achieved by local administration in the eye under the therapeutic conditions in the treatment of glaucoma. Repeated administration may differ from a single administration, and the question of free versus bound betaxolol is also an issue. The vasodilation produced by betaxolol could be associated to blockade of voltage-dependent calcium channel.

**Dr. Flammer**: Thank you, Dr. Langer. I would like to comment that we did a study in humans in which we applied single dosage of timolol and of betaxolol and placebo in the dosage that is used to treat systemic hypertension, and we measured blood flow in the finger, and all three improved the blood flow, but betaxolol did it significantly more than the others. We are repeating the study again now with capillomicroscopy, at that time we did it with the laser Doppler. So I think we can confirm *in vivo* your results.

**Dr. Quigley**: Why would placebo improve the blood flow?

**Dr. Flammer**: I do not know. Psychological effect, I do not know.

**Dr. Quigley**: Did they know which one was the placebo, or they thought they were getting something active, I guess, is what you are saying.

**Dr. Flammer**: They did not know what was the placebo.

**Dr. Quigley**: Was there an effect of timolol and betaxolol that was greater than the placebo?

**Dr. Flammer**: Oh yes, clearly. Now, timolol was very close to placebo, but betaxolol very clearly did more.

**Dr. Siesjö**: I was wondering, does betaxolol have any effect in the intrinsic noradrenergic system of the brain, and is there any inference on cerebral blood flow?

**Dr. Langer**: Betaxolol crosses the blood–brain barrier and is present in significant concentrations in the brain. Nevertheless, after many years of betaxolol being sold in many countries, the incidence of side effects, because it is beta-1 selective, is very low. It appears that CNS side effects due to beta adrenoceptor blockade are pronounced or more relevant if there is a beta-2 component in the molecule. As far as blood flow, cerebral blood flow, I do not know.

**Dr. Alm**: There is one thing I am not quite sure I understand, that is, if you compare the pigmented and the albino rabbits and look at the concentration of the topical application, I can understand that you have higher concentrations in the choroid, but why do you have it in the retina? Is the pigment epithelium included in the tissue sample, or ...?

**Dr. Langer**: I assume that might be the case, but again, I think Lou DeSantis may have a more precise answer than myself.

**Dr. DeSantis**: These are the numbers. I do not have an exact answer for you. I mean, these are the data from using the radiolabeled drug. I believe, personally, that the drug gets to the back of the eye both through the eye, because we could find drug in the vitreous humor, and certainly some of the drug is getting there through the circulation, because there is a definite but lower concentration in the contralateral undosed eye of the rabbit, but I do not know the exact route by which the drug can get there. I think it has been postulated that there are ways for drugs to arrive at the retina through, maybe through the peripapillary region. I think Dr. Anderson has proposed that as a potential route for drug entry from the choroid to the optic nerve head. And again, these are rabbits.

**Dr. Flammer?**: How many doses and what kind did you give, in a multidosage...?

**Dr. DeSantis**: We studied it in several fashions. We first started with single instillation to determine the kinetics of the removal of drug from the tissue. Later, in the pigmented rabbit studies we gave nine doses, giving a half-percent drug twice a day for nine doses. In the albino we gave five doses. Based upon the half-life from the single instillation, we felt that with nine doses we were achieving a steady state distribution of the drug in the tissue, so this is why we chose that number of doses.

**Dr. Flammer**: If I may add something to that. The reason why I am asking is that in clinical treatment with betaxolol we had some indication, it is really only a suggestion, that the improvement of the visual fields came only after weeks or months. So could it be that it takes such a long time to get these concentrations in the back of the eye? By applying just twice a day betaxolol?

**Dr. DeSantis**: Well, that is possible, but within five or six half-lives, if you just give doses over five or six half-lives of a drug, you should reach a steady state. I think that eventually you would expect to saturate the pigment binding and that subsequent doses are going to be more bioavailable to the receptors, and to the ion channels. I think that because betaxolol is so lipophilic, and it has such a persistence in tissues, that it is going to find its way to the ion channels. We have to consider that there will be binding to receptors and also the calcium channels that are in the blood vessels. So I do not think it is too far removed from the possibility that this effect is occurring. Besides your own studies, but bringing the relevance to the eye, there are data from a couple of laboratories using the Langham instrument that show a positive effect of betaxolol on choroidal blood flow. I think that the effect of betaxolol is probably going to be more prominent in the choroidal blood flow than perhaps in the retinal blood.

**Dr. Alm**: Well, I think you misunderstood my question. I was not asking you in which route the betaxolol reached the retina, I am just surprised that you have higher concentrations in the retina, in pigmented rabbits than in non-pigmented rabbits, and my question was, did you include the retinal pigmented epithelium in the retinal samples?

**Dr. DeSantis**: Yes.

**Dr. Alm**: Did you have higher concentrations also in the vitreous of the pigmented rabbits compared to non-pigmented rabbits?

**Dr. DeSantis**: Not markedly so, but you know, the eye of the pigmented rabbit is substantially smaller than that of the albino rabbit.

**Dr. Quigley**: We have been hearing a little bit about the data of actual measurements of blood flow, and I think that while it is important to have surrogates, such as what the concentration is in the back of the eye, it is really the retinal or the optic nerve blood flow that we would like most to hear about. There are direct methods of looking that Grunwald and Riva have used. There are laboratory methods of measuring blood flow. The indirect methods of measuring the ocular pulse, as Dr. DeSantis says, measure choroidal blood flow, and I am not sure we are terribly interested in choroidal blood flow. It may not be relevant to glaucoma, although of course any data is data. So what do we know about retinal or optic nerve blood flow with various beta blockers? We have a roomful of experts, I was hoping somebody knew some answers.

**Dr. Langer**: To my knowledge, there is very little. I would like to add, however, one point. When we saw the vasodilating properties of betaxolol in different vascular beds, we did not think first of calcium antagonist mechanisms, because many betablockers have affinity for 5-HT receptors sometimes. Therefore our main concern at the time is that we missed an effect of betaxolol on 5-HT receptors. We explored carefully this possibility, but betaxolol has no affinity for any of the multiple 5-HT receptor subtypes, even the more recent ones. So this is a mechanism that we very carefully excluded. But coming back to your question, I think that specific studies need to be carried out if the appropriate techniques are available to establish the relevance.

**Dr. Quigley**: I wonder if anybody wanted to talk about what we should be doing. You know, we do not have these data; if one drug is better than the other, by all means let us demonstrate it with direct means.

**Dr. Ransom**: I may have missed this. Are there any direct electrophysiological studies showing calcium channel blocking activity of this drug?

**Dr. Langer**: Yes, you can show it by electrophysiological techniques, the same as you can show the competition for the nitrendipine binding site. But again, you are in a concentration range which is micromolar, and by the way, one of the questions that we face in these electrophysiological studies was whether it was a stereoselective effect, because betaxolol is a racamate and is available in the *r* and *s* forms, and only one of the enantiomers is the one that possesses the beta-blocking properties. But both enantiomers in our hands possess the so-called calcium antagonist property.

**Dr. Ransom**: When you say electrophysiological, are you talking about single..?

**Dr. Langer**: Action potential in the heart.

**Dr. Ransom**: But how about single channel? I mean, ultimately, if you want to know that something is a calcium channel blocker, you have to go back and look at single calcium channels. Because there are curious interactions that can take place at different sites. Is there anything about the structure of this molecule that would suggest it ought to interact at the calcium channel?

**Dr. Langer**: Absolutely, not with my limited medicinal chemistry knowledge, but some chemists will be very imaginative and tell you there is something. In our organization, we did not manage to establish a structure activity relationship at all.

**Dr. Alm**: In response to Harry Quigley, what we should do. First of all, the effect of isoproterenol was studied on the uveal blood flow in cats 20, 25 years ago, and there was no effect, and I could not find any effect on retinal blood flow injected into the artery. Then the study that Grunwald did with timolol has shown a slight increase in the human eye, but that is a small increase of about 10 or 15%. We could not exclude that this is maybe due to some indirect effect, I mean, you could expect that perhaps a beta blocker could have an effect on retinal metabolism or something. So we still have not settled the question of whether there are beta receptors or not. So I think that what should be done is to try to use molecular biology to find out if there are relevant beta receptors in the vascular smooth muscles of the eye, and then maybe someone should try to measure directly blood flow with betaxolol and timolol.

**Dr. Langer**: But the point is that the blood flow effects are unrelated to actions mediated by beta-1 or beta-2 adrenoceptor effects. Because they are, in other vascular beds, resistant to blockade by propranolol. Consequently the presence or absence of beta receptors may not be a crucial point, if mechanistically it is the presence of L type calcium channels that may be the relevant question.

**Dr. Alm**: Well, if you have receptors, you have to go to high doses, the betaxolol I would guess is not that selective for beta-1, you would have an effect on beta receptors also, so you would have both calcium channel and a beta receptor effect.

**Dr. Langer**: Yes, there is, depending on the tissues, a 100- to 200-fold difference. But the question for vasodilatation, as I see it, would be only dependent on beta-2 partial agonist action, and not blockade.

**Dr. Alm**: What I am saying is, we could solve these discussions by measuring blood flow. Whatever the mechanism. And we have had it for five or 10 years now, and maybe it is time to measure it.

**Dr. Langer**: I could not agree more. Yes, absolutely.

# 21. OPTIC NERVE BLOOD FLOW

DOUGLAS R. ANDERSON, M.D.

**Dr. Flammer**: We are coming to the last, and surely the most interesting part of the session, Dr. Anderson is going to summate all this and make it relevant to the back of the eye, and to glaucoma.

**Dr. Anderson**: I guess we will try to bring this all together. I do not know what to do, because most of what I had planned to say has at one point or another already been said. What we have been talking about together, I think, is a broad speculation about any conceivable mechanism of damage to the optic nerve in glaucoma, perhaps with an eye toward giving us ideas for what we might do scientifically in the future in order to learn something that we do not presently know. I think a lot of what I am going to say will therefore be in the form of questions: what do we want to know, are we asking ourselves the right questions, and in what direction should we go?

I can begin by refreshing our memory about the vascular anatomy, since we are talking in this session about blood flow. Remember that the central retinal artery comes in, and although it gives some branches to the core of the optic nerve outside the eye, we presume this part of the nerve is not relevant to our present discussion. The central retinal artery does not give branches as it enters the lamina cribrosa or passes through the optic nerve head, but further in its course gives off branches to the retina. Its primary job is to supply the retina, but it does give some capillary branches to the most superficial part of the optic nerve head.

The second vascular supply is via the posterior ciliary arteries, whose primary job is to supply the choroid, but some of the branches enter into the optic nerve head. While the arterial source for the optic nerve head is from the posterior ciliary artery, the capillary bed is quite separate from the capillary bed of the choriocapillaris. They are anatomically separate capillary beds, different branches supply the choroid and the optic nerve head, and their microanatomies are quite different in nature. The optic nerve capillaries are central nervous system type vessels, which have tight junctions between the endothelium and are lined with pericytes. They are in fact a continuous capillary network with retinal vessels anteriorly and optic nerve vessels posteriorly. From the retina you can walk through the capillary bed and without leaving capillaries end up in the capillary bed of the optic nerve head, and from there walk down to the capillaries behind the eye. So this is one continuous capillary bed. You could not arrive at the choroid without going back up to an artery and then back out a different arterial branch to the choroid. In contrast to the optic nerve head microvasculature, the choroid capillaries have leaky endothelium with fenestrations in the endothelium, and an incomplete covering of pericytes and so it is a different vascular bed.

**Dr. Kaufman**: If the capillaries from the posterior ciliary circulation in the nerve head are continuous with the capillaries from the retinal circulation, what is the actual arterial supply, where are particular nutrients coming from?

**Dr. Anderson**: Yes, I think your question contains some implications. Since we have an anastomotic connection at the capillary level, if one arterial source became con-

*Optic Nerve in Glaucoma, pp. 311–331*
*edited by S.M. Drance*

stricted or inadequate in some way, then it might be that an adjacent artery expands its area of responsibility. The boundary between the regions served by two arterial branches might change depending on whether one becomes less adequate than the other, and that could very well happen. How far could that happen? You can not cut off one entire arterial supply and expect the other to take over completely without there being some anastomoses at the arterial level, because the resistance in the capillary bed is very high in actual fact. They are very small vessels, so there is a limit to how far one arteriole could take over another arteriole's responsibility.

I would now like to try to separate cardiovascular physiology components that are global, systemic, maybe even regional, from the blood flow components and control mechanisms that are very local. Thus, control of blood flow to the orbit is different from the control of blood flow in the optic nerve head. The retina and the choroid are also separately controlled.

I would like to talk first of all about the global cardiovascular physiology and what its functions and purposes are, not that they are relevant to the local control that I want to get to, but I want to hear from the physiologists present whether or not I have the right perspective on this. I view that one of the main functions of global cardiovascular physiology is to maintain blood pressure. That is to say, that there is a blood pressure that must be maintained, and I view then that the capillary bed is tapping into this pressurized source. Each local bed may at any moment tap into the pressurized source in a large way or in a small way depending on its needs at the moment, and another bed may also tap into it in a large way or a small way depending on its needs, but there has to be a pressurized reservoir for each local bed to tap into.

A very relevant question, it seems to me, is, where is the relevant gate that taps into it? It might be that that is at the very small vessels, the 20-μm or the 30-μm vessels that are tapping into this pressurized source. Clearly there is a resistance between the major arteries. In the carotids, the ophthalmics, central retinal artery, even posterior ciliary artery there is some resistance that accounts for the fact that there is a fall in pressure as you enter into the capillary bed.

I want to point this out in the context of Dr. Flammer's patient yesterday, when he was talking about the low blood pressure. What really happens is that you have the cardiac output being distributed to all the various microvascular beds. The driving pressure through a particular bed may simply be the difference between the pressure at the inlet of this tap and the pressure in the vein, not the pressure from the brachial artery or the aorta or the ophthalmic artery. It might very well be that an individual who has a low blood pressure, has a low blood pressure because, throughout his body, his intermediate bed of "resistance vessels" are all generally dilated. The cardiac output, that is, the volume of flow going throughout the whole body, maybe the same in a person who has higher central pressure as in a person who has lower central presure of generally in the end arterioles (or "resistance vessels", the gateway into the capillaries). There is a high resistance between the high pressure arterial bed and the capillaries. After all, blood pressure is determined by the cardiac output and the total resistance between the arteries and veins. If you have less resistance in these intermediate level vessels, you may have low blood pressure, which is not to say at all that there is necessarily reduced perfusion in any of the local beds. Nor is it true that raising the pressure in the central vat is going to do anything with regard to improving the blood flow, if that higher pressure is achieved by increasing the resistance in all of the intermediate beds, which is, of course, the only way you could possibly achieve a higher blood pressure without increasing cardiac output. At a given cardiac output, the blood pressure is determined by the summated capacity of all the intermediate segments. As far as any little local segment is concerned, it is tapping into a pressure of 30 mmHg, because separating it from the mean arterial pressure of 80 mmHg. is a certain resistance in the case of a low blood pressure person, but separating it from 110 mmHg. a higher blood pressure person is a greater resistance. But this local bed does not know the difference, so that raising systemic blood pressure does not necessarily affect the volume of flow that might go into a particular bed.

Now, we must add to the global functions not only the maintaining of blood pressure, but also the allocation of the cardiac output to various organs and tissues. Again this function does not reside in the smallest vessels, but in the somewhat larger vessels. They determine that, at some moment, the brain needs a little more blood than the gut. I see a tiger, I need to run, I need to be alert, and so there is a hormonal and a neural input that gives preference to a region of tissue, or a type of tissue, by changing the vascular caliber in larger vessels. Under another circumstance, we just had a nice lunch and our intestines seem to have some needs, and we are not seeing tigers at the moment, so we feel sleepy, our brain is taking less nutrition, and our gut is getting more. These are rather global effects with the same cardiac output, perhaps. Now, there may be circumstances in which we also have to increase the cardiac output, with exercise or different things, and we do that too.

What I am doing is taking cardiac output, blood pressure, and regional distribution of blood flow away from what I finally want to talk about, which is the local control of blood flow. Some of what we have been talking about at this meeting, in terms of the pharmacology and physiology, has to do with this function of determining what happens to the cardiac output after it has been generated by the heart, and where does it go.

Finally I should mention that an important global function is to produce a stable state of mid-dilation. There was talk at this meeting of nitric oxide, the thing that produces this function. You must have all the vessels in a mid-dilated state, so that they are capable of dilating when there is a physiologic signal that says, I need dilation, and likewise capable of constricting. If the vessels are maximally constricted or maximally dilated, you can not have control. You have to maintain the vessels in a mid-state. Importantly, nitric oxide produced by the endothelium actually maintains this mid-dilation state. Nitric oxide also participates in vascular physiology as a mediator in the response to certain hormones which may cause an increase or decrease in nitric oxide production. Thus nitric oxide, as an intermediary, participates in endothelium and mediates hormone effects on the smooth muscle of the larger arteries, and perhaps the microvascular bed as well. But in the absence of any hormonal modulation, a basal level of nitric oxide production is important in keeping the vessels in a state of non-spasm.

So the image I have tried to create is that the major elements of the cardiovascular system are responsible to maintain a pressurized source of blood into which local microvascular beds can tap. I hope that that is a reasonable perspective. I would want that, if this is not a perspective that is correct, some of the people here who are knowledgeable about general physiology in the cardiovascular system to correct this notion. And the point to which I am leading is that each locality can have considerable local control of its own blood flow by the degree to which it taps into the pressurized source.

**Dr. Drance**: Although you said that the blood pressure level, for instance, need not completely determine what happens at the local level, it might have influence. In other words, an individual whose pressure is, for instance, 80/50 continuously, is he not more likely to have a lower perfusion pressure in any local microvascular bed given whatever local circumstances or control is superimposed.

**Dr. Anderson**: Right. The concept that I have of that is that the blood pressure is there to be tapped into. If the local signal is that you need more perfusion, if the vessels can dilate locally but there is a limit to the flow that can be achieved if you do not have a big enough pressure head, and so that there may be a limitation there.

On the other hand, I would say that if you were to use a drug to raise the central pressure in an effort to improve perfusion, the manner in which it would do that is by constricting some vessels. If it constricts the right ones, the ones in the skeletal muscle, while leaving the ones to the central nervous system relatively undilated, you have enhanced the dynamic range into which the local nervous system vessels can tap. But if you use a different agent, one that raises blood pressure by constricting arterioles leading to the vascular bed in which you are trying to improve blood flow, you may, in fact, have been counterproductive in your efforts, and actually shunt the cardiac output into other tissues. So simply raising the blood pressure *per se* is not the way to think about it. The way to think about it is what differential effect does it have on the various local vascular beds. Thus in Dr. Flammer's patient, raising the blood pressure with a vasoconstrictive agent might have an adverse effect on the optic nerve.

And, of course, the notion of using a general vasodilator to enhance blood flow in an arteriolar vascular bed is equally fallacious. If you dilate all vessels, the blood pressure will be lowered. Additionally, only if the vascular bed in question is *preferentially* dilated will its blood flow be enhanced. If other localities are more strongly dilated, the blood will actually be shunted away from the tissue you are trying to help.

**Dr. Lüscher**: May I just add, and really I think Dr. Baumbach would be the one to address this point, that if we talk about perfusion of the tissue with blood flow, it comes down to the question of whether you have autoregulation or not. And not all vascular beds have autoregulation, number one, and the second point, coming back to Dr. Drance's question, is it more dangerous to have 80/50 than 120/80, is actually a good question, because your autoregulatory range ends somewhere. And so if you are at the lower range of autoregulation and then you have a further drop in blood pressure, let us say at night, then you may run into troubles, while if you are in the higher normal range or middle normal range, you have more buffer, so to speak, to maintain your flow.

**Dr. Anderson**: You are thinking faster than I am presenting it, because of course that is exactly correct. I do want to make the careful distinction between global or central cardiovascular control which I have just talked about, and autoregulation, which I want to address now. Autoregulation is defined differently by different people. So I would like to define autoregulation as I intend to use it in this context today. My use of the word "autoregulation" differs from that of Dr. Zeiher (Chapter 17) for instance. By autoregulation I think it makes sense to specify that the stimulus that has initiated the response is local, as opposed to the situation in which the stimulus that initiated the response is remote. So if you have something that causes your adrenal gland to put out a lot of sympathetic stimulation, you are talking about a global reaction to something that is happening elsewhere in the body. But in autoregulation, local stimuli could cause the local blood flow to change without affecting the rest of the body. "Auto" implies that the tissue regulates the blood flow within itself, and that means the stimulus that causes the regulation arises there, and then there is also a local response. Now, it may be mediated through some of the same mediators as global responses: there may be adrenergic agents involved, there may be nitric oxide involved, there may be cyclic AMP involved. Some of the same systems may become involved in the response, but as a definition for today's purpose, the *local* initiation of a *local* response is what I would like to call autoregulation.

There are a number of local signals for a local response. One is stretch, that is to say, when the vascular muscle is stretched, it may contract as a reaction. Stretch of the muscle is separate from shear stress on the endothelium. It is visualized that the stretch response that might participate in controlling blood flow. In other words, you get too much blood pressure coming in, because the aorta is presenting too high a blood pressure to this vascular bed, and the vascular bed would be overperfused unless every vessel locally reacts by a constriction in response to stretch. We see that, in people with high blood pressure their retinal arteries constrict, for example.

However, in addition to controlling blood flow, the stretch response also controls the level of intraluminal pressure in the capillary bed, which is an important thing to control. It is a delicate balance, because there must be adequate perfusion, which is determined by the pressure difference and total resistance between veins and arteries, but the intracapillary pressure must be proper so that you do not get edema. So not only blood flow, but also capilliary intravascular pressure, has to be regulated, somehow, and the stretch response, I presume, must play a role. I am thinking teleologically and very hypothetically in all of this, of course, but I presume that this stretch response in arterioles is in part protective of excessive intraluminal pressure downstream.

Now, a second stimulus was described already in this meeting, and that is the stimulus of the blood flow shearing against the endothelium, which produces through nitric oxide a relaxation response so that the vessels are responding to the linear rate of flow going through the vessels, and that is a local response because nitric oxide does not travel very far, so wherever there is a high shear, there is a high response.

And then finally, the metabolic state is a local stimulus. And again, I noticed Dr. Zeiher earlier separating this from autoregulation, which he viewed as a response to intraluminal pressure only. Yet to me this is still autoregulation, viewed as a local response to local conditions, but an autoregulation of a different variety. In that sense, the separation of this from myogenic autoregulation as defined by Dr. Zeiher is important. Well, no matter what you call it, the local metabolic state affects circulation. That is to say that the vessels react to whether or not the tissue at the moment has a high enough oxygen tension, too high a carbon dioxide tension, inadequate amount of glucose, too much adenosine, etc. Whatever the signals might be, there is something about the local metabolism that tells the vascular bed, I am getting enough or I am not getting enough of some substance or I am getting too much or too little in the way of blood flow. Each of these is a local signal that you would like to have initiate a local response, and to convey, for example, that this microvascular bed now needs to dilate a little bit and provide a little more blood flow from this pressurized central source.

And so, maybe too simplistically, I am separating local control from the global neural and hormonal influences. Local control, by whatever mechanism, I would like to call autoregulation in the present context, if you will permit me.

Now, what happens in glaucoma. In glaucoma, the intraocular pressure (IOP) is elevated. This is certainly a challenge to the blood flow in the area whether or not reduced blood flow is the mechanism by which damage occurs is something that we can debate and discuss, but at least intraocular pressure is a challenge to the blood flow. One of the challenges is that it raises the intraluminal pressure in the veins as they exit from the eye. If the venous pressure, for example, is only 8 or 10 mmHg and the intraocular pressure is 18 mmHg, naturally it is going to collapse the walls. The walls of the veins are not rigid and at some point, near the exit point of the eye, the furthest downstream (with the lowest pressure) the wall is compressed, restricting the lumen and producing resistance and raising intravascular pressure upstream. Just upstream from that the pressure inside the vein has to be high enough to maintain its lumen against the external force of the intraocular pressure. So there is some point just upstream from the compression at which the venous pressure is just a little higher than intraocular pressure. As intraocular pressure rises, even, within the physiologic range, where the intraocular pressure might be 15 or 18 mmHg, which is higher than the venous pressure outside the eye, this physiologic change will occur, and the higher the intraocular pressure is, the higher the venous pressure will become. Without a regulatory mechanism, the flow would be reduced, but there is an autoregulation that allows the flow to be maintained in this vascular bed.

Dr. Alm has shown that in the optic nerve head and the retina, as the perfusion pressure decreases, with the intraocular pressure increasing and the venous pressure increasing, the blood flow is maintained over a range until at some point the ability to autoregulate is exceeded. When the range of the autoregulation is exceeded, then the blood flow drops.

In our studies, while there was some decline over the range of autoregulation, it was not as great as it was when it got to a critical pressure after which blood flow fell rapidly. At this point where capacity for maintaining flow was exceeded, the perfusion pressure was such that intraocular pressure was approaching diastolic arterial pressure. In these studies, the blood pressure is in the remote ophthalmic artery, femoral artery, or brachial artery. The relevant blood pressure is probably the blood pressure in the central retinal artery or at the arterial branches of the posterior ciliary artery just before entering the capillary bed. That might be something that is more like 30 mmHg or so, anyway.

**Dr. Siesjö**: Could you explain to us, please, what the technique is for measuring blood flow here?

**Dr. Anderson**: In my experiment, and this is not necessarily the important one, it was done with iodoantipyrine, but other people used different techniques, and all demonstrated an autoregulation capacity within the optic nerve head. We measured the response to elevating intraocular pressure. Other people have documented regulation by showing the response to blood pressure. Raising the blood pressure does not cause an elevation in flow, because there is a regulation to keep it from happening and vice versa. Yet other people have shown, and this is an important point, that there is a metabolic autoregulation, so that if you put a flashing light into the eye, which increases the neural activity, there will be an increase in the blood flow to meet that new metabolic demand in the optic nerve head, because the many axons going through the area have a higher firing rate. And so we can say that there is at least a metabolic component to this, even if stretch (myogenic) or shear stress is also probably occurring.

**Dr. Zeimer**: The graph of your results suggests autoregulation of the choroid. Is that the first evidence there is regulation, in the choroid?

**Dr. Anderson**: Very observant. The graph includes the choroid, in addition to the retina and optic nerve. I should have pointed out that while the choroid seemed to show an autoregulation, what you really see is that the graph is truncated at the top end because there is a maximum level of blood flow that the iodoantipyrine method can measure. At low intraocular pressure, the choroidal blood flow is so high that it exceeds the level that the method will measure. One could extrapolate that curve up as if the choroid did not autoregulate.

**Dr. Flammer**: You mentioned the increase of blood flow after flickering by light. This might not be due to an increased demand. It might be a direct effect on the vascular bed, because a light effect does occur in isolated vessels, because light might directly induce the increase in nitric oxide production. Thomas Lüscher might comment on that, if there could be a direct influence of light on the vessel.

**Dr. Anderson**: Dr. Lüscher, could you respond to Dr. Flammer's comment?

**Dr. Lüscher**: Yes, actually Dr. Furchgott has done it all in the '60s, as usual, and he has demonstrated already then that if you expose blood vessels to light, that they do relax. And a Greek group has recently shown that light can increase nitric oxide production from endothelial cells in culture, so it may well be that this is a stimulus for the ophthalmic circulation.

**Dr. Quigley**: I would have to look up the paper, but I am fairly sure that that was flickering light compared to constant light of the same total magnitude. So while the light level may in fact be another factor in ocular blood flow, it probably was not in that particular experiment.

**Dr. Anderson**: Was it done with UV light, or were you referring to flickering light, which increases neural activity? We will have to look and see whether or not an experiment that might well be worth doing is whether a steady light does the same thing and then we have to go back to the vascular literature to find out if there is a difference between flickering and steady light directly, as opposed to mediated by metabolic needs. You suggested a good experiment for us to do, and I thank you.

Let us accept for the moment that the optic nerve head vascular bed is autoregulated, and now begin to talk about the location of this response. If the choroid is not autoregulated, and the optic nerve head is, then you assume that this regulatory response is not occurring in the posterior ciliary arteries and vessels of that size, but presumably in vessels of smaller size. As opposed to regulation in a global or even regional sense, which might be mediated by arteries of 100 μm to 50 μm, autoregulation, as I define it, may be a function of even the smaller vessels in the local region. It might be the very smallest of the arterioles, for example. There are small arterioles that enter into the optic disc, through the choroid, yes, through the sclera, yes, branches from the posterior ciliary artery, yes, but it is not those arteries that are relevant, but is the very smallest arteriole at its entry point to the optic nerve that could be controlling the blood flow in the optic nerve head. Now, there are not very many of those branches, and they are quite small, but they are at a place of potential control. And we will have to think about that as one of the possibilities for site of autoregulation control.

A second possibility derives from the fact that the vascular bed of the optic nerve head, in fact, is mostly capillaries, or at least arterioles that are so small that they can not really be distinguished morphologically from capillaries. Once in a while you can find some small vessel that looks like it might be an arteriole that is entering, but mostly the optic disc has only a capillary bed, which starts outside the eye, passes through the lamina cribrosa and the optic nerve head, continuing into the retina. There is continuity of the capillary bed occurring between the retina and the optic nerve head.

**Dr. Flammer**: Obviously, the way from the artery to the vein must be longer, because we have just capillaries. Could these make it more vulnerable for this reason?

**Dr. Anderson**: I do not know the average length from artery to veins through this capillary bed in comparison to the length through other beds such as in the retina, where there may be also a fairly long course, I suppose. I do not know.

**Dr. Siesjö**: I was wondering, in this optic head, what is the intercapillary distance, the average intercapillary distance, and what its metabolic rate?

**Dr. Anderson**: I do not know that, I presume they match. Does Dr. Quigley know that?

**Dr. Quigley**: If you have perfused the tissue with a balanced salt solution and fixative, so that you have probably produced maximal dilation if these capillaries change in size, and you measure the volume of the tissue that is made up of capillary lumens, it is about 2½% of the volume is made up of capillary lumens. My reading of the central nervous system literature is that that is very similar to the total volume of tissue. The intercapillary distance varies depending on whether you are in the superficial part of the optic nerve head or you are down in the connective tissue part. But the longest distance is across the bundles, since the bundles of nerve fibers do not have capillaries within them. So what you are really asking in the relevant area here is, the bundle width, and the bundle width is in a range between 50 μm and 200 or 300, 400 μm across. So that is the diffusional distance, and that should not be a problematic distance for oxygen, from what I know of oxygen diffusion, in gray matter. This is, in effect, a gray matter tract. We do not know the metabolic rate in this tissue, that I know of, but Albert has measured it, at least with deoxyglucose, so he must know something.

**Dr. Alm**: I was not involved in that study, and I am trying to remember, but I think that in the optic nerve behind the eye, the metabolic rate is as in white matter in the brain. I think that it is a little bit higher in the optic disc, but that is explained by the absence of myelin, so it is about the same as in the brain gray matter.

**Dr. Ransom**: I feel a little bit uncomfortable referring to an unmyelinated tract as gray matter. If it has no synaptic machinery in it, if it has no neuronal cell bodies, if it has no demand because of protein synthesis and genetic activity, etc. etc., I think the metabolic demand is probably pretty close to what you would find in a so-called white matter tract, that is, axonal pathways that are purely myelinated. There is no reason to think that the metabolic needs are greater just because it does not have myelin. The distribution of sodium channels winds up being smeared out and the demands of maintaining transmembrane ion gradients are probably similar.

**Dr. Anderson**: Well, I do not know if I am in a position to agree or disagree with that, but might the metabolic need be intermediate in this sense, that in white matter tracts really the only place that has to be repolarized after depolarization (because of the saltatory conduction) is at the nodes of Ranvier, where you find mitochondria congregated, whereas in between the nodes there are very few? In this unmyelinated nerve fiber region that we are talking about, mitochondria are quite numerous. With conduction of action potentials, there is a need to repolarize continually the entire membrane, there may be a high metabolic demand. The number of mitochondria in the region presumably reflect the metabolic need. So it may be that it is a region that while it is not synthesizing protein, it has other functions that require ATP.

**Dr. Ransom**: Well, I can not say very much about the numerous mitochondria, but it turns out that when you look at saltatory conduction you have to take into account that there is a tremendous aggregation of ion channels at the nodes of Ranvier. When you finally look at the amount of transmembrane ion gradient degradation that takes place in a myelinated versus an unmyelinated tract, there is zero difference, so the amount of energy necessary to recreate the previous gradient is essentially the same based on just thermodynamic considerations.

**Dr. Anderson**: I have learned something. I thought there were two advantages to the myelinated nerve, and saltatory conduction. One was that it was faster, because the impulse went faster from node to node, but secondly I thought it was more efficient because the metabolic demand for repolarization is less, but you are telling me that that is not the case.

**Dr. Siesjö**: I think if you have a high density of mitochondria in that area, that would be at least circumstantial evidence that there is a high metabolic rate. But on the other hand, if the intercapillary distance is say, 50 to 200, that would not imply that there is a high metabolic rate. If it would be high metabolic rate, then the cells would be at risk with these very high intercapillary distances, so I think it would be better to assume that we may have a low metabolic rate. What do you think, Albert, I mean, would you agree that this is the metabolic rate of white matter than of gray matter in the brain?

**Dr. Alm**: Of course, it is white matter. But if you look at blood flow, and measure blood flow as flow per weight, you have about the same flow in the optic nerve as in white matter. But in the optic nerve head let us say it is in between white and gray matter. This is, of course, in anesthetized animals, you have very little activity in gray matter in the brain, I guess.

**Dr. Hoffman**: The density of mitochondria in the initial segment of the axon may be a little bit misleading in terms of metabolic activity. There is some evidence that the mitochondrial genome is preferentially expressed in the cell body along with the nuclear genomes, so that there may be the assembly and synthesis of mitochondrial proteins and mitochondria in the cell body, and all the mitochondria in the axon further downstream have to get there by way of transport through the initial part of the axon. So that you may be seeing an area where there is a relatively high density of mitochondria simply because they are getting into the distal part of the axon through that pathway, and it does not necessarily imply that that is an area of increased metabolic activity.

**Dr. Anderson**: That would be so if there was a high turnover rate for mitochondria, which I do not know...I mean, if there is a low turnover rate, then there would not be a crowding...

**Dr. Hoffman**: I do not think anybody knows. But it is the pathway by which they get into the axon. We do know that things that move rapidly that are the size of mitochondria move in a very saltatory way, so it is possible that the mitochondria that are residing in more distal parts of the axon are sitting around, whereas the ones that are getting into the axon, and they move bidirectionally, so it is very hard to know...

**Dr. Quigley**: Your answer might be true if the mitochondria are at their highest concentration near the cell body and their lowest concentration distally.

**Dr. Hoffman**: No, I think that my statement is that it is hard to interpret the metabolic activity from the density of mitochondria, because there may be places where mitochondria preferentially accumulate, for instance in the terminals or maybe in the area of the nodes. But it is clear that the ones that are going to accumulate in the axon all have to get into the axon by flowing along that initial segment, so that may be the wrong place to look and make an inference about metabolic activity.

**Dr. Quigley**: But the people who have done this stereologically showed that in the area right in the lamina cribrosa there are more mitochondria than on either side. That is, up toward the cell body on the one hand and down into the myelinated nerve on the other hand. And I believe it is Mark Tso's work, or Don Minkler and Mark Tso's, Doug may remember better than I. Maybe this is the first node of Ranvier, this area, and maybe that is why it has a concentration of mitochondria.

**Dr. Zeimer**: Doug, maybe another evidence that there is a high metabolic activity of the axons is that, if you look with eccentricity on the macula at the number of capillaries, you see that the number of capillary beds increases with the thickness of the nerve fiber layer. See, apparently these nerve fibers do require a lot of blood flow. And the density of capillaries next to the nerve fiber layer is pretty much similar to what you have deeper inside the retina. So apparently these axons require as much nourishment as the synaptic regions.

**Dr. Anderson**: I think we have spent enough time on metabolism...

**Dr. Hoffman**: One comment about Harry's, it is an excellent point that Harry suggested that maybe this is analogous to the first node. And the evidence for that would be in the case of the IDPN intoxication. With IDPN intoxication, neurofilaments preferentially accumulate proximal to the first node with initial intoxication, and that is exactly where they accumulate in the eye with IDPN, so that from the standpoint of that toxin, Yes, the laminar area is analogous to the first node.

**Dr. Anderson**: Continuing to consider the potential location of the local regulation. We have talked about arterioles as they enter into the optic nerve head being a potential location. We can consider precapillary sphincters which are another seeming mechanism for local control in some tissue beds. Such sphincters are more obvious in some tissues than others, where precapillary sphincters may actually completely close off one capillary at a time of low metabolic need, and therefore the space between perfused capillaries can be larger and still supply the needs, and the opening and closing may rotate through capillaries in a tissue. This has not been demonstrated in the retina. The retina anatomically does not have these sphincters, and there is not a migratory opening and closing of vascular beds. It seems that all retinal capillaries are perfused all the time. If you think that the vascular beds that are continuous with one another should be alike in this way, one could say that the optic nerve head probably does not have them either, though anatomically it is a much more difficult bed to study, to see whether they exist. But at least they have not been observed here. And I think it might be a reasonable assumption that they do not exist and do not really play a role here.

Now, there might be some semantic argument as to whether the last arteriole as it enters the optic nerve head is the equivalent of a precapillary sphincter, and whether that is or is not what is being observed when Dr. van Buskirk shows that just at the optic nerve edge there is a constriction in response to endothelin, I do not know. But this observation suggests that in the terminal arterioles there is the potential for some control mechanism that would respond to local conditions. That is to say, some lack of oxygen or excess of carbon dioxide might be perceived by this vessel, which is at the edge of the optic nerve head, and then it would open up a little bit.

I have been interested in another possibility, the potential role of capillaries themselves in regulating the flow, because they seem to be so dominant here in a tissue that is, after all, autoregulated. Capillaries, as was mentioned yesterday, are endothelial tubes lined by an outer cell just as arteries are lined by smooth muscles. The outer surface of the capillary endothelium tube is lined with pericytes, which for all the world morphologically look like smooth muscle cells to me. The main difference perhaps is that they are not united to each other by gap junctions, so they are more independent rather than being a syncythium. By morphology it seems that while following the transition from artery to capillary, the smooth muscle cells finally become a unilayer, then pretty soon you begin to call the vessel a capillary, and you call the cell that is around it a pericyte instead of a smooth muscle. Now, there are certainly differences. There are some antigenic differences, which allow you to distinguish between pericytes and smooth muscles in culture. They are not exactly the same cell type, but there are certainly a lot of resemblances. These pericytes around the capillaries have been shown to be responsive to neurotransmitters, to various hormones, and to paracrine mediators. Nitric oxide was mentioned as something that Ivan Haefliger recently had studied in our laboratory. Response to forskolin implies that cyclic AMP as well as cyclic GMP will cause relaxation. And the question is, will they respond to the metabolic state? We have preliminary evidence that carbon dioxide levels affect pericyte contractile tone. We are going to study this in more quantitative ways, but it seems that if you increase the carbon dioxide level in the atmosphere of pericytes in culture, they relax, and when you decrease it, they constrict. And so they are capable of responding to the local metabolic state. And that being my definition of autoregulation means that the capillaries themselves can change their diameter in response to local metabolic state and participate in autoregulation

So I have been interested in the fact that the capillaries too participate. They potentially have an important role, because they are very high resistance vessels. The reason they do not contribute very much to controlling blood pressure is because there are so many of them, and their total cross-sectional area is large through the body. If you are considering where the blood pressure falls and which size vessels are responsible for the difference between arterial pressure and capillary pressure, why, that is not due to capillaries. The responsible resistance is a little further upstream, because capillaries are so numerous in parallel that they do not contribute to producing the total net resistance to the flow represented by the cardiac output that generates the systemic blood pressure. But for local control, the capillaries could have a large role, because they are very high resistance vessels having such a small caliber, with the resistance relating to the fourth power of the radius inversely.

**Dr. Zeimer:** Doug, could I add one more comment regarding the caliber of the capillaries and the resistance? There is evidence that if a capillary decreases its diameter by 1 μm, that would be enough to stop the blood flow, especially if you have white blood cells trying to get through that blood vessel. So when you mentioned that it is proportional to $r$ to the minus 4, that does not apply to capillaries. In capillaries one pericyte constricting with a white blood cell caught in the lumen, that would be enough to stop the blood flow. Now, if you have on top of that sticky white blood cells, or sticky particles, that would be even more drastic, so I just want to reinforce your point that the resistance could be dramatic and could also be very, very local.

**Dr. Anderson**: Being a physicist, you pointed out that it is really not just water that is flowing through these vessels. Particulate things can clog up the vessels if they get too small, and that could include white cells or red cells, either one. However, there are some actual measurements to show that the resistance in these small vessels goes according to the inverse of the fourth power of the radius.

**Dr. Hoffman**: Does this imply that there is a resting tone to the pericytes, so that the vessel is at sort of a mid-dilated range, so that if you relax the pericyte you can increase flow?

**Dr. Anderson**: Well, so far it seems that when you study the cells in isolation, they pretty much behave very much like vascular smooth muscles. One has to assume that they are in mid-dilated state, so that there can be some range of control. For example, they do respond to nitroprusside, a donor of nitric oxide, with a relaxation. Therefore, if the endothelium is producing nitric oxide, the vessels are in a state of active dilation that is presumably partial dilation, if you have the right amount of nitric oxide present. And that makes them subject to control. They can dilate further or they can constrict.

Well, now, in glaucoma, one of the dilemmas that we have is that if we think that vascular things have something to do with optic nerve damage, but that the blood flow is autoregulated with respect to intraocular pressure, so that you can change the intraocular pressure with only a little effect on blood flow, well then, how can damage occur? Terry Ernest a long time ago suggested there might be an individual variability with regard to the capacity for autoregulating, which now we have to be careful to define, as I brought out earlier today. Are we talking about the upper limit, or are we talking about the amount of change per stimulus, or what are we talking about when we talk about deficiency of autoregulation? But let us say that as a general concept, that some kind of deficiency, some kind of inadequacy of response in some people might explain why those people suffer harm at normal levels of intraocular pressure or somewhat elevated levels, whereas in other people the blood flow remains adequate despite its considerably elevated intraocular pressure. The concept is that the intraocular pressure, along with a deficient autoregulation in some way, is what results in the damage. There is in fact some evidence of reduced autoregulation in people with glaucoma, but it is not compelling evidence, only suggestive. The reason it is not definitive is that most of the measurements really are not dealing with measurements of blood flow *per se* in the relevant vascular bed of the optic nerve, but some surrogate such as the visual cortical electrical response to light. For example, when you elevate intraocular pressure, people who have glaucoma behave differently from people who do not with regard to how high you can raise the pressure before the cortical electrical responses to light begin to fade or disappear. Others have looked at the color of the optic nerve head, and how it changes when you raise the intraocular pressure, and the compensatory recovery immediately thereafter. These are not direct measures, but they are all suggestive that there is a difference in these reactions between people who have glaucoma and those who do not, adding to the interest in the hypothesis that somehow a deficiency of autoregulation might be relevant for glaucoma.

Now, how might you develop a reduced capacity for autoregulation? And here I can think of a variety of possibilities. Maybe we can consider "inadequate autoregulation" to be something like a common final pathway, or, what did we have yesterday, a death funnel? The physiologic manifestation may be an inability to regulate (dilate) adequately to meet the metabolic need. For instance, if you had an upstream arterial obstruction, this was already mentioned earlier today, some kind of atheroma, what would happen downstream is that the vessels would dilate so that the total resistance along the pathway remains the same and the volume of flow remains pretty good, and we know that the carotid artery can become stenosed quite a bit before blood flow in the brain is reduced. However, when you go from a mid-dilated state to 95% dilated, you have used up most of your reserve regulation, and if you add another challenge such as elevated intraocular pressure you may not have enough remaining to meet that challenge. This would be considered, with respect to ability to respond to an elevated intraocular pressure, a deficiency in autoregulatory capacity. That is one way that a deficiency might occur.

**Dr. Siesjö**: I am fascinated by this. Let me go back 20 years to an article that we published on autoregulation. That was at a time when I also dealt with vascular things and not neurochemistry. What we did was to reduce blood pressure in normocapnic animals. When you came below the autoregulatory range, you could see that the venous $pO_2$ in the sagittal sinus was being reduced. And when you come down to a venous $pO_2$ of about, say, 19, 20, then you could see that the ATP started falling in the tissue. Now, in another series of experiments, we induced hypercapnia first with a $pCO_2$ of about 60, so we dilated the vessels in the tissue and now reduced the arterial blood pressure, and much to our fascination we found that at a blood pressure of say, about 40, you had a venous $pO_2$ of 60, 70 mmHg and yet only two-thirds of the ATP left in the tissue. There was only one thing we could conclude from this, tentatively, and that was that, if you will dilate the peripheral microvessels and you now reduce the pressure supplying them, you get a preferential perfusion of blood through some of them to the exclusion of others. The preferential perfusion would explain why you have a higher than normal venous oxygen tension and the low ATP would be explained by the non-perfused vessels.

**Dr. Anderson**: Yes, you get into a problem of a steal by one vascular bed from another, in fact another way that the residual capacity for autoregulation in a particular vascular bed might be impaired. I have been interested in yet another mechanism, which I will bring up now, and that is that if the vessels are in a vasoconstricted state under some external influence, they may then lose their ability to dilate fully because of that external influence. I think of vasospasm as possibly acting this way. For instance, let us say that vessels are vasospastic and the person has been exposed so they got their hands cold. If this vascular bed in the optic nerve head participates in a general vasospastic response, but is now called upon to dilate by the metabolic need, it might not be able to do so because there is something keeping it constricted. In a sense you have reduced its ability for autoregulatory dilation.

We happened to come upon an experimental model that showed this. We were trying to decide whether or not this whole problem of intraocular pressure-induced nerve damage was vascular or non-vascular in the first place. And we decided that if we raised the blood pressure in the animal, we might protect the optic nerve from damage from elevated intraocular pressure, because it would have a better potential for perfusion. If it was simply a fact that the lamina cribrosa was being pushed back mechanically, and this was kinking the axons and causing an interruption of axonal transport, which is the thing we were measuring as our physiologic endpoint, why, the blood pressure would be quite irrelevant. So we anticipated that with higher blood pressure we would find that there would be a protection if it was vascular. We chose a drug which does not have a vasoconstrictive effect on central nervous system vessels, because we did not want to interfere with the vascular bed we were studying. We chose angiotensin, which is said not to constrict the central nervous system vessels. To our surprise, we found the opposite result, that when we raised the blood pressure the optic nerve became *more* susceptible to axonal transport blockade when you elevated the intraocular pressure than if you had not raised the blood pressure. And we were quite puzzled by that. It was as if we had had a damaging effect of elevated blood pressure instead of a protective effect or a neutronal effect. Then we read more carefully what it said in the book about angiotensin. It said angiotensin does not constrict blood vessels in the central nervous system, except where there is a defect in the blood–brain barrier, and therefore angiotensin has bioavailable access, because it can get out of the vessels and have access to the external coat and cause constriction. We realized that that is what happens in the optic nerve head, because there is no barrier between the choroid, which is a leaky vascular bed, and the optic nerve head, which is not a leaky vascular bed. So angiotensin is retained within the lumen of the vessels in the optic nerve head all right, but is not retained in the lumen in the choroid, and it could potentially diffuse into the optic disc. And we thought, well, maybe that is the explanation for our observation. Obviously we are making up something to explain our observation. But the finding suggested that a vasoconstrictor, having access to the vessels at the optic nerve head and causing spasm, might reduce its ability to dilate when it is challenged by the elevated intraocular pressure. This is potentially another way, then, to limit autoregulation that the vessels are under some vasoconstrictive influence, and that limits their ability to vasodilate.

Earlier today we heard about vessels that become, shall I say, sclerotic. They were remodeled, and they had collagen that becomes more solid and prevents the vessels from dilating very well. Thus, in arteriosclerosis after hypertension, if vessels become sclerotic and can not dilate they might not be able to autoregulate, because they are physically prevented from doing so by a disease that is more prevalent with age. Now, this sort of thing happens in, I guess, the arterioles of moderate size but perhaps not the very smallest one, which does not have much collagen in the first place, as was pointed out earlier today. But atherosclerosis is on the list of potential causes for a limitation for autoregulation reserve.

All I am trying to do is to point out that there are a number of different ways by which autoregulation might become inadequate in glaucoma, and you have a reduced capacity for a dilation response. Another way that regulation might become inadequate is if there is a situation where there is a vascular steal, as Dr. Siesjö suggested earlier, and here the choroid becomes very important to us. We like to think of the choroid as being a surrogate for what is happening in the optic nerve, and a lot of people have measured choroidal blood flow, thinking it reflects what is happening in the optic nerve. But it could be the inverse, could it not. It could be that when the choroid vasodilates under the influence of some physiologic or pharmacologic circumstance, that the blood is in essence stolen from the optic nerve head, which is then required to autoregulate by dilating in order to maintain its flow, thereby reducing its ability to meet a further challenge. And so just to say that you increased blood flow in the eye or the choroid does not say that you have provided any help to the optic nerve. You may in fact do the opposite, because you have caused the optic nerve to have to use up some of its capacity for autoregulation, and now it can not meet an additional challenge as well as it could before.

We talked about calcium channel blockers as if they are an entire group, but they are all different. Those that dilate vessels, or even selectively some vessels including optic nerve vessels and improving their flow, may not improve their ability to regulate. It may be their ability to regulate rather than the amount of flow, that is relevant. For example, let us say that what you have is periods of hypotension when you sleep, or you have some other challenge that combines with that of intraocular pressure, and there are times when you must really dilate your optic disc vessels. But if you have somehow changed the cardiac output, changed the blood pressure systemically, or changed regional relative redistributions of blood flow in such a manner that the optic nerve has had to use up some of its ability to regulate, and it does not have enough, it can not meet those additional challenges as well. So vasodilation is not necessarily good, if you are talking about something that causes vasodilation everywhere. Getting rid of vasospasm is not necessarily good if you are talking about getting rid of vasospasm everywhere. You may or may not have helped the optic nerve, which has to be studied as its own entity, I think. We must consider what is happening in the optic nerve, as opposed to looking at surrogates. Dr. Flammer posed a question yesterday of, should he raise the blood pressure in his patient, and well, I do not know whether that would help his patient or not. But now we can ask the question, should he remove the vasospasm from his patient, will that help or not. Well, it depends on the relative degree to which some beds get more and some beds get less, and which of the two happens for the optic nerve in that circumstance. Dr. Flammer has a comment.

**Dr. Flammer**: Because we sometimes saw improvement after calcium channel blockers even in cases with marked drop in blood pressure, and I think I totally agree with you. It depends also on the local action. They may even reduce the perfusion pressure and still be of help, but in some people it was the other way round.

**Dr. Anderson**: That is right, you lower the blood pressure by arteriolar dilation and you may have better flow, but on the other hand if it happens that this person had an atheroma on that particular side, in balance he might have ended up with less flow. So it may be different in different people whether you get a benefit or not, and it is very hard to predict from fundamental principles. I think that as clinicians we too often just think that vasodilation is likely to be good. I am going to give my patient a vasodilator, without realizing that vasodilation is not all the picture. Whether cardiac output is affected and how it is redistributed is very important. At the limit of effective vasodilation, if all the vessels dilated you would have a low blood pressure and you die.

**Dr. Lüscher**: I have a question as a non-expert in this area. I mean, in the coronary circulation we know that whole structural changes which we relate to atherosclerosis in the broadest sense sort of stop once the vessels enter the myocardium and become intramyocardial vessels. What sort of changes do we see in the ophthalmic circulation, and in what size blood vessels is there atherosclerosis, and if so, does this relate to this group of patients? I would suspect that if they have low blood pressure they have very little changes, if at all, in these blood vessels.

**Dr. Anderson**: I do not have accurate or detailed knowledge of that, but I can give you what my impression is, namely that the central retinal artery branches, which are really arterioles, do have a layer of collagen between the smooth muscle and the endothelium, but it is not very much. Those vessels do become sclerotic with chronic hypertension, if the vessels have been kept for a long time in a contracted state. On the short term, raising of blood pressure will contract, and then lowering it will dilate the retinal arterioles, but after a while they become sclerotic and they can not dilate anymore. But the smaller vessels, and in particular the ones that we are interested in in the optic nerve head, the smooth muscle and the pericytes are apposed onto the endothelium, so there is not a connective tissue space to become sclerotic, so to speak. Therefore, I think that the very smallest vessels are not subject to sclerosis, but the central retinal arterial branches, the larger ones, which are still small in terms of what many people are talking about in vascular physiology, but for us they are the largest ones, they do have some amount of sclerotic capacity. Dr. Hoffman?

**Dr. Hoffman**: I do not know if I am remembering my pathology correctly. But maybe it is helpful to look at what happens in diabetes. Do not diabetics have a loss of pericytes in the retinal vessels?

**Dr. Anderson**: Yes, they do, and interestingly, I will point out to you, they also lose their ability to autoregulate the vessels.

**Dr. Hoffman:** And could that be in some way related to the microinfarcts that they get, on the basis of probably altered regulation of their retinal circulation?

**Dr. Anderson**: It is conceivable. They also become leaky vessels, which means that some of the intravascular vasoconstrictors might become extravascular and cause constriction of both arterioles and capillaries, but the lack of a pericyte in particular capillaries may allow the wall to be weak enough to develop the microaneurysms. The total function of pericytes in general is another interesting topic. There are a lot of interesting findings in diabetes that may relate to the glaucoma problem.

**Dr. Caprioli**: Doug, this comment is actually prompted by your remarks about a vascular steal. I think it is important to at least consider the nutritional contributions from the choroid to the nutrition of the optic nerve head. In fact, one of the problems with measuring optic nerve head blood flow with the diffusable tracers is that these tracers really pour in from the peripapillary choroid, fairly rapidly. So while you showed that the capillary beds are quite separate, there is certainly some nutritional supply to the optic nerve head from the peripapillary choroid, I would think.

**Dr. Anderson**: This includes at least oxygen, because the oxygen levels in the optic nerve head near the choroid are much higher than they are toward the center and higher than are necessary, because the choroid is overperfused and has a very high oxygen level. Now, whether that is true of other needed nutrients, like glucose, I would have to depend on somebody who knew about diffusion of those things, and whether they also would be oversupplied from the choroid, or even adequately supplied by the choroid alone. But there must be some nutritional need for capillaries in the optic nerve itself, perhaps to carry away carbon dioxide.

**Dr. Siesjö**: Can I come back to the possibility of a preferential perfusion? If you have lost your autoregulation of individual microvessel areas within a tissue like the optic nerve head, then some of the capillaries may be perfused just because they are straight, and rheologically they are very easy to perfuse, and others may be tortuous and difficult to perfuse, and there you would have a stoppage of flow. Is there any information on the perfusion of individual capillaries when you raise the intraocular pressure? Can you see if all the capillaries are being perfused or not?

**Dr. Anderson**: The answer to that is no, we do not have information on that. This is a very small region of tissue, less than 1 mm in diameter, that we are talking about, and maybe half a millimeter high. Techniques to really measure accurately are just lacking, and individual capillaries can not be well visualized. Even measuring blood flow at all in the tissue has been incredibly difficult. Dr. Alm will attest to that.

**Dr. Siesjö**: Kochinsky and his collaborators in Heidelberg have used techniques in the cortex which may be applicable to the optic nerve head. What they have done is to inject Evans blue 5 or 10 seconds after decapitation of their experimental animals, then visualize by microscopy where the Evans blue is, and then they have taken these sections and stained them a bit for enzymes which are localized to the microvessels. And they have a lined dissection, so they can see if the vessels which they observe have been perfused.

**Dr. Anderson**: I will have to get the details of that technique and maybe we can use it to advantage.

**Dr. Quigley**: I believe Dr. Anderson has forgotten an experiment. We studied a series of monkeys, in which we had elevated the eye pressure by raising of reservoir connected to the anterior chamber. We looked at the effect on the nerve head by elevating the pressure acutely in both eyes, but also the animals had one eye that had had chronic pressure elevation with damage to the optic nerve head in 10 or 11 monkeys. We contrasted the blood flow with tritiated iodoantipyrine in the elevated pressure eye to the eye that did not have a chronically elevated pressure. This molecule, because we were using tritium, permits resolution on the autoradiographs, I think, that if there was a lack of perfusion of, say, two bundles across, 200 or 300 µm, you would be able to detect that. There is no local lack of radioactivity in the tissue under these conditions in an experimental animal that is anesthetized. There is no sign that there is a local lack of perfusion to eye pressures that are up to the range we were talking about before. If we get to perfusion pressures of 25 mmHg or less, then you begin seeing a generalized decrease, and in fact, even local, losses of perfusion to the tissue. Now, of course, the experiment is open to all sorts of criticism. But the experiment does exist.

**Dr. Anderson**: But local in the sense that this tissue is unperfused, whereas an adjacent one is perfused. And you are saying that within the optic nerve head tissue, you could not find some locations perfused and others not.

**Dr. Quigley:** Correct.

**Dr. Siesjö**: That is clearly an interesting experiment, but I can not see how you can use antipyrine and come down to the resolution of the individual capillaries, simply because before you have gotten your tissue dissected out, you have got diffusion of antipyrine across large distances.

**Dr. Quigley**: Well, the distances, as Joe was saying and as I mentioned myself, the distance it goes in the approximately minute and 15 seconds it took us to freeze the tissue from the termination of circulation to the freezing of the eye, it could conceivably go some distance, that is absolutely right. It does not, however, go a great distance into the vitreous cavity, for example. If you look at the vitreoretinal interface, in the same sections of tissue, the iodoantipyrine is not sort of going everywhere. There are dramatic differences between the perfusion in the retina and the perfusion in the immediately adjacent choroid, so this molecule may go very rapidly through neural tissue, but one sees reasonably localized differences. So the spatial resolution is not so poor that the experiment is worthless, it is somewhere in the middle.

**Dr. Anderson**: Let me go on and conclude here, since the time is running out. The final thing I was going to point out is that damage may not all be due to a regulatory inability. There is some evidence, and Michael Schulzer and Stephen Drance are responsible for this evidence, that there may be some mechanism that is not due to pressure-induced challenge to the circulation. It is conceivable that there is something wrong with blood coagulation or the platelets so that microthrombi form in some of the small vessels, and it was pointed out, when you get them constricted in a certain way, a certain red cell or something else might obstruct it, since they are not opened and closed by precapillary sphincters, or maybe fibrinolysis is inadequate, or some other problem exists that creates small lesions with marginally adequate blood flow.

In any event, there seem to be two sets of glaucoma patients, according to this preliminary, but suggestive study. In those people who have vasospasm, and might be then subject to some of the things that I have been talking about earlier, the level of intraocular pressure correlates with the amount of damage which is present in the eye. But in another set of patients, who do not have vasospasm, but they have recognizable biochemical abnormalities related to platelet and fibrin and fibrinolysis, who have glaucomatous damage to the optic nerve, the level of intraocular pressure in those patients does not correlate with the amount of damage that occurs. We call them glaucoma, maybe normal-tension glaucoma, maybe they happen to have elevated intraocular pressure, but the pressure level may or may not be relevant. The suggestion is that we have a pressure-independent mechanism for producing harm. Now, this is a hypothesis that needs some confirmation by a more direct study, there may be some selection bias in the patients who enter this study and so on and so forth and so on. They were individuals who were in trouble in some way, and therefore they were put in the hospital in order to make all of these studies to try to sort out what was going on. So there certainly is a selection bias, and we do not know what proportion of patients might have this. But there is some suggestion, and I think we would be remiss if we did not mention it, that there is a group of people who have what looks like glaucoma, may or may not have elevated intraocular pressure, in whom the intraocular pressure is not necessarily part of the mechanism for the damage, and that it is due to some other kind of vascular inadequacy that occurs. Now, maybe these thrombi, through releasing platelet factors, are indirectly affecting or causing vasospasm in a local sense, rather than vasospasm of the kind that we have been thinking about, and there really is very much a similar condition. But I simply want to point out that the problem is complex, and there is, possibly, a microvascular occlusion, pressure-unrelated mechanism at play in some cases.

**Dr. Zeimer**: Doug, before you finish or we run out of time, could you explain, building to your model explanation, why we see an excavation, an enlargement of the scleral canal, or an excavation that is typical to glaucoma. How does that fit into your model?

**Dr. Anderson**: I wish I understood that. I wish I understood what makes the clinical presentation of ischemic optic neuropathy different from the presentation of glaucoma. They look different, and that is a piece of evidence that suggests that the intraocular pressure or weakness of the collagen is part of the picture in glaucoma, whereas it is not in this other. It is a puzzle. You point out a true paradox.

**Dr. Zeimer**: May I suggest something? I am bothered by the differentiation between the first day and the last day of this meeting. Why could not we have a deformation of the tissue that supports the optic nerve head, which then causes, among other things, deformation of the blood vessels? In which case, if you have, everything that is presented here fits extremely well in a patient that already has a susceptibility because the tissue is deformed. Now, if you have deformed the tissue and the capillaries are not well regulated, or the capillaries have an obstructive abnormality, or there is stealing by another bed. All the phenomena that you described here, would be an enhanced susceptibility to a tissue that is already deformed. So it would fit very nicely.

**Dr. Anderson**: Yes, thank you very much for the synthesis. I have heard Harry Quigley express the same idea. It fits very well in the death funnel concept, too, in the sense that you could translate kinking a blood vessel in a weak support tissue as causing some kind of local high resistance which causes some vasodilation somewhere else in order to compensate, which uses up some of the reserve of autoregulation, which means that some additional challenge, like elevated venous pressure, can not be met. And so if you put in the entire picture, the discrepancy between the first and the last day is only seeming, but not real. They all must somehow come together into a final clinical manifestation and in trying to create a final common pathway I have said, well, I will describe it in terms of vascular insufficiency due to autoregulation deficiency. But, then you asked the question, how is it different from ischemic optic neuropathy, and well, who knows, I do not know. Maybe if it is an ischemic problem it has to do with how the ischemia is produced, namely by weakness of the collagen as opposed to occlusion of the posterior ciliary arteries, that makes a difference in the clinical presentation.

**Dr. Caprioli**: Also, Doug, in terms of the difference between ischemic optic neuropathy, you have to consider the rates of damage and the bulk of the tissue that is involved at any one particular time. With ischemic optic neuropathy, of course, you really have something like a stroke of the majority of the optic nerve head.

**Dr. Anderson**: Some neuro-ophthalmologists are beginning to talk about chronic ischemic optic neuropathy as a separate entity which has, as its clinical appearance, a pale disc which is not excavated. Anyway, whatever theory I think you choose, I point out also it has to explain why the disc is susceptible, and not the retina and choroid, because they seem not to be. And there is something anatomic, something peculiar about this location that makes it susceptible. And secondly, whatever theory you come up with has to explain why people are different from one another. And I would say that any theory that someone wants to propose should look at why this is so.

**Dr. Drance**: We have unfortuntately reached the end of our time. Doug has brought together the highlights of the meeting, and we are not able to address ourselves, unfortunately, to some of Joseph's questions which he posed or wanted to pose, and we are not able, unfortunately, in spite of the three days, to have a debate with the questions that you raised, which all need to be discussed much further. This really means that even three days are not enough for this subject; we could be doubling the time. We have learned so much from each other that I think we must have altered some of our preconceived ideas and concepts.

Finally, I want to thank a number of people. I want to thank the three moderators for having got together a group of very exciting people who have helped us at least to concentrate on what is a very complex disease. I think they were all excellent. I am sure that we will benefit from the transactions.

I want to thank Johan Przydryga and through him Alcon for the fact that they remain long-sighted enough to support us in this way.

I would like to thank Geoffrey Crewe for the excellence of the arrangements. As you saw, he brought on the floods yesterday for us, a spectacular highlight to the meeting, and it is only a person like he who can then stop the flooding and have sunshine on your final day. Thank you all for joining us.

# INDEX OF AUTHORS